MELTZER

INTENSIVE CORONARY CARE

a manual for nurses

FIFTH EDITION

MELTZER'S
INTENSIVE
CORONARY CARE

a manual for nurses

FIFTH EDITION

Kathleen Dracup, RN, DNSc
Professor
University of California, Los Angeles
School of Nursing
Los Angeles, California

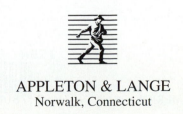

APPLETON & LANGE
Norwalk, Connecticut

Prentice Hall International (UK) Limited, *London*
Prentice Hall of Australia Pty. Limited, *Sydney*
Prentice Hall Canada, Inc., *Toronto*
Prentice Hall Hispanoamericana, S.A., *Mexico*
Prentice Hall of India Private Limited, *New Delhi*
Prentice Hall of Japan, Inc., *Tokyo*
Simon & Schuster Asia Pte. Ltd., *Singapore*
Editora Prentice Hall do Brasil Ltda., *Rio de Janeiro*
Prentice Hall, *Englewood Cliffs, New Jersey*

Library of Congress Cataloging-in-Publication Data

Dracup, Kathleen.
    Meltzer's intensive coronary care : a manual for nurses. — 5th
ed. / Kathleen Dracup.
      p.   cm.
    Rev. ed. of: Intensive coronary care : a manual for nurses /
Lawrence E. Meltzer, Rose Pinneo, J. Roderick Kitchell. 4th ed.
c 1983.
    Includes index.
    ISBN 0-8385-4276-X (p. : alk. paper)
    1. Cardiac intensive care—Handbooks, manuals, etc.
2. Cardiovascular system—Diseases—Nursing—Handbooks, manuals,
etc.   3. Coronary heart disease—Nursing—Handbooks, manuals, etc.
4. Coronary care units Handbooks, manuals, etc. I. Myocardial
Infarction Intensive coronary care. II. Title. III. Title:
Intensive coronary care.
    [DNLM: 1. Coronary Disease—nursing. 2. Coronary Care Units
nurses' instruction. 3. Arrhythmia—nursing. 4. Myocardial
Infarction—nursing. WY 152.5 D757m 1995]
RC684.I56D73   1995
616.1′2—dc20
DNLM/DLC
for Library of Congress   95-5351
                                            CIP

Acquisitions Editor: Sally J. Barhydt
Production Editor: Jennifer Sinsavich
Production Assistant: Jeanmarie Roche Hoover
Designer: Mary Skudlarek

ISBN 0-8385-4276-X
90000

9 780838 542767

Contents

Preface

The fifth edition of this textbook reflects the many changes that have occurred in coronary intensive care since the fourth edition was published in 1983. Readers familiar with previous editions will find that the textbook is completely reorganized and that many chapters have been rewritten or added. For example, most of the material in the first seven chapters is new to this edition.

This book is intended for nurses and student nurses who are beginning their careers in coronary intensive care. It can also be used by nurses caring for patients with cardiac disease who work in other acute care areas, such as the emergency department or telemetry unit. Readers who have had extensive clinical experience outside of cardiology may also find it a helpful review to prepare them to care for acutely ill cardiac patients.

Although excellent reference books are available on various aspects of critical care, their encyclopedic content can be overwhelming to the beginning clinician. This text was originally written by Dr. Meltzer and colleagues to provide a framework for the practice of coronary intensive care, and after several decades it continues to serve this important function.

At the time the first edition was written, coronary intensive care units were relatively unknown to most physicians and nurses. Their philosophy and protocols had to be explained in some detail. Now the importance of coronary intensive care is undisputed, and the collaborative philosophy underlying the relationships of nurses, physicians, and other staff working in critical care is well established. Chapters describing the organization of the coronary intensive care unit have been replaced by chapters describing the ideal physical environment and the type of physiological and psychological patient problems commonly seen in patients admitted to the coronary care unit. A new chapter on monitoring has also been added.

We have learned a great deal about the pathogenesis of coronary heart disease and its consequences over the past decade. These developments in our understanding are described in Chapters 4 through 7. Here the role of thrombolytics and other interventions to increase myocardial oxygen supply and reverse the process of infarction are detailed. Heart failure, which affects millions of Americans each year, is described along with the latest approaches to its treatment. Two new chapters have also been added on the treatment of arrhythmias, including the most recent guidelines for advanced cardiac life support.

The chapters requiring only minimal revision are Chapters 8 through 14 on electrocardiography and arrhythmias. These have been updated to reflect new knowledge provided by electrophysiology studies and clinical trials of antiarrhythmics, but they generally remain unchanged from the elegant description provided by Dr. Meltzer many years ago.

This textbook was my introduction to coronary intensive care. In large part, Dr. Meltzer was responsible for my choosing cardiac nursing as a specialty some 25 years ago. His description of the philosophy of coronary intensive care and his visionary role for nurses in this important specialty was clear and compelling. It has been a privilege and a pleasure to revise this text for yet another generation of nurses.

Kathleen Dracup, RN, DNSc
Professor
University of California, Los Angeles

Foreword

Nearly 30 years have elapsed since the first edition of this book was published. The objective of the book was to describe a new system of care we designed to reduce the extraordinary hospital mortality from acute myocardial infarction and, perhaps more importantly, to define the nursing role demanded by this system of care. It was our premise from the outset that intensive coronary care was essentially a form of specialized nursing care. In this system, nurses were placed, for the first time, in a responsible decision-making role, able to act on their own when the situation demanded. This concept represented a radical departure from traditional nursing. Remember, recording blood pressure was considered outside the scope of nursing until World War II. Moreover, as late as 1960, only one percent of hospitals had any intensive care facilities at all. Many nurse directors were convinced that nursing would be pushed beyond its scope if this nurse-centered system of care was even attempted. But attempted it was. With the insight of a few nurse leaders, one of whom, Dr. Faye Abdellah, Chief Nurse Officer and Assistant Surgeon General of the United States, the program was carefully studied at the Presbyterian-University of Pennsylvania Medical Center. *Intensive Coronary Care: A Manual for Nurses* was a product of this research experience.

The book became an immediate success, reflecting the unparalled acceptance of coronary care and the upheaval of nursing practice that accompanied this plan. Well over one million copies of the book are in print in English as well as translations in French, Dutch, Spanish, and Japanese.

The next three editions brought the book up to date with changes in medical concepts and expansion of the nursing role. This fifth edition differs greatly. None of the original team, including myself, have been able to keep pace with nursing education and practice or the ever-growing nursing role. A fresh breath of air was needed.

To our delight, Dr. Kathleen Dracup has taken up where we left off. I can think of no one more suitable or better qualified than Dr. Dracup to handle the task of updating this book. Not only has she worked diligently in a coronary unit, but she is clearly aware of where coronary care nursing stands today, having served as editor of *Heart & Lung,* currently as editor of *American Journal of Critical Care,* and in her present capacity as Professor, University of California, Los Angeles, School of Nursing. With this new fifth edition, we pass the baton to this extremely talented educator and researcher.

Lawrence E. Meltzer, MD
Philadelphia, Pennsylvania

Chapter 1

The Coronary Care Unit: Philosophy, Design, Equipment, and Nursing Staff

A coronary care unit (CCU) is a specially designed and equipped facility intended to provide optimum care for patients with severe cardiopulmonary disease. The original intent of the CCU was the monitoring of patients with suspected or confirmed acute myocardial infarction. Over the past three decades the admission criteria for the CCU have broadened to include patients with diverse cardiovascular pathophysiology. Admission criteria usually include one or more of the following diagnoses: suspected, evolving, or confirmed acute myocardial infarction; unstable angina; life-threatening arrhythmia with or without a previous cardiac arrest; severe congestive heart failure; cardiogenic shock; pulmonary embolism; acute respiratory distress syndrome; acute endocarditis or myocarditis; and severe cardiac complications related to a systemic illness or trauma (eg, Marfan's syndrome, collagen vascular disease, myocardial contusion, etc). Patients who are not in acute crisis may also be admitted for specific monitoring or treatment (eg, hemodynamic monitoring, elective pacemaker insertion, or mechanical ventilation).

The construction of cardiac stepdown units that have telemetric monitoring capabilities and smaller patient-to-nurse ratios than do general medical–surgical units has reduced the number of patients admitted to the CCU for observation. In today's CCU, patients are often in severe physiologic crisis and require an intensive range of technologic support and skilled nursing care. The object of this chapter is to discuss the philosophy, design, equipment, and staff of an effective CCU.

PHILOSOPHY OF INTENSIVE CORONARY CARE

Intensive coronary care is a system of care designed primarily to prevent morbidity and mortality from the complications of coronary heart disease, particularly acute myocardial infarction and heart failure. As with any effective system, its optimal function depends on the interrelationship of its various components; individually the components are not self-sufficient and cannot achieve the desired result. Many components go into the system of coronary care, but the key players are the nurses, physicians, patients, and patients' families.

When coronary intensive care was first conceived three decades ago, the structure of working relationships in all hospitals was hierarchical (Figure 1–1). Coronary care departed from that system by the *amount of responsibility* that physicians delegated to the nursing staff. Physicians wanted nurses working in the first coronary care units to be able to anticipate complications, assess each problem as it arose, and above all to assume a *decision-making* role. It was recognized that unless nurses were delegated authority to make and execute therapeutic decisions on the basis of their own observations and judgment, the coronary care system would be ineffective.

However, in the intervening years, nursing has emerged as a scientific discipline with an independent sphere of practice related to patient care. Nurses and physicians have come to realize the importance of collaboration in patient care, and have moved to models of shared governance in developing policies

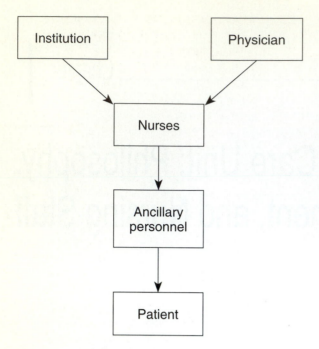

Figure 1–1. The traditional hierarchical model of coronary intensive care.

and procedures for the CCU and in decisions related to patient care.

Consumerism and advance directives are other trends that have changed the relationships within coronary care. Patients are no longer passive. They, along with their families, expect to have a voice in their treatment program and to determine the level of care they will receive at the end of life.

Although individual CCUs may lurch between the old hierarchical model and the newer collaborative model, the philosophy of coronary care is now expressed in Figure 1–2. The interrelationships of the nurse, physician, and patient/family are based on assumptions of mutual respect, trust, and shared authority. Effective communication is required for this system to work, since many decisions have to be made instantaneously.

While nursing and medicine are key to the delivery of coronary care, other health-care personnel are often involved in caring for the patient in the CCU. Respiratory therapists, dietitians, social workers, unlicensed personnel (to assist with nursing duties), and psychiatric liaisons contribute to the treatment program in important ways. Mechanisms must be in place for coordinating these efforts and enhancing communication between the many individuals involved in a treatment program.

From the foregoing description of the coronary care system, it is readily apparent that *the nurse is the key to the success of the entire system of coronary care.* This is not to say that nursing practice alone determines the effectiveness of intensive coronary care, but it does indeed mean that without specially educated, highly skilled nurses the system can never achieve full effectiveness. In fact, without specialized

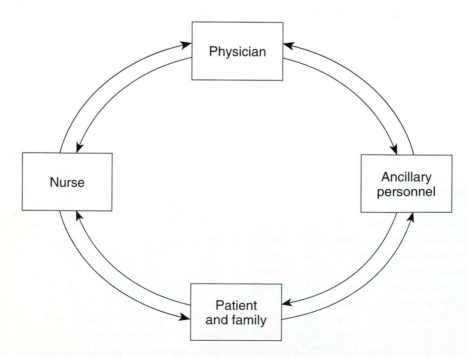

Figure 1–2. The structure of collaboration in coronary intensive care.

nursing practice, intensive coronary care is no more than a token gesture.

It should also be emphasized that the use of monitoring equipment alone, regardless of its sophistication or elegance, must not be construed as constituting intensive coronary care. Monitoring is only one component of the total system and can never be self-sufficient. In the absence of a skilled nursing staff, monitoring equipment by itself does not even warrant its expense.

DESIGN OF THE CORONARY CARE UNIT

Almost every hospital in the United States with over 50 beds has a CCU or combined medical intensive care unit (MICU)/CCU. Some of these are still "first-generation" units that were built when the primary purpose of the CCU was the observation and monitoring of patients at risk for life-threatening arrhythmias. First-generation units were constructed in the form of a single large room containing a centrally located nursing station with cardiac monitors, from 4 to 20 patient beds, and movable curtains to provide a degree of privacy to patients. Although observation is optimal in such a physical design, the environment (with its high noise level, unchanging light, lack of orienting windows and clocks, and clear views of other patients) can cause severe psychological stress in patients admitted for observation and treatment. This stress can result in one or more environmentally related nursing diagnoses, such as altered orientation (specifically confusion and disorientation), altered memory (particularly impaired short-term memory), altered neurosensory processes, sleep-pattern disturbance, and impaired physical mobility. However, a number of strategies can be used in the design of a CCU to reduce the incidence of these deleterious patient responses and provide an environment that facilitates recovery.

Nurses and other health professionals in the CCU need to be active participants in the planning and construction of new CCUs and the remodeling or relocation of old units. Many architectural firms that specialize in hospital design and construction include nurses on their design team. Nonetheless, experienced CCU nurses need to insure that the design of a new or remodeled unit is consistent with research findings on intensive-care-unit (ICU) psychosis.

The following design factors have been documented to reduce the emotional stress experienced by patients in early CCUs, and to decrease the incidence of delirium.

1. The unit should consist of a series of individual private rooms located around a central nursing station. An open ward with curtains or partitions between beds is unsuitable for providing the quiet and serenity required for the recovery of patients with heart disease. In one study, researchers documented noise in an open ward CCU that was consistently above 70 decibels (dB) over a 24-hour period (comparable to the hospital cafeteria at noon). When looking at specific sounds, they found that a cardiac monitor alarm registered 71 dB, an MA-1 respirator alarm 92 dB, and an AVCO balloon pump 74 dB. Three physicians talking at the patient's bedside resulted in a 68-dB noise level. These levels are in dramatic contrast to the International Noise Council's recommendations that noise levels not exceed 45 dB during the day, 40 dB during the evening, and 20 dB during the night. Appropriate levels of quiet can only be insured if patients have individual rooms with floor-to-ceiling walls, doors to the unit that close, and appropriate insulation in ceilings, walls, and floors.

2. Direct visual observation is an integral part of coronary care nursing, and it is never adequate to rely on computerized monitor surveillance as the prime means of patient assessment. Therefore, all beds must be directly visible through glass windows from a central nursing station. Patient privacy during physical examinations and procedures can be maintained by drawing curtains over the windows of the patient's rooms. Nurses need a place from which to observe patients when reading or writing in the patient chart, using the telephone, or discussing a case with other members of the health-care team. The nursing station needs to be centrally located and have good visibility (ie, no walls). Large units with more than eight beds may require more than one nursing station.

3. Lighting and temperature need to be controllable from within each room rather than centrally, so that adjustments can be made for individual patient needs. Lights should be dimmed at night to facilitate patients' sleeping. Day/night patterns are maintained by having an outside window in each patient room. Windows must be located in an appro-

priate wall so that patients can look outside (ie, not at the head of the bed), and at an appropriate eye level for patients lying in bed.

4. Many patients hospitalized in the CCU are alert during all or part of their stay. Rooms can be personalized with bulletin boards to provide a place for family pictures and cards. Clocks and calendars are important to help patients remain oriented to time despite the 24-hour schedule of care.

5. Patient rooms should be large enough to accommodate at the very least an electric bed, bedside commode, intraaortic balloon pump, respirator, several infusion pumps, and a chair for a family member or nurse. Many units were built when the equipment requirements in caring for critically ill patients were far smaller than today. Small patient rooms are a nightmare for nurses, particularly in times of emergency. Since nursing staffs are wisely moving to unrestricted visiting policies within many CCUs, rooms need to be large enough to allow the nurse to provide care to the patient without having to ask a family member to leave. The minimal size for a CCU patient room is 12×15 feet.

6. It is beneficial to locate the CCU at a site contiguous with the hospital's other critical-care units. This arrangement allows for sharing of certain basic facilities and services (eg, utility rooms, kitchens, storage areas, fluoroscopy units, a conference room) that would otherwise be duplicated for each unit. It also has the advantage of allowing staff to cross-train for more than one intensive-care unit (ICU), thus facilitating flexible staffing patterns and broadening the scope of clinical nursing experience. However, it is generally disadvantageous to combine the CCU with another specialty unit (eg, medical intensive care) because the environment and pace of the two units are very different.

7. In the design plan it is worthwhile to provide certain additional rooms near the CCU for purposes other than direct patient care. Providing these rooms in close proximity to the CCU gives families and staff a physical location outside the unit in which to hold conversations

that would be potentially disturbing to patients. Of special importance are the following areas:

a. *Waiting room for families.* Because of the abrupt and critical nature of cardiac emergencies it is understandable that families gather and remain near the patient for prolonged periods. Moreover, patients interviewed after hospitalization in a critical-care unit list social isolation as one of their greatest stressors. Families need an area that is physically close to the CCU and in which they can talk with each other and rest. The waiting room should have adequate telephone facilities both for making outside calls and for communicating with the nursing staff in the CCU.

b. *Nurses' lounge.* Because nursing and nonlicensed personnel must be in continuous attendance in the CCU, it is important that a lounge be included within the unit for the nursing staff. This lounge should include bathroom facilities, lockers, comfortable furniture, and telephones.

c. *Physicians' lounge.* In medical teaching centers, interns and residents need sleeping quarters close to the CCU.

d. *Conference room.* A room that can be used for conferences and team meetings, with appropriate educational resources, is useful to all members of the health-care team.

8. Effective air conditioning and ventilation systems are mandatory, not only for patient and personnel comfort, but for proper upkeep of the monitoring equipment. Many computer systems are heat sensitive and proper room temperatures must be maintained to ensure satisfactory function. Multiple, separately fused electrical outlets are absolutely essential and should be considered in the early stages of planning. Patient equipment may require as many as 15 electrical outlets at one bedside. Electrical grounding within the unit must have unquestionable integrity. Unless true and effective grounding is provided, there is danger of patient electrocution, particularly when several electrical devices are used simultaneously. No compromise can be made with the need for a proper

grounding circuit. Because of the increasing use of major electrical equipment within units (including portable x-ray machines and fluoroscopy), 220-volt lines should be included in the electrical system. An emergency power supply should also be available in the event of electrical failure of the primary circuit.

9. Effective communication and alarm systems are of great importance. The objective of the system should be to permit the nursing staff to summon help instantly and directly. Bedsides need to be equipped with emergency alarms so that a nurse can summon help instantly. The hospital communication system needs to include an emergency page system so that help can be summoned to the unit without the usual circuitous chain of dialing a page operator.

EQUIPMENT FOR A CCU

Cardiac Monitoring System

The most important detection instrument in the CCU is the cardiac monitor, which is used to identify arrhythmias on a continuous basis. A separate monitor, consisting of an oscilloscope, rate meter, alarm mechanism, and recording device is required for each patient. (The specific details of cardiac monitoring are discussed in Chapter 3.) Today most monitoring systems are computerized and provide an automated strip-chart recording of aberrant rhythms. The optimal arrangement for most CCUs is to have an individual monitor (with an oscilloscope, rate meter, and graphic recording device) at each bedside, along with a central oscilloscope, alarm system, and recording module at the nursing station. When the nurse is away from the bedside, alarm sounds should be heard only in the nursing station, in order to avoid patient anxiety and reduce the noise of false alarms.

Electrocardiographic Machine

In addition to the monitoring system, the CCU requires one or more electrocardiography (ECG) machines for obtaining 12-lead ECGs for diagnostic purposes. The machine is also used to document arrhythmias seen on the cardiac monitor when the site of the arrhythmia is unclear (eg, supraventricular versus ventricular tachycardia).

EQUIPMENT FOR ASSESSMENT

Hemodynamic Monitoring

To assess the clinical status of patients with cardiogenic shock or congestive heart failure, it is often necessary to measure pressures directly in the heart and arteries (Figure 1–3). Equipment for this purpose should be on hand in the CCU. This equipment includes manometers, transducers, catheters, and appropriate tubing. Digital-readout devices, oscilloscopes, and strip-chart recorders are usually shared with the cardiac monitoring system.

Although noninvasive measures of cardiac output can be obtained quite reliably through such means as Doppler ultrasonography and transthoracic electrical bioimpedance measurement, these methods are used relatively rarely. Both methods require extensive operator training to insure reliable and valid measurements. In patients with relatively normal heart function, both techniques provide accurate estimates of cardiac output; however, bioimpedance measurement provides inaccurate estimates of cardiac output in patients with a low ejection fraction, ventricular septal defect, aortic insufficiency, or heart rate above 150 beats per minute.

Assessment of Arterial Oxygen Concentration

The "gold standard" in the measurement of arterial oxygen concentration is arterial blood-gas analysis. Blood-gas analyses are used to assess tissue oxygen consumption and metabolism, particularly in the presence of circulatory failure. Nurses usually collect blood specimens for this purpose from the femoral artery or through arterial lines. The arterial blood specimen is placed in a heparinized collection tube to prevent clotting, and is transferred to the laboratory in a container of crushed iced. Some CCUs are experimenting with the continuous measurement of arterial blood gases.

Two other measures of oxygen concentration commonly used in the CCU are pulse oximetry and continuous monitoring of the oxygen saturation of mixed venous blood (SVO_2. The pulse oximeter (Figure 1–4) provides a noninvasive measure of arterial oxygen saturation. It can be placed on any extremity (ear lobe, finger, toe, nose), but is most accurate when placed on a patient's finger. It provides continuous data about the patient's oxygenation without the risks involved in arterial blood gas measurement.

Continuous SVO_2 monitoring involves invasive measurement of the oxygen saturation of mixed venous blood returning to the heart. It can provide an estimate of the patient's oxygen utilization, but requires the placement of a pulmonary artery catheter and therefore carries the same risks as pulmonary

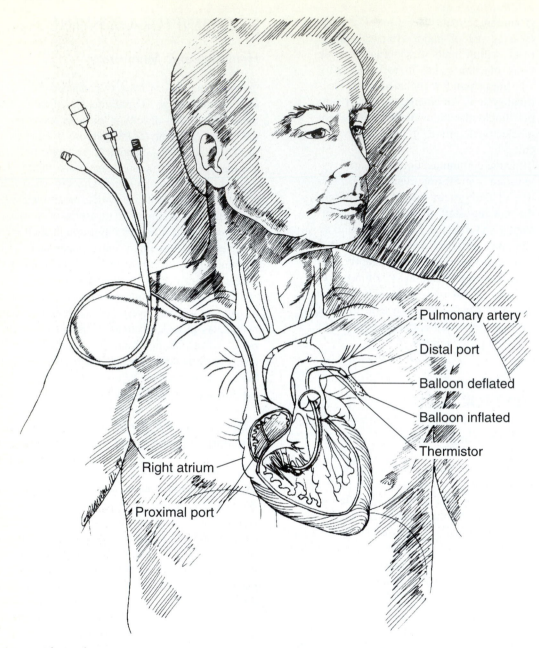

Figure 1–3. The pulmonary artery catheter. (Redrawn with permission from Dennison, RD. Making sense of hemodynamic monitoring. *Am J Nurs*. August 1994 p. 25.)

artery catheterization (eg, sepsis, arrhythmias, pulmonary artery infarction).

EQUIPMENT FOR TREATMENT AND RESUSCITATION

Defibrillator/Cardioverter

A defibrillator must be available at all times, in the CCU, and must be readily accessible to each patient.

Larger CCUs will require more than one defibrillator unit. If the hospital has a biomedical engineer, the latter is usually responsible for ensuring that the defibrillator unit is in constant working order. In hospitals that do not have a biomedical engineering department, the CCU nurses are responsible for checking the defibrillator on a daily basis. A portable, battery-operated defibrillator must also be available for terminating ventricular fibrillation that may develop while patients are being transported to or from the CCU.

Each defibrillator also has a cardioversion func-

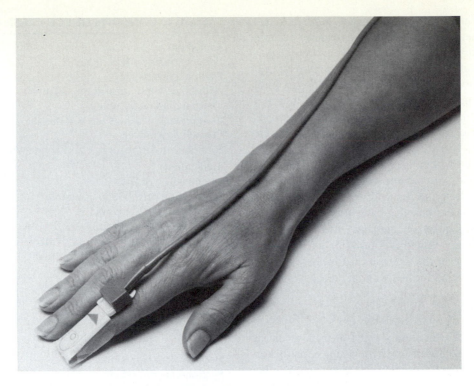

Figure 1–4. The pulse oximeter.

tion that is used to terminate certain rapid-rate arrhythmias (such as atrial fibrillation or ventricular tachycardia). Since the delivery of a large direct electrical current during the vulnerable period of the cardiac cycle can cause ventricular fibrillation, special electronic circuitry is required to deliver the shock within the period of the electrocardiographic QRS complex, when the heart is not susceptible to ventricular fibrillation. All defibrillators have a facility for synchronized cardioversion, eliminating the need for two machines.

Pacemakers

Battery-operated, external (transcutaneous) pacemakers for temporary cardiac pacing must be readily available to the nursing staff in the CCU. Many of the new defibrillators include a built-in transcutaneous pacemaker and a single pair of anterior–posterior chestwall electrodes for pacing and defibrillation. External pacing is valuable during cardiac arrest or while transvenous pacing is being established.

A transvenous pacemaker system has the following three components:

1. An electrode(s) that makes contact with the endocardium or myocardium for transmission of the electrical stimulus into the heart and transmission of cardiac electrical activity to the pulse generator for sensing;

2. Electronic circuitry to sense the electrical activity of the heart and to time and deliver the electrical stimulus to the heart; and

3. A power source or generator for the system. Since temporary pacemaking wires may be inserted transvenously from the unit during emergency situations, an assortment of different-sized pacing wires and generators is also required.

Many types of temporary pacing are now available, including ventricular demand (VVI), atrial demand (AAI), AV sequential (DVI), dual-chamber pacing and sensing (DDD), and atrial tracking (VDD). They are discussed in Chapter 15.

Respiratory Equipment

Respiratory support equipment should be kept permanently in the CCU. Of the many types of mechanical respirator now available, the pressure-cycled machine, which inflates the patient's lung until a preset pressure has been reached, is the most commonly used. Because they provide more efficient gas distribution, respirators that provide pressure-controlled inverse-ratio ventilation are also used, often for patients with acute respiratory distress syndrome (ARDS).

Patients may require emergency intubation and immediate mechanical respiratory assistance because of a respiratory arrest or rapid disintegration of pulmonary function. Ambu bags and tubing must be kept at each bedside to provide respiratory support until the patient can be intubated and connected to a mechanical ventilator. Emergency trays with a laryngoscope, nasotracheal tubes, and endotracheal tubes are also required. Every bedside should have a suction device mounted within the wall at the head of the bed so that a nurse can suction nasotracheal secretions from patients being mechanically ventilated.

On rare occasions the patient cannot be intubated and will require an emergency tracheostomy. A sterile tray, complete with various size tracheostomy tubes, should be in the CCU at all times so that the procedure can be performed without delay.

Oxygen Supply

A dependable oxygen supply piped in from a central source to each bedside is mandatory. Face masks and nasal cannulas for oxygen delivery, along with humidification bottles and flow meters, should be available for each patient. Because patients often remove their face masks while eating, drinking, or talking, nasal cannulas are most frequently used for patients who are alert and do not have special respiratory needs.

Crash Cart

A mobile cart that contains all supplies, equipment, and drugs needed for cardiac emergencies and resuscitation attempts must be ready for use at all times in the CCU. This cart should be easily movable and constructed of heavy-gauge stainless steel, with a low center of gravity to prevent tipping. Most crash carts are equipped with a flat board that is used to provide support under the patient's back during cardiopulmonary resuscitation.

Preferably the crash cart should contain three or more shelves, the topmost of which serves as a work area. The cart's content is listed in Table 1–1. Drugs should not be "borrowed" from the cart in nonemergency situations. Some CCUs have adopted a system in which all drugs are kept in a locked box on the cart. Once opened, the box is returned to the pharmacy and refilled. This plan assures that all appropriate drugs will be available in an emergency.

Prepared Trays and Infusion Pumps

As in other critical-care units, a stock of prepared trays for various procedures should be kept in the CCU. The procedures most frequently seen in a CCU include venous cutdown, urinary catheterization, tra-

TABLE 1–1. CONTENTS OF CCU CRASH CART

Equipment
Portable monitor/defibrillator
External pacemaker
Ambu bag with tracheostomy adapter
Oxygen mask with tubing
Oxygen tank with wrench and regulator
Oxygen flow meter
Suction canister, regulator, and connecting tubing

Medications
Atropine (0.1 mg/mL)
Epinephrine 1:10,000 (0.1 mg/mL)
Lidocaine 2% (20 mg/mL)
Lidocaine 0.8% (8 mg/mL)
Sodium bicarbonate 7.5% (0.89 mEq/mL)
Adenosine (3 mg/mL)
Bretylium (50 mg/mL)
Calcium chloride 10% (100 mg/mL)
Dextrose 50% (500 mg/mL)
Diazepam (5 mg/mL)
Dopamine (80 mg/mL)
Epinephrine (30 mg/30 mL)
Heparin (1000 units/mL)
Hydrocortisone sodium succinate (50 mg/mL)
Isoproterenol (0.2 mg/mL)
Magnesium sulfate (500 mg/mL)
Naloxone (0.4 mg/mL)
Norepinephrine (1 mg/mL)
Phenylephrine (10 mg/mL)
Procainamide (100 mg/mL)
Propranolol (1 mg/mL)

Prepared Trays from Central Service
Intubation tray
Cut-down tray
Cardiac-arrest tray (for open thoracotomy)
Pulmonary artery catheter insertion tray

Supplies
Foley catheter insertion tray
Airways (small, medium, large)
Intravenous solutions
Serum albumin (50 mL and 250 mL)
Sterile water and sterile saline (30 mL)
Heparin locks and intravenous catheters
Needles and syringes
Laboratory supplies [blood sample tubes, tourniquets, povidone/iodine (Betadine), alcohol wipes]
Gauze pads and tape
Sterile towels and gloves
Intravenous tubing
#16 Levine tube
Suction kits
Yankauer suction tip
ECG monitoring leads
ECG paste

cheostomy, right-heart catheterization, use of a temporary pacemaker, arterial pressure monitoring, and insertion of an intraaortic balloon pump.

Nurses working in the CCU also need a large number of intravenous infusion pumps. Many of the intravenous drugs given to cardiac patients have to be carefully titrated. Infusion pumps ensure that the patient will receive the appropriate quantity of a drug safely; they are absolutely required in the case of vasoactive drugs. In this cost-conscious age of care, it falls to the individual CCU nurse to see that such pumps are not used needlessly.

Drugs for the Coronary Care Unit

Because medications usually have to be administered at a moment's notice in cardiac emergencies, all necessary drugs and fluids must be immediately available in the CCU. Although a wide variety of drugs are available for the treatment of cardiac emergencies, the drugs kept in stock in most CCUs do not vary greatly at different hospitals.

THE STAFF OF THE CORONARY CARE UNIT

It is absolutely essential that the care of patients in a CCU be delegated to a *team* of nurses, physicians, respiratory therapists, nonlicensed assistive personnel, social workers, and dietitians. Historically, the team approach distinguished coronary care from other types of care. Because all members of the team understand the aim of care and recognize their respective responsibilities and functions, the effectiveness of the system is markedly enhanced. Furthermore, a team effort develops clarity of communication and a mutual respect among the individual members of the team. Unless the physicians and nurses in a CCU function as part of this organized team, the ultimate result of the entire program will prove very disappointing. Therefore, the ideal structure of a CCU includes two co-directors, a physician and a nurse, who have equal authority but different areas of responsibility.

Nurse Director

The nurse director of the CCU is responsible for the administration, monitoring, and evaluation of patient care provided within the CCU on a 24-hour basis. Optimal preparation for this position consists of a masters degree in nursing and at least 3 years of recent clinical experience, at least one of which includes a required administrative component. The nurse director has management, clinical, and leadership responsibilities related to the nursing staff in the

CCU and the delivery of patient care. The general duties and responsibilities of the nurse manager are to: (1) actively participate on nursing service and hospital committees that establish policies and procedures to improve patient care and nursing practice; (2) establish, in collaboration with the medical director, basic policies of the unit regarding admission, transfer, and discharge criteria for patients in the CCU, clinical procedures, and other administrative matters; (3) develop and implement a quality-assurance program that incorporates the goals and objectives of patient care in the CCU and conforms to standards set by the Joint Commission on the Accreditation of Health Care Organizations; (4) participate, in cooperation with the clinical nurse specialist or unit educator, in the orientation and ongoing educational activities of the unit; (5) select appropriate equipment and supplies in collaboration with the medical director; (6) serve as a liaison between the CCU nursing staff, medical staff, hospital administration, and other support departments; (7) participate in planning, administering, and monitoring a CCU budget; (8) coordinate nurse staffing on a 24-hour basis; (9) recruit, hire, evaluate, and (when necessary) terminate CCU nursing staff; (10) periodically evaluate the effectiveness of the unit in collaboration with the medical director; and (11) serve upon request as a clinical consultant to the nursing staff.

Clinical Educator/Clinical Nurse Specialist

Many hospitals now employ clinical educators or clinical nurse specialists who are based in the CCU and who are primarily responsible for the professional development of the CCU nursing staff. The clinical nurse educator usually holds a bachelor's degree in nursing, while the clinical nurse specialist must hold a master's degree in nursing. Both serve as clinical experts and role models for the nursing staff. In collaboration with the co-directors of the CCU, the clinical nurse specialist or educator assesses the educational and developmental needs of the nursing staff and implements formal and informal educational programs to meet these needs. The nurse specialist or educator also assesses the clinical competencies of staff members and provides specialized knowledge and skill to assist the staff with the management of difficult patient and/or family problems. The clinical nurse specialist often assumes the role of a case manager, carrying a caseload of patients and acting as a hospital-wide resource for nurses caring for patients with cardiovascular problems. The nurse specialist also facilitates research studies conducted in the CCU and ensures that research findings are utilized in the development of clinical protocols and pathways for the CCU.

Acute-Care Nurse Practitioner

Nurse practitioners have traditionally focused on providing health care in outpatient settings. Recently, schools of nursing have begun offering master's degrees with a specialization in acute or critical care. Nurses with such a specialization are unit based and provide a variety of services to patients. They may be prepared to perform such procedures as intubation, pacemaker insertion, placement of arterial lines, chest tube removal, and insertion of pulmonary artery catheters. They may serve as case managers, working with other members of the nursing staff to facilitate the timely discharge of patient from the CCU. They are also prepared to take patients' histories and perform physical examinations at the time of admission, to manage resuscitative efforts, and order routine laboratory tests. Their role is evolving and currently differs from one hospital to another.

Nursing Staff

The success of the CCU depends above all on the competence of the nurse members of the CCU team. As already noted, unless nurses are adequately prepared for their role and given the authority to make and execute therapeutic decisions based on their own observations and judgment, the entire intent of a coronary intensive care program will be thwarted.

For optimum effectiveness, a CCU should maintain a ratio of one professional nurse to every one to two patients at all times. Thus, a six-bed unit will usually require three or four nurses per shift, or a total nursing staff of approximately 20 professional nurses for full coverage (including relief during staff illness, vacations, and days off).

Most hospitals supplement their nursing staffs with specially trained ancillary personnel (eg, monitor technicians, intraaortic balloon-pump technicians, physician assistants, licensed vocational nurses, nonlicensed personnel, and unit secretaries). None of the programs in which this is being done have been systematically evaluated, but in a time of budgetary constraints, such personnel are being used with increasing frequency. No matter what the philosophy of the individual hospital regarding the use of ancillary personnel in critical care, it is vitally important that CCU nurses not misuse their considerable expertise by completing paperwork, filling in for members of the housekeeping staff, or hunting for needed supplies. The nursing co-director needs to assess the degree of support given to CCU nurses for their role in patient care, and to provide the resources and procedures required to enable nurses to remain at the bedside with critically ill patients and their family members.

All CCU nurses must be graduates of an accredited school of nursing, preferably with a baccalaureate program. Most hospitals require at least one year of clinical experience in general medical-surgical nursing prior to transfer to the CCU. A nurse who has not had previous experience in a CCU or in critical care will need to be prepared to assume this challenging role.

Nurses in the CCU must provide expert nursing care to acutely ill patients, many of whom are at high risk for sudden death. Surveillance and monitoring have long been the hallmark of CCU care. However, with the advent of cardiac transplantation and thrombolysis, CCU nurses are now caring for patients who have such minimal cardiac function that they cannot be discharged from a critical-care unit while awaiting a heart transplant, or who are in the midst of an aborted myocardial infarction. Patients may require mechanical ventilation, intraaortic balloon pumps or ventricular assist devices, complicated pharmacologic regimens, and a variety of other supportive measures. No matter how complicated the disease or treatment requirements, CCU nurses are expected to assess patients, develop a comprehensive plan of care, and implement and evaluate that plan in a highly skilled manner. Moreover, given the nature of the CCU team, its nurse members need to communicate with its other members and attain a consensus about the priorities of care.

Medical Director

Ideally, the medical director of the CCU is a cardiologist or an internist who has the knowledge, dedication, interest, and interpersonal skills to be a successful leader. The general duties and responsibilities of the medical director are to: (1) establish standard medical procedures to be followed in the unit; (2) establish, in collaboration with the nurse director, basic policies of the unit regarding patient admission, transfer, and discharge criteria, and procedures, physicians' privileges, and other administrative matters; (3) participate in cooperation with the clinical nurse specialist or unit educator in the orientation and ongoing educational activities of the unit; (4) collaborate with the nurse director in selecting appropriate equipment for the CCU; (5) serve as liaison between the attending staff, hospital administration, and members of the CCU team for problems that arise in or affect the CCU; (6) direct the medical care of patients in critical situations if the attending physician is not immediately available; (7) periodically evaluate, in collaboration with the nurse director, the effectiveness of the unit; and (8) serve as a consultant to attending physicians upon request.

In some hospitals the overall responsibility for the proper functioning of the CCU is shared by a committee consisting of the medical and nurse directors, representatives from other nursing services (eg, the associate director of critical care), hospital administrative personnel, and medical staff members. The advantage of this plan is that all parties participate in making decisions that may affect their respective departments.

Attending Physicians

It is generally agreed that the medical care of the patient in the CCU should be directed by his or her own physician in collaboration with the nursing staff and other members of the CCU team. However, it is essential that attending physicians transfer certain authority to the nursing staff of the CCU so that they can assume a decision-making role on their own when the situation demands. The essence of the physician–nurse relationship in the CCU is collaboration, not delegation.

The relationship of the attending physician to other physicians varies considerably among hospitals. In some institutions it is understood that any physician who happens to be present at the time of an emergency may assume command (eg, directing a code). In other hospitals the director of a unit (or a committee of physicians) is empowered to act not only in the event of emergencies but also if the general treatment program prescribed by the attending physician fails to meet the care standards of the unit.

Attending physicians should participate in a hospital's ongoing educational program for its nurses and house officers. Their presence at team conferences is especially important when the patients to be discussed are under their care.

The Intern and Resident Staff

In teaching hospitals, interns and resident physicians become part of the coronary-care team as delegates of the attending physician. It should be recognized that these house officers are in training and that their primary function is not to replace the attending physician in the direct care of patients; their assignment to the CCU is meant to be an educational experience.

It is customary practice for a house officer to be notified when the CCU nurse detects a change in the patient's clinical status or the patient develops a life-threatening problem. The decisions the house officer makes at these times often mean the difference between life and death. In many instances the house officer has time to confer with the attending physician or the unit medical director before deciding on a course of action, but in catastrophic situations the resident physician alone makes the ultimate decision about

treatment. Consequently, his or her role is vitally important to the success of an entire coronary-care program. Certain aspects of house officers' responsibilities are worth considering, so that nurses can assist them in clearly seeing their role in the CCU team.

The medical and nursing co-directors of the CCU should carefully explain to the house officers, during the first day's orientation, the unique role and status of the nurse on the CCU team. As might be anticipated, the nurse assumes a high degree of responsibility for the care of the patient. Not infrequently, because of their constant exposure to the problems related to the care of acutely ill cardiac patients, CCU nurses become extremely competent in the detection and management of a variety of cardiac complications, and the wise house officer will recognize the value of their judgment and experience. On the other hand, nurses need to be sensitive to the anxieties of physicians in training, and communicate their concerns and recommendations in a way that leaves the self-respect of the house staff intact.

The patient assignments of house staff and their on-call schedule should be posted in a conspicuous manner so that the nurse knows which physician to call for advice or for emergencies during each shift. In catastrophic situations, calling for a specific physician is more effective than having the nurse sound a general alarm that may be answered by any physician who happens to be nearby. General alarms tend to create confusion, with the sudden assemblage of several members of the house staff but without one person responsible for making decisions.

House officers and the nursing staff should join in making daily patient rounds in the CCU. In this way patient problems that may not be apparent to individual members of the team may be identified and solved. It is important that the primary nurse caring for the patient actively communicate information about the patient's status and seek clarification about the treatment plan. This form of communication is fundamental to effective care and can be an important learning experience for new members of the house staff in terms of the collaborative role of physicians and nurses in critical care.

PREPARATION OF THE CORONARY CARE UNIT NURSE

As mentioned previously, a nurse cannot function effectively in a CCU solely on the foundation of a basic nursing education program or previous general nursing experience. A hospital has a responsibility to provide all of the nurses working in its critical-care units with the necessary specialized knowledge they require. Many hospitals, as part of the general orientation to a unit, offer a general critical-care course to all nurses who do not have extensive experience in critical care. Such courses combine and integrate classroom instruction and clinical experience, with the latter being under the supervision of a nurse preceptor. The courses usually last approximately 6 weeks, and the entire orientation may last from 1–6 months, depending on the previous clinical experience of the staff nurse.

Because the background and previous experiences of the students in a critical-care course may vary considerably, the design and objectives of the course must be tailored to meet the diverse needs of the participants. Moreover, such courses need to be based on adult learning theory, with optimal opportunities for the CCU orientee to be an active participant in the learning process. Instructional aids used in many CCU orientations include audiotapes, computer-assisted instruction, heart-sound simulators, videotape simulations and lectures, and programmed instructional books. The terminal objectives of the orientation reflect minimal safe practice in critical care.

More advanced knowledge and skills can be obtained through a hospital-based advanced course in critical care or through one of the many commercial courses designed to prepare nurses to take the critical-care certification examination sponsored by the American Association of Critical-Care Nurses. Nurses are not eligible to sit for the certification examination until they have worked full-time in a critical-care setting for 2 years.

Nurses preparing to work in the CCU have special learning needs, related to the care of the acutely ill patient with cardiac disease, that have to be met outside a standard critical care course. For example, CCU nurses need a knowledge of cardiac-rhythm analysis that goes far beyond what might be required in another critical-care specialty. The following constitutes a sample list of classes that might supplement a basic critical-care course in preparing for CCU nursing.

Topics for Classroom Instruction and Discussion

1. Introduction to the concept of CCU: rationale, collaborative approach, shared governance
2. Anatomy and physiology of the cardiovascular system: cardiac chambers and valves; coronary circulation; cardiac hemodynamics; electrical conduction system
3. Cardiac auscultation: auscultation techniques, normal and abnormal heart sounds
4. Electrocardiography: basic principles, 12 surface leads and monitoring leads, normal ECG, ischemic changes
5. Cardiac diagnostic tests: laboratory tests, echocardiography, cardiac catheterization and angiography, radionuclide studies, electrophysiology
6. Coronary heart disease: incidence and prevalence, risk factors, pathophysiology, diagnostic procedures, counseling to promote life-style changes, angioplasty
7. Acute myocardial infarction: signs and symptoms, diagnostic tests (including cardiac enzymes), common nursing diagnoses, clinical course, thrombolysis, complications, psychological adaptation, patient and family teaching
8. Arrhythmias: classification, drug treatment, elective cardioversion, temporary cardiac pacing, permanent cardiac pacing, automatic implantable cardioverter-defibrillator, patient and family teaching
9. Cardiac and respiratory arrest: advanced cardiac life support
10. Heart failure: etiology, clinical assessment, hemodynamics, common nursing diagnoses, pharmacologic treatment, patient and family teaching
11. Cardiogenic shock: pathophysiology, clinical assessment, hemodynamics, pharmacologic treatment, intraaortic balloon pump
12. Cardiomyopathy: etiology, signs and symptoms, cardiac transplantation, immunosuppressive regimen
13. Oxygenation and respiratory therapy: indications, modes, complications, blood-gas interpretation, pulse oximetry, continuous $S\bar{v}o_2$ monitoring, weaning procedures
14. Cardiac rehabilitation: philosophy, patient and family education, stress testing, exercise prescription

In the CCU, the clinical nurse specialist or clinical educator usually plans the content of coursework that is supplemental to a more general critical-care course as part of the orientation program. The medical co-director or other physicians may be asked to lecture on various disease states, emphasizing their pathophysiology and current medical and surgical treatment. Nurse experts would be asked to lecture on the nursing diagnoses and treatment plans specific to a CCU patient population. Again, a team approach to the orientation of nursing staff personnel underscores the importance of a collaborative approach to the care of the CCU patient. This same team approach should also be used in the orientation of new medical house staff, with nurses lecturing on the human responses that are most frequently seen in a CCU patient population.

The presentations should build on what is usually presented in basic nursing programs and a beginning critical-care course. The lectures and discussion should be planned at an advanced, in-depth level.

Clinical Experience during Orientation

Clinical experience in coronary-care nursing is obtained primarily by having new orientees assigned to clinical nurse preceptors. The latter are experienced CCU nurses who are recognized by their peers as being outstanding models for nurses new to the CCU environment. The match should not be made on the basis of scheduling (ie, which nurses are scheduled to work in the unit), but rather on the expertise of the potential preceptor and his or her willingness to serve in this valuable role. The preceptorship requires the systematic provision of clinical experiences, with opportunities for the orientee to observe and practice necessary skills. Because the orientation program should be individualized to the unit, not all of the items on the checklist given in Table 1–2 may be appropriate; the items to be included should depend on the technology used in a particular unit.

TABLE 1–2 CLINICAL SKILLS CHECKLIST FOR CCU NURSES

Patient history

Physical examination
Examination of arterial pulses
Examination of jugular veins
Cardiac auscultation
Lung auscultation

Cardiac monitoring
Arrhythmia interpretation
12-lead ECG recording and interpretation

Hemodynamic monitoring
Pulmonary artery catheter measurement
Pulmonary wedge pressure measurement
Cardiac output measurement
Pulmonary artery catheter removal

Transthoracic electrical bioimpedance

Arterial pressure monitoring

Left atrial pressure monitoring

Assessment of oxygen delivery
Arterial blood-gas measurement
Pulse oximetry
Continuous mixed venous oxygen saturation
Respiratory therapy
Mechanical ventilation
Suctioning (tracheostomy and endotracheal tube)

External temporary pacemaker

Intraaortic balloon pump

Chest tube management

Cardiopulmonary resuscitation

Extracorporeal membrane oxygenation

Ventricular assist devices

Patient and family teaching

Chapter 2

Coronary Care Nursing

Intensive coronary care is an area of nursing specialization in which the number of lives saved is directly related to the competence of the nursing staff. To define this specialized nursing role clearly, it is appropriate first to outline the overall duties and responsibilities of the CCU nurse and then consider specific aspects of nursing care from the time of admission to discharge from the unit.

NURSING RESPONSIBILITIES IN CORONARY CARE UNIT

The primary goals of coronary care are to preserve life, prevent complications, and restore the patient to his or her maximum functional capacity (physical and emotional). To achieve these objectives the nurse members of the CCU team assume the responsibilities discussed in the following sections.

CONTINUOUS ASSESSMENT OF THE PATIENT'S CLINICAL STATUS

Direct Observation of the Patient

The patient is observed for any signs of circulatory compromise. This process includes an overall assessment of the patient's physical status as well as a focused examination of the patient's skin, extremities, pulses, blood pressure, heart sounds, and lung sounds. The purpose of the physical examination is to identify the patient's baseline cardiopulmonary status upon admission to the CCU, and then to note any change in cardiopulmonary status as a result of complications or therapy.

Skin. The skin is an important barometer of cardiopulmonary function. The nurse needs to assess the patient's skin color, turgor, temperature, and moisture. Although the range of normal variation in skin condition is immense, a number of acute physical conditions also affect the qualities of the skin. Therefore, the assessment of the patient's skin primarily involves changes from its baseline characteristics.

Pallor is a pale skin tone that is best seen in the creases of the palm of the hand and the conjunctiva. It reflects a decreased oxyhemoglobin concentration secondary to anemia, hypovolemia, low cardiac output, or infective endocarditis. During anxiety, or if the ambient temperature is cold, the skin may also appear pale because of vasoconstriction, but the color will improve as soon as the patient becomes less anxious or his or her temperature normalizes.

Cyanosis is a blue hue of the skin that reflects an increased quantity of deoxygenated hemoglobin. Central cyanosis (seen in the mucous membranes and tongue, as well as peripherally) occurs only when the concentration of deoxygenated hemoglobin in the blood is greater than 5 gm/100 mL. It can be seen in patients with congenital heart disease, chronic obstructive lung disease, or pulmonary hypertension. Its sudden appearance in a patient recovering from an acute myocardial infarction may signal a ventricular septal rupture (resulting in a left-to-right shunt) or pulmonary embolism. Peripheral cyanosis (seen in the extremities, particularly the nail beds, and the lips) is a sign of decreased peripheral perfusion. Like pallor, it may result from vasoconstriction caused by cold temperatures, but in the setting of a CCU can also be an important sign of low cardiac output.

Skin turgor reflects skin elasticity and fluid status. The turgor of the skin decreases with the normal process of aging, but also decreases when the patient is dehydrated (eg, from excessive diuresis) because of water loss from subcutaneous tissues.

The skin should be warm and dry. Cold and clammy skin is one of the hallmarks of cardiogenic shock, and occurs because of stimulation of the sympathetic nervous system. Patients with an evolving myocardial infarction or severe angina can also become cold and clammy, both as a response to the attendant chest pain and to the sudden reduction in cardiac output that occurs in both conditions.

Extremities.

The extremities are examined to reveal any evidence of edema, clubbing, cyanosis, inflammation, or peripheral emboli. The volume of interstitial fluid increases in congestive heart failure and is usually seen first as edema of the lower extremities when patients are not at bed-rest. When patients are primarily in a semi-Fowler's position, the edema may first appear in the sacral area. Edema is usually classified on a 1+ to 4+ scale by the amount of depression that remains when the nurse gently presses a finger on the edematous area for approximately 5 seconds, with 1+ being a 2 mm indentation, 2+ a 4 mm indentation, and so forth.

Clubbing occurs in a variety of disorders, many of which are not cardiac. However, in patients with low arterial oxygen saturation (eg, cyanotic congenital heart disease), clubbing is almost always present to some degree. The physical signs of digital clubbing are bulbous fingertips, nails that are thickened and hard, a nailbed that feels spongy to the touch, and a straightening of the nail angle (normally 160 degrees).

Patients at bed-rest in the CCU for more than a few days are at high risk for venous thrombosis in the lower extremities. This risk increases in those patients who also have a low cardiac output. Because of the threat of pulmonary embolism, it is important to identify immediately any inflammation, pain, or swelling in the lower extremities, thighs, or pelvic area that could signal a thrombosis so that treatment can be initiated.

A final note should be made of any petechiae seen on the ankles and wrists or under the nails, as well as any nodes on the pads of the fingers and toes (called Osler's nodes). These findings are seen in approximately one fourth of patients with endocarditis and are thought to be due to a vasculitis that occurs in response to circulating immune complexes.

Pulses.

Examination of the arterial pulses provides valuable information about the status of the left ventricle, aortic valve, and the arteries themselves. Pulses are palpated to determine the rate, rhythm, amplitude, and contour of the pulse wave. Pulse amplitude is usually rated on a 0 to 4+ scale, with 0 being the absence of a pulse, 2+ a normal pulse, and 4+

a bounding or hyperkinetic pulse. Seven pairs of pulses are assessed: the carotid, brachial, radial, femoral, popliteal, posterior tibial, and dorsalis pedis. The last, which is felt on the dorsum of both feet, is absent normally in about 15% of the population.

If the patient does not have a pulmonary artery catheter, examination of the jugular veins in the neck can provide information about the volume and pressure in the right side of the heart. Veins are assessed by inspection rather than palpation, since pressing on the jugular pulse obliterates it. The neck veins are best examined with the patient at a 30- to 45-degree angle. At this angle one would expect the venous pulsation to be seen at 1 to 3 cm above the sternal angle (the right atrial pressure equivalent of 6–8 cm H_2O). A venous pulsation at a level more than 3 cm above the sternal angle is the result of increased volume and pressure in the right atrium, usually secondary to right ventricular failure, tricuspid regurgitation, or pulmonary hypertension.

Blood Pressure.

Blood pressure is determined primarily by two factors: cardiac output and the elasticity of the arterial walls. Therefore, changes in blood pressure provide important clues to the cardiovascular status of the patient, and can be used as a partial guide to much of the therapy that patients receive in the CCU.

Hypertension (defined as a diastolic blood pressure above 90 mm Hg) is not often seen in the setting of the CCU. Hypotension (defined as a persistent blood pressure of less than 95/60 mm Hg) is much more of a concern because patients who have it frequently experience dysrhythmias (which negatively affect cardiac output and therefore blood pressure). Severe hypotension is also a sign of severe ventricular failure or cardiogenic shock. Patients also receive a number of vasoactive and diuretic drugs that can produce hypotension as a side effect. Hypotension is treated by correcting its cause (eg, normalizing the cardiac rhythm or giving the patient volume-expanding fluids) or treating a low cardiac output (eg, with inotropes, an intraaortic balloon pump, or a ventricular assist device).

Examination of the Heart and Lungs.

Normally the examination of the thorax involves a methodical assessment of the lungs and heart by inspection, palpation, percussion, and auscultation. In the CCU setting, where the patient's cardiopulmonary status is evaluated by numerous different (and often continuous) measures, the nurse's physical examination is quite focused. The purpose of the examination is to evaluate any change in the patient's condition that represents a response to therapy (for better or worse) or a worsening of the patient's disease (eg, extension of a myocardial infarction).

The lung fields are auscultated to identify the

development or disappearance of rhonchi, wheezes, or rales. Because these auscultory findings appear approximately 24 hours before changes are seen in a chest X-ray, frequent evaluation of breath sounds is an important strategy for identifying beginning pulmonary congestion. Lung sounds are auscultated by using the diaphragm of the stethoscope and asking the patient to take a deep breath and cough. Following this maneuver, the patient slowly inhales and exhales while the nurse systematically listens to each lung, beginning at the base.

The heart is usually auscultated to identify abnormal sounds that indicate a change in the patient's condition. The most important of these for a CCU nurse to identify are a third (S_3) and/or fourth (S_4) heart sound, a pericardial friction rub, and a mur-

mur(s). S_3 and S_4 are soft, low-pitched sounds heard best at the apex with the bell of the stethoscope. These sounds result from the vibration of the ventricular walls when blood rushes into the ventricles. S_3 occurs during early diastole with the rapid filling of the ventricle when the atrioventricular valves first open. S_4 is heard in late diastole when the atria contract, resulting in a forceful ejection of blood into the already distended ventricles. S_3 and S_4 become audible when the ventricles lose their compliance, such as immediately following an acute myocardial infarction or in patients with chronic hypertension. The sudden appearance of S_3 or S_4 can signal a change in the patient's clinical status (eg, new myocardial ischemia or heart failure).

A pericardial friction rub is caused by the two sur-

TABLE 2–1. COMMONLY HEARD HEART MURMURS

Murmurs	Valve	Auscultory Technique	Quality of Sound	Variables
Holosystolic murmur	Mitral regurgitation Tricuspid regurgitation Ventricular septal defect	Diaphragm at apex, radiates to left axilla or base	High pitch, harsh blowing quality	Thrill may be palpable at base; S_1 decreased; S_2 increased with P_2 often accentuated; S_3 often present
				If mild, late systolic crescendo murmur present; if severe, early systolic decrescendo murmur and summation gallop present
Systolic ejection	Aortic stenosis	Bell over third intercostal space; right sternal border	Medium pitch, coarse with crescendo-decrescendo pattern	May radiate to apex and to cartoid; S_1 may be followed by ejection click
	Pulmonic stenosis	Bell over third intercostal space, left sternal border; radiates left to neck	Same as for aortic stenosis	S_1 usually followed by ejection click; S_4 common if right ventricular hypertrophy present
Diastolic murmur	Mitral stenosis	Bell at apex with patient in left lateral-decubitus position	Low rumble, more intense in early and late diastole	P_2 commonly followed by opening snap. Decreased arterial pulse
	Tricuspid stenosis	Bell over tricuspid area	Similar to mitral stenosis but louder on inspiration	Decreased arterial pulse. Jugular pulse prominent, especially a wave; v wave falls slowly
	Aortic regurgitation	Diaphragm, with patient sitting and leaning forward	High pitch, blowing in early diastole	Early ejection click may be present. Wide pulse pressure
	Pulmonic regurgitation	Same as aortic regurgitation	Same as aortic regurgitation	

faces of the pericardial sac rubbing together. It is heard when the parietal and visceral surfaces of the pericardial sac became inflamed (pericarditis). The friction rub is a rough, scratchy noise that increases with inspiration and is usually heard best at the left sternal border in the third and fourth intercostal spaces.

Finally, many patients are admitted to the CCU with cardiac murmurs, usually related to incompetence or stenosis of one or more of the heart valves. A summary of these murmurs is presented in Table 2–1. In the CCU setting, nurses are usually less concerned about identifying preexisting murmurs and more concerned about assessing any change in a murmur. For example, in a patient recovering from a recent acute myocardial infarction, the sudden appearance of a high-pitched, blowing murmur at the apex could represent the rupture of one or more papillary muscles of the mitral valve, and may signal the onset of acute congestive heart failure or cardiogenic shock.

Electrocardiographic Monitoring

Patients admitted to the CCU are, by virtue of their cardiac disease, usually at high risk for sudden death and/or arrhythmias that severely compromise their ability to maintain tissue perfusion. Therefore, the hallmark of CCU nursing care has been surveillance. Nurses must be able to identify arrhythmias, assess their relative danger, and decide what action to take. (ECG monitoring is discussed in Chapter 3 and arrhythmias are discussed in Chapters 8 through 14.) Heart rate and rhythm are monitored continuously in all patients in the CCU, and nurses in the unit operate under the auspices of standing clinical protocols to treat life-threatening arrhythmias as soon as they develop. In the absence of house staff, the nurse must also identify candidates for thrombolytic therapy by obtaining a 12-lead ECG from patients with chest pain of new onset.

Hemodynamic Monitoring

In patients with severe ventricular failure, it is often necessary to measure cardiac venous and arterial pressures repeatedly in order to assess the severity of the problem and the effects of treatment. Hemodynamic monitoring can mean anything from taking a patient's blood pressure to measuring pulmonary artery pressure and cardiac output. The latter is an invasive technique that requires catheterization of the right side of the heart, most often through the internal jugular or subclavian veins. When possible, the procedure is conducted with the aid of fluoroscopy.

Several catheters with two or three lumens (or openings) have been developed for hemodyamic monitoring. One lumen permits measurement of pressure in the right atrium as well as providing a port through which to inject fluid for measurement of the

cardiac output. A second lumen measures the pressure in the pulmonary artery. When a balloon is inflated in the pulmonary artery catheter, the lumen measures the pressure in the left ventricle. Cardiac output can also be measured by the thermodilution technique, using a catheter equipped with a thermistor. A third lumen is available for administering drugs or intravenous fluids. A special fiberoptic pulmonary artery catheter provides a continuous measure of the mixed venous oxygen saturation ($S\bar{v}o_2$), a value that reflects the patient's overall oxygen utilization. (See Chapter 3 for the normal ranges of the parameters measured.) Pulmonary artery catheters may also contain a pacemaker wire that can provide temporary pacing of the heart in an emergency situation.

Invasive hemodynamic monitoring is an integral component of any CCU because it provides a direct means of quantifying a patient's cardiac status and response to therapy. (The technique is discussed in greater depth in Chapter 3.) CCU nurses use the information provided by hemodynamic monitoring to titrate drug dosages and make other treatment decisions. Hemodynamic monitoring is almost always used for patients who have developed serious complications following a myocardial infarction (eg, heart failure, cardiogenic shock, ventricular septal defect, pericardial tamponade).

ANTICIPATION AND PREVENTION OF COMPLICATIONS

Patients admitted to a CCU are at high risk for a number of complications related to their cardiac disease and accompanying psychological stress. By anticipating these complications, nurses can intervene to minimize or prevent their occurrence.

Decreased Cardiac Output Related to Arrhythmias or Mechanical Factors

One of the fundamental objectives of coronary care is to prevent ventricular fibrillation and standstill by treating warning arrhythmias. CCU nurses are authorized to treat arrhythmias with appropriate intravenous drugs (eg, lidocaine or adenosine) under standing protocols. All patients should have an intravenous line or heparin lock for emergency intravenous drug administration.

Conduction defects also lead to decreased cardiac output. CCU nurses should document the occurrence of any conduction defect so that the CCU team can consider the possible need for inserting a temporary transvenous pacemaker. Patients with temporary or permanent cardiac pacemakers require careful and continuous assessment. An abrupt failure of a pacemaker (eg, as the result of battery failure or a disconnected wire) can be disastrous. Nurses sometimes can prevent these failures by noting early failure of the pacemaker to capture the ventricles, or noting other changes on the cardiac monitor that suggest pacemaker malfunction.

Derangements in the mechanical forces that affect stroke volume (ie, preload, afterload and myocardial contractility) are the second most frequent cause of alterations in cardiac output in CCU patients. Patients at risk for heart failure need to have their hemodynamic status constantly monitored and vasoactive medications titrated to maintain their preload (as reflected by the pulmonary capillary wedge pressure) and afterload (as reflected by systemic vascular resistance) within a therapeutic range.

Impaired Gas Exchange/Ineffective Airway Clearance

Oxygen tension (PaO_2) is measured by arterial blood gas analysis on admission to the CCU. If the patient's oxygen tension is normal, supplemental oxygen may be omitted. Hypoxemic patients and patients with intermittent ischemic chest pain are usually started on oxygen at 2 to 4 L/min by mask or nasal cannula for the first 2 to 3 days following a myocardial infarction.

In the patient with ventricular failure and high pulmonary capillary pressures, alveolar-capillary gas exchange will be compromised. The patient will have to be monitored closely to detect signs and symptoms of impaired ventilation and perfusion. Frequent physical examinations (including lung auscultation), serial arterial blood gas analysis, chest X-rays, hemodynamic monitoring, continuous $S\bar{v}O_2$ monitoring, and/or pulse oximetry all provide important information toward preventing further compromise of a patient's respiratory status. Oxygen therapy by mask or nasal cannula will be required to correct hypoxemia and hypercapnia, and the nurse should be prepared to assist with intubation and mechanical ventilation if the patient's respiratory status deteriorates.

Patients requiring mechanical ventilation who have aspirated gastric material into their lungs (eg, during a cardiac arrest) or who have acute or chronic pulmonary disease need frequent pulmonary hygiene to maintain clear airways. Nurses will need to suction these patients frequently and provide chest percussion to prevent further deterioration of the respiratory system.

Fluid-Volume Excess or Deficit

The body responds to a reduced cardiac output by increasing its secretion of aldosterone and antidiuretic hormone (described in Chapter 7) in a regulatory mechanism that increases cardiac output by increasing intravascular volume. This increase in intravascular volume in the face of a reduced cardiac output results in fluid-volume excess. To reduce the possibility of pulmonary edema patients' fluid intake and output must be scrupulously measured and the sodium content of their dietary intake and intravenous fluids must be severely restricted (usually to 2 or 3 grams or less of sodium each day in patients with ejection fractions below 40%).

CCU nurses must monitor the patient's clinical status for any signs of fluid-volume excess (eg, weight gain, dependent edema, crackles and wheezes over the lung fields, jugular venous distention, tachypnea, or the appearance of a third heart sound). Volume overload must be treated with diuretics and fluid restriction. Because intravenous medications often involve the administration of large volumes of fluid over a 24-hour period, intravenous drips given to patients with advanced heart failure and hypervolemia should be as concentrated as possible.

Patients can also experience hypovolemia (too little blood volume) if they have been given excessive diuretics or had fluid withheld for long periods. Signs of volume deficit include thirst, poor skin turgor, a high urine specific gravity, and hypotension.

Sleep-Pattern Disturbance

The nature of medical and nursing care in any ICU frequently leads to high levels of noise and light and many interruptions in the patient's sleep. Patients are therefore prevented from sleeping for any extended period, and suffer the effects of sleep-pattern disturbance within a few days of admission. In one study conducted in a respiratory ICU for example, only 50% to 60% of patient sleep occurred at night, and no patients completed natural 90-minute sleep cycles. Sleep-disturbing events occurred on an average of every 20 minutes. Patients at greatest risk for sleep-pattern disturbance are the elderly, because of the normal changes in the quality of sleep that accompany aging.

Nursing interventions to prevent and/or treat sleep-pattern disturbance are based on a thorough assessment of the patient's normal sleep pattern, including the duration of sleep, pattern of daytime naps, customary rituals surrounding sleep, and use of hypnotics. All noise and lighting on the CCU need to be minimized, and beds must be physically screened from the rest of the unit. Because changes in sound and light levels can create documented electroencephalographic arousal and sleep-stage transitions without actually awakening the patient, the bedside environment needs to be controlled as much as possible. Probably the most important nursing intervention with regard to sleep is to allow the patient to sleep unless some disturbance is absolutely required.

Nursing care in the CCU should be carefully reviewed and planned so that patients can have optimal sleep patterns. No routine nursing activities or diagnostic tests should be performed at night, during patients normal sleeping hours. The need for routine monitoring of vital signs should be assessed and orders altered to provide for uninterrupted sleep whenever possible. Many CCU patients are inappropriately assigned a schedule of having their vital signs measured every 2 hours, which ensures sleep deprivation ("routine vital signs" are not a justification for awakening a patient who is sound asleep and whose monitor remains unchanged). Finally, when possible, nurses should evaluate hemodynamic parameters without disturbing the patient. Pulmonary artery pressures and cardiac output measurements can, for example, be accurately obtained in a variety of supine positions ranging up to 60 degrees of headrest elevation. Patients do not need to be awakened and repositioned each time these measurements are made.

Anxiety

Patients are naturally anxious upon admission to the CCU. Given the meaning of heart disease to most individuals, and the stress of being hospitalized in a CCU, much of this anxiety cannot be prevented. However, the arousal of the sympathetic nervous system that occurs with anxiety can markedly increase myocardial oxygen consumption in a patient who can ill afford it. Therefore, it is important that nurses do whatever they can to minimize a patient's anxiety by providing the patient with an appropriate orientation to the unit (both to the personnel and the routines), giving information about the events the patient has experienced and what they mean, preparing patients beforehand for any diagnostic tests or procedures, using appropriate sedation, and involving the family as fully as possible in the patient's care. This last intervention deserves amplification.

According to several national surveys conducted in the 1980s, the majority of CCUs and ICUs allow only structured, limited visiting hours (ie, 10 minutes every hour for immediate family only), even though research reported over the past two decades suggests an inverse relationship between patient anxiety and family visiting in the CCU. Comparisons of patient stress responses in three types of CCU interactions—family/patient; nurse/patient when the nurse was performing a patient-care task; and nurse/patient when the nurse was conversing with the patient—have found no change in patient cardiovascular parameters during any of these interactions, but have found that the measured vocal stress of patients decreased during family visits. Patients whose families are allowed unlimited visiting are frequently less anxious and less likely to become confused than when visiting is severely restricted. A policy of open visiting hours allows the primary nurse to contract with patients and their families for the amount of time they will spend together and the families' degree of involvement in the physical care of the patient. For some patients and families the optimal arrangement may be to have a relative at the bedside at all times, while for other families a restricted visiting schedule would be best for all concerned.

Another source of patients' anxiety is their transfer from the CCU, which represents a form of "separation anxiety" for patients who have become accustomed to the security of constant monitoring and of established relationships with the CCU nurses. A number of interventions can be implemented to reduce the stress surrounding transfer from the CCU. Preparation for transfer from the CCU to a stepdown unit or general ward should include both patients and their families.

Patients in the CCU often experience a sense of powerlessness related to their disease. This feeling can be accentuated by the enforced immobility required during hospitalization in an intensive care unit, which can quickly erode a patient's sense of control. Much of today's physiologic monitoring requires that the patient remain attached to machines. Nonetheless, nurses and physicians can compound the problem of limited mobility by choosing sites for intravenous and intraarterial lines that require arm boards and wrist restraints (ie, in the antecubital fossa), or which prevent the patient from standing or sitting at the bedside (ie, the groin or ankle). Promoting a patient's mobility in the ICU therefore, involves minimizing the use of restraints and armboards, encouraging the patient to get out of bed and sit at the bedside, and allowing the patient to go out of the unit whenever possible (particularly in the case of chronically, critically ill patients who spend weeks or months in the CCU).

Ineffective Coping

A problem experienced by many patients in the CCU is ineffective coping. The stress that these patients experience in relation to their illness and/or hospitalization is often more than they can tolerate. Patients feel incompetent to meet their new situation, whether it be in the CCU itself or in the anticipated future, with their usual coping mechanisms or resources.

Ineffective coping is manifested in a variety of behaviors, including denial, anxiety, anger, and depression. These can be normal responses to the losses imposed by illness or hospitalization, but when experienced to a severe degree they can reflect a patient's inability to incorporate the loss(es) and sense of crisis that admission to the CCU has triggered.

The stress experienced by the newly admitted CCU patient is extraordinarily high. The patient may feel a sense of imminent death and total dependence on others for survival. If the precipitating event was a first myocardial infarction, the patient probably experienced pain that is severe and ominous, and unlike anything previously experienced. If the event that precipitated admission to the CCU involved a life threatening arrhythmia (aborted cardiac arrest), the patient may wake up to the terrified looks of family members or co-workers and not remember any of the events that preceded the collapse. The patient can spend days in the CCU wondering what would have happened had the event not been witnessed and help called, or contemplating what lies ahead. If the diagnosis is pulmonary edema, the patient may experience terrifying breathlessness.

The subjective experiences that bring an individual to the emergency room or CCU are compounded by the rites of hospital admission. Monitoring electrodes are attached to the chest, an intravenous infusion is started, oxygen is administered, injections are given, blood samples are drawn, and unfamiliar nurses, physicians, and technicians hurriedly enter and leave the cubicle where the patient lies. The thought, "Am I dying?" often runs through the patient's mind. The strangeness of the CCU environment, with its monitors, machines, and noises, contributes to the burden of the patient's fear. Patients often cannot mobilize their internal resources to reduce their stress response because they are focusing on simply surviving.

The intensity of the emotional reactions to a cardiac emergency can be reduced if these reactions are anticipated. It is helpful for patients to know that the emotions they experience are normal and are experienced by most patients who have cardiac disease. Some reactions, such as mild depression or denial, are physiologically helpful to the patient because they reduce blood pressure and heart rate (in the case of depression) or minimize the sympathetic response to an emergency (in the case of denial). Both reactions prevent an increase in myocardial oxygen consumption. Patients need not be confronted with their behavioral response. If they can articulate their feelings, it can be helpful to them if the nurse listens attentively and tries to clarify areas of misconception. Patients usually do not retain information provided in the CCU about heart disease and the course of their hospitalization, but such information is helpful in supporting a positive, problem-solving attitude.

Social Isolation

Unlike patients in other intensive-care specialties, patients in the CCU are often fully alert. When admitted to the CCU for observation and monitoring, most are frightened and lonely. One of the most effective measures for preventing a sense of social isolation is open visiting, in which patients can see their families and friends. Primary nursing is also a powerful weapon to combat feelings of alienation, since this system of care encourages the patient to identify one or two nurses who become well-known and trusted.

Nurses can minimize the patient's sense of social isolation through a number of individual strategies, none of which are dramatic. These include identifying themselves by name when they approach the bedside, using consistent eye contact during conversations, calling the patient by name (after asking the patient how he or she prefers to be addressed), and not discussing the patient in the third person within the patient's hearing range.

Alterations in Comfort

Patients in the CCU have many reasons for feeling pain and discomfort. Some have pathologic processes, such as myocardial ischemia or pericarditis, that can cause intense pain. Their pain needs to be treated immediately to prevent the sympathetic nervous response to pain that translates into increased myocardial oxygen consumption.

Unfortunately, nurses and physicians also create pain in the course of treating a patient. Suctioning through endotracheal tubes, venipuncture, and the insertion of pulmonary artery catheters, to name but a few routine procedures, are all accompanied by some degree of pain. If control of pain is truly a mutual patient–staff goal, the nurse must work with the patient to relieve pain before it becomes unmanageable, and to prepare the patient for procedures so as to minimize the pain they incur. Patients need to receive analgesia one half hour before any activity that will result in pain, and must be instructed in strategies that have been shown to augment the pharmacologic approach to pain control, such as the relaxation response, biofeedback, imagery, and distraction.

Patients who are on ventilatory support and are given a neuromuscular blocking agent such as pancuronium bromide (Pavulon) to allow better synchronization of their breathing with the ventilator still require analgesia. Paralyzing agents do not reduce pain or alter a patient's level of consciousness. Patients who are paralyzed in this way can become quite terrified. *Paralyzing agents should never be administered without concomitant sedation, pain control, and reassurance. It is the role of the nurse to ensure that patients who are paralyzed are also sedated adequately and remain pain free.*

EMERGENCY AND RESUSCITATIVE TREATMENT

Despite all efforts at preventing them, unexpected catastrophes can and do occur in patients with acute myocardial infarction. In these circumstances, survival hinges on split-second decisions and actions. Not only must the nursing staff itself be prepared for such emergencies, but it is absolutely essential that all resuscitative equipment and supplies be ready for instant use. Machines—particularly defibrillators—should be tested regularly to verify that they are functioning properly.

Cardiopulmonary Resuscitation

When sudden death impends because preventive treatment is ineffective or cannot be accomplished in time, the final hope for survival is cardiopulmonary resuscitation by means of external cardiac compression and mouth-to-mouth ventilation. This technique maintains the circulation until corrective procedures can be instituted. Every nurse must be proficient in performing effective cardiopulmonary resuscitation. Because resuscitation skills quickly decay, even when they are used frequently in clinical practice, the staff of the CCU requires biannual certification in advanced cardiac life support (ACLS) and annual certification in cardiopulmonary resuscitation (CPR).

Defibrillation

Although preventive measures certainly reduce the risk of ventricular fibrillation, the fact remains that this lethal arrhythmia can develop at any time. The preservation of life after the onset of ventricular fibrillation depends in nearly all instances on the ability of the CCU nurse to recognize the arrhythmia and terminate it immediately by means of precordial shock (defibrillation). The nurse applies a large direct-current (DC) shock without synchronization, usually 200 J. The earlier the shock is applied after the onset of ventricular fibrillation, the more likely it is that normal sinus rhythm can be restored.

Assisted Ventilation

Mechanical ventilators are sometimes needed to provide adequate tissue oxygenation in the treatment of advanced circulatory failure. Although, respiratory therapists operate and maintain this equipment in most hospitals, the CCU nurse must be familiar with the ongoing operation of mechanical ventilators and must be able to recognize problems that occur during their use. Nurses must also know how to use manual breathing bags effectively during periods of cardiopulmonary arrest (prior to intubation) and during patient transport.

COMMUNICATION

As the only member of the CCU team who constantly attends the patient, the nurse must communicate with the patient and the patient's family, with physicians and other nurses, and with other CCU and hospital personnel. The specific responsibilities involved in this communication are:

1. To explain to the patient (and a family member whenever possible) the objectives of coronary intensive care, the reasons for various procedures, and how these procedures are accomplished. Above all, the nurse should answer questions about the patient's illness in direct, understandable terms.
2. To apprise the family of the patient's clinical condition and progress, allay their fears, and enlist their cooperation.
3. To serve as a liaison between the physician(s), the patient, and the family, particularly in clarifying misconceptions about the plan of care and in clarifying the patient's and family's desires for treatment.
4. To advise the physician of the patient's clinical status and to report any meaningful changes as soon as they occur.
5. To present succinct, comprehensive reports to the other members of the nursing staff about the condition of each patient, so that there will be effective continuity of care. This communication occurs at each change of shift, but the patient's condition and treatment plan also need to be summarized in a nursing-care plan that is updated on a daily basis.

COLLECTION AND RECORDING OF DATA

Nursing History

A sometimes tedious but always important nursing responsibility is to obtain and record pertinent information about the patient's personal health habits, dietary and elimination patterns, problems with activity and sleep, social history, and other facts that influence nursing care.

Nursing-Care Plan

It is essential that the information obtained in the nursing history be summarized in a nursing-care plan, so that the patient's baseline nursing diagnoses can be established and a plan of care instituted.

Documentation of Arrhythmias

Whenever a significant arrhythmia is observed, the nurse should document it by recording an ECG from the cardiac monitor. Other cardiac rhythms are recorded and analyzed at regular intervals (eg, at the beginning of each shift) and placed in the patient's record to provide a baseline and serial record of the patient's rhythm. These tracings can be useful in detecting progressive changes in arrhythmias.

Drug Therapy

The dosage, time of administration, and effects of all drugs must be specifically noted. This information is extremely important in assessing whether changes are necessary in a patient's treatment program. (The actions of commonly used cardiac drugs are described in Appendix A.)

Nursing Notes

Progress notes written by both nurses and physicians provide an ongoing account of the patient's illness and are an important communication tool within the CCU team. The nurse should record all pertinent clinical observations, interventions, future plans, and other information pertaining to nursing care. In many hospitals, notes written by both nurses and physicians are recorded in combined progress notes, using medical and nursing diagnoses to identify the patient's problems and the SOAP format (subjective and objective findings, assessment, and plan of care) for their management. Physiologic data, medications given, and fluid intake and output are often summarized on separate flow sheets (Figure 2–1) or entered directly into a bedside computer (as discussed in Chapter 3).

EDUCATION

Students

An important responsibility of all CCU nurses who work in institutions involved in educational programs is to teach nursing and medical students knowledge and skills specific to the care of cardiac patients. Experienced nurses serve as preceptors for nursing students. They also can help medical students to attain various critical-care skills (eg, starting intravenous infusions, measuring cardiac output, interpreting cardiac arrhythmias) and apply theory to individual clinical situations. By generously sharing their knowledge and respecting the learning needs of the students who rotate through the CCU, nurses continue the tradition of mutual interdisciplinary collaboration that has been the hallmark of coronary care.

Staff Nurses

New staff nurses are usually assigned to a single clinical preceptor during their orientation to the CCU. To be fully integrated into the CCU team, new orientees need time to learn the policies and procedures of the individual unit. Obviously, orientees who are new graduates, will require a longer time to become safe and effective practitioners. Not only does the preceptor's teaching benefit others, but it also enhances the preceptor's own learning.

Patient and Family Members

Although detailed, structured teaching of patients and their family members is not usually attempted during the acute phase of a patient's illness, there is much that the CCU nurse can do in assessing the readiness of the patient and family to learn, and in providing information that is appropriate at the time. Research has shown that patients remember very few facts taught in formal teaching programs in the hospital; however, they do benefit from clear and direct answers to questions and from simple explanations about what they can anticipate while in the CCU and after they are discharged from it. By responding to the patient's and family's questions or cues in a simple but informative manner, the nurse can start an educational process that can be developed throughout the course of the patient's hospitalization.

The main object of patient education is to dispel common misconceptions about heart disease and its consequences. The patient's concept of a heart attack is often grossly distorted, and many of his or her fears are therefore unrealistic and unwarranted. For example, patients commonly believe that even if they recover from a heart attack they will have to take medication for the rest of their lives, or curtail their sexual activity. To combat these fears the nurse should offer repeated explanations about various aspects of myocardial infarction, and should identify and clarify any misconceptions the patient may have. It is important to answer the patient's questions in a forthright manner. By avoiding a question the nurse can indirectly intensify a patient's anxiety (as well as block any further discussion).

The family should be included in all explana-

PATIENT PROBLEM/NURSING DX	STANDARD/PROTOCOL	EVALUATION

UCLA Medical Center
DEPARTMENT OF NURSING
CRITICAL CARE FLOW SHEET

DAILY USE ITEMS

- SOFCARE MATTRESS
- SHEEPSKIN
- INCENTIVE SPIROMETER
- PULSATILE STOCKINGS
- TRAY/TYPE
- MONIT. KIT/TYPE
- URINE METER
- SUCTION CANISTER SET
- OXIMETER PROBE
- BURETROL
- TED HOSE
- BP CUFF
- FOOTBOARD
- SPECIAL BED
- AQUAPAD
- COOLING BLANKET
- OXIMETER
- COMMODE CHAIR
- IV PUMP:TYPE   NO.
- THROMBOGUARD MACHINE
- EXERCISE BIKE
- OVERHEAD FRAME

PATIENT TEACHING

TOPIC	P F	WRITTEN MATERIAL	VERBAL EXPLANATION	DEMO GIVEN	EVALUATION/ RETURN DEMO

NURSE TO PATIENT RATIO DOCUMENT

07-19: 2:1☐   1:1☐   1:2☐   OBS☐
☐OFF   ☐ON
☐CONTINUING

19-07: 2:1☐   1:1☐   1:2☐   OBS☐
☐OFF   ☐ON
☐CONTINUING

CRITERIA: (FOR 2:1 or 1:1)
☐ HEMODYNAMIC INSTABILITY
☐ PULMONARY INSTABILITY
☐ NEUROLOGIC INSTABILITY
☐ INFECTION/ISOLATION
☐ TOTALLY DEPENDENT; POTENTIAL FOR HARM
☐ SPECIAL TRIPS/PROCEDURES
☐ OTHER:

PROCEDURAL CHECK LIST

NURSING PROCEDURES	TIME INIT.	TIME INIT.	TIME INIT.	TIME INIT.	TIME INIT.	TIME INIT.	TIME INIT.
BATH							
SKIN CARE							
FOLEY CARE							
TRACH/ETT CARE							
MOUTH CARE							
RESTRAINTS							
WOUND CARE/ DRESS CHANGE							

INVASIVE MONITORING AND IV LINE CARE	DAY NO.	CONDITION OF SITE
ARTERIAL LINE		
PA CATHETER		
CENTRAL VENOUS CATHETER		
OTHER:		
OTHER:		
OTHER:		

Figure 2–1. Flow sheet for charting in coronary intensive care unit.

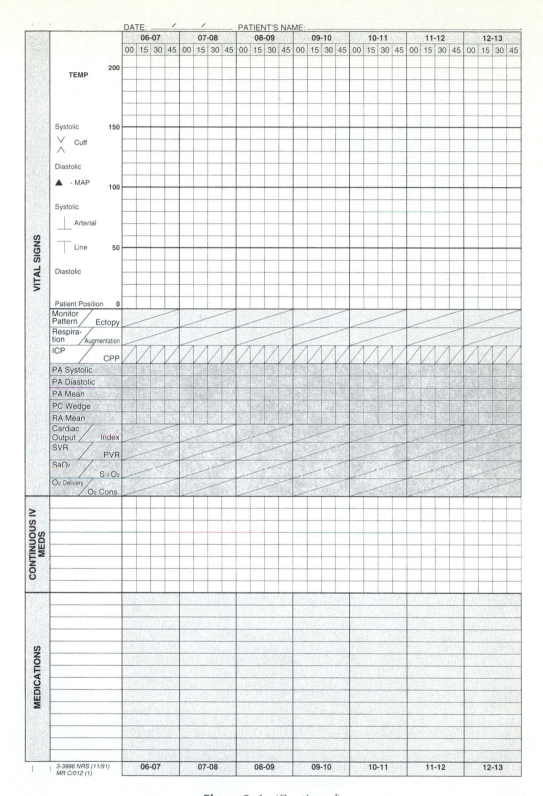

Figure 2–1. (Continued).

SHIFT ASSESSMENT	TIME

NEURO:
Corneal R___ L___   Babinski R___ L___   Cough___   GAG ___   CSF color_____
Ventriculostomy/Camino   Level:_____ Head dressing/drainage_____ /_____

CARDIOVASCULAR:
Heart sounds: S1 S2 S3 S4   clear   distant   rub   Murmur: Systolic   Diastolic   Pacer: Type:___ Settings: MA:___ Rate:___
Edema: pitting   non-pitting   Location:_____ JVD___ Radial Pulses: R___ L___   Demand Asynch.
Chest pain:___ Location:_____ Intensity: (1→10)_____   Quality: sharp   dull   heavy pressure   burning   radiation

PULMONARY:
Respiratory pattern: regular   shallow   deep   other:_____   Complaints: dyspnea   orthopnea
Bilateral chest expansion: Breath sounds   bilateral other:_____ Location of: crackles____   rhonchi____   wheeze____
Cough: productive   non-productive   Sputum consistency/color_____ ETT/Trach: Size:_____   Position: R L   Cm_____
Chest tube: location _____ suct.___ WS clamped   Chest tube: location_____ suct.___ WS clamped

GASTROINTESTINAL/GENITOURINARY:
NG tube:_____ Placement verified___ Suction: I C Drainage _____ Tube feeding:_____
pH _____ Abdomen: distended soft flat rigid tender obese   Location of tenderness _____
Bowel Sounds: normal   absent   hyperactive   hypoactive
Drainage tubes: (1) type/location/drainage _____   (2) type/location/drainage _____
                (3) type/location/drainage _____   (4) type/location/drainage _____
Stool: last BM ____ Appearance:_____   Incontinent   collection system_____
Urine: foley condom voiding Appearance: _____
Vaginal discharge: _____

INTEGUMENTARY:
Skin color/condition: WNL flushed cyanotic pale jaundice cool warm moist dry location:_____
Skin integrity: intact ecchymosis decubitus lacerations rash other_____ Location/description_____
Wounds/incisions/location _____ dressing/drainage _____
Wounds/incisions/location _____ dressing/drainage _____
Wounds/incisions/location _____ dressing/drainage _____

PSYCHOSOCIAL:
Emotional state: calm anxious crying withdrawn agitated combative other: _____
Thought Content: delusions hallucinations suicidal ideation normal other:_____ Family: visiting telephone

PAIN: location/description: _____

Comments: _____

Nurse/Hours of Care _____ / _____   Nurse/Hours of Care _____ / _____

SHIFT ASSESSMENT	TIME

NEURO:
Corneal R___ L___   Babinski R___ L___   Cough___   GAG ___   CSF color_____
Ventriculostomy/Camino   Level:_____ Head dressing/drainage_____ /_____

CARDIOVASCULAR:
Heart sounds: S1 S2 S3 S4   clear   distant   rub   Murmur: Systolic   Diastolic   Pacer: Type:___ Settings: MA:___ Rate:___
Edema: pitting   non-pitting   Location:_____ JVD___ Radial Pulses: R___ L___   Demand Asynch.
Chest pain:___ Location:_____ Intensity: (1→10)_____   Quality: sharp   dull   heavy pressure   burning   radiation

PULMONARY:
Respiratory pattern: regular   shallow   deep   other:_____   Complaints: dyspnea   orthopnea
Bilateral chest expansion: Breath sounds   bilateral other:_____ Location of: crackles____   rhonchi____   wheeze____
Cough: productive   non-productive   Sputum consistency/color_____ ETT/Trach: Size:_____   Position: R L   Cm_____
Chest tube: location _____ suct.___ WS clamped   Chest tube: location_____ suct.___ WS clamped

GASTROINTESTINAL/GENITOURINARY:
NG tube:_____ Placement verified___ Suction: I C Drainage _____ Tube feeding:_____
pH _____ Abdomen: distended soft flat rigid tender obese   Location of tenderness _____
Bowel Sounds: normal   absent   hyperactive   hypoactive
Drainage tubes: (1) type/location/drainage _____   (2) type/location/drainage _____
                (3) type/location/drainage _____   (4) type/location/drainage _____
Stool: last BM ____ Appearance:_____   Incontinent   collection system_____
Urine: foley condom voiding Appearance: _____
Vaginal discharge: _____

INTEGUMENTARY:
Skin color/condition: WNL flushed cyanotic pale jaundice cool warm moist dry location:_____
Skin integrity: intact ecchymosis decubitus lacerations rash other_____ Location/description_____
Wounds/incisions/location _____ dressing/drainage _____
Wounds/incisions/location _____ dressing/drainage _____
Wounds/incisions/location _____ dressing/drainage _____

PSYCHOSOCIAL:
Emotional state: calm anxious crying withdrawn agitated combative other: _____
Thought Content: delusions hallucinations suicidal ideation normal other:_____ Family: visiting telephone

PAIN: location/description: _____

Comments: _____

Nurse/Hours of Care _____ / _____   Nurse/Hours of Care _____ / _____

Figure 2–1. (Continued).

tions. The patient's illness and hospitalization affects the family in a major way, and family members also need information and clarification regarding any misconceptions they may hold. Providing them with clear explanations of the patient's medical condition and the anticipated hospital course gives family members the information they need to plan for the future, and is an important source of reassurance. In many CCUs the family is given prepared brochures that describe the purpose of the CCU, the monitoring equipment it contains, visiting hours, and other information pertinent to the patient's stay in the unit. The American Association of Critical Care Nurses also has a brochure that can be given to family members of patients hospitalized in a critical-care unit. Written information is helpful since, like the patient, the family members may be so emotionally upset that they have difficulty understanding verbal communication. Despite this difficulty, it is important that nurses communicate verbally with the family to help them understand their role in the patient's recovery. Every effort should be made to enlist their cooperation and understanding. Reassuring the family is every bit as important as reassuring the patient.

Chapter 3

Monitoring in the Coronary Care Unit

In the history of coronary care, continuous electrocardiographic monitoring of the heart was long the key to patient management. Indeed, the CCU was set apart from other units in the hospital by its nurses' ability to detect warning and lethal arrhythmias and treat them immediately. During the past three decades other types of monitoring have been added. Of these, the continuous monitoring of a patient's hemodynamic status has become as important as ECG monitoring in a subset of patients (particularly those with advanced heart failure). Continuous monitoring of a patient's oxygenation status is now also possible with pulse oximetry and $S\bar{v}O_2$ monitoring. Monitoring of the ST segment of the ECG is used to assess a patient's response to thrombolysis. Most recently, clinical-information systems have been introduced into many CCUs to integrate the vast array of patient data gathered by nurses.

In this chapter we will focus on the two most commonly used types of monitoring: cardiac and invasive hemodynamic monitoring. We will also briefly discuss the exciting potential and the frustrating problems of clinical-information systems.

CARDIAC MONITORING

Central to the concept of coronary care is continuous electrocardiographic monitoring of the heart. Indeed, without the ability to detect warning and lethal arrhythmias, intensive coronary care would have little advantage over regular hospital care. Therefore it is essential that all coronary care nurses fully understand the principles and methods of cardiac monitoring, and be able to utilize this technique to its fullest advantage.

Cardiac monitoring is based on the fact that each heartbeat is the result of an electrical stimulus. This stimulus, which normally originates in a specialized area of the right atrium called the sinoatrial node, is conducted as an impulse through a network of fibers within the heart (the conduction system) and finally stimulates the myocardium to contract. This same electrical force spreads outward from the heart and reaches the surface of the body, where it can be detected with electrodes attached to the skin. The purpose of the cardiac monitor is to pick up the electrical signals generated by the heart and display them on a screen (oscilloscope) in the form of a continuous ECG. Analyzing the wave forms in the ECG permits any disturbance in cardiac rate, rhythm, or conduction to be identified (as explained in subsequent chapters).

MONITORING EQUIPMENT

Dozens of different types of cardiac monitors are available currently. While these machines vary in size, design, dependability, elegance, and cost, their fundamental components are the same. A basic monitoring system works in the following way:

1. Electrodes applied to the patient's chest wall pick up the electrical impulses initiated by the heart.
2. These original waves are too small to be seen on the monitor screen, and for this reason are directed through an amplifier where their amplitude (height) is increased about 1,000 times.
3. The amplified impulses pass through a magnetic field (galvanometer), where

they are transformed into a series of wave forms. These deflections, reflecting each phase of the heart's electrical activity, comprise an ECG.

4. The ECG is then displayed continuously on an oscilloscope screen (similar to a small television screen). The size, position, and brightness of the ECG can be adjusted as necessary to obtain the clearest "picture" of the patient's cardiac rhythn. Many monitors (dual channel) allow the simultaneous display of the pattern detected by two ECG leads.

5. The monitor also counts each heartbeat and displays the average heart rate per minute on a rate meter. (Actually, the machine counts the electrical waves associated with ventricular depolarization, called R waves, and not the ventricular contractions themselves.) With each heartbeat a light (pulse light) flashes and a sound ("beep") is heard. (The monitor sound may be turned off if it is annoying.)

6. Integrated with the rate meter is an alarm system that sounds a loud audio signal and causes a light to flash if the patient's heart rate falls below or exceeds a preset level. For example, if the lower-limit alarm is set at a heart rate of 50 beats per minute (bpm) and the upper limit at 120 bpm, any decrease or increase in the heart rate beyond this particular range will cause the alarm to be triggered. This permits the onset of slow-rate or fast-rate arrhythmias to be recognized immediately, even though the nurse may not be observing the monitor at the time.

7. A direct recording mechanism provides a printed record of the ECG seen on the oscilloscope. This documentation (in the form of a rhythm strip) permits precise identification of an arrhythmia, and is also valuable for comparing ECG changes over a period of time. The recording can be obtained on demand as well as automatically (whenever the alarm system is triggered.)

A basic cardiac monitor is shown in Figure 3–1. In addition to the fundamental components described above, cardiac monitors may also include a variety of accessory devices. Perhaps the most useful of these additional devices are those designed to enhance the detection of early warning signs of lethal arrhyth-

mias. (As noted previously, one of the underlying themes of intensive coronary care is to prevent lethal arrhythmias by recognizing and treating warning arrhythmias.) That it may be difficult to specifically identify a transient warning arrhythmia from the electrocardiographic pattern seen on an oscilloscope screen can be readily appreciated: the ECG moves across the screen rapidly, and the observer has only one fleeting glance at the pattern with no chance to analyze it in detail. The most popular mechanisms used to facilitate the detection of arrhythmias are memory systems and components that hold or "freeze" the oscilloscopic pattern for closer inspection.

Memory systems are designed to store and play back the ECG of the preceding 15 to 60 seconds (or more). This "instant replay" technique is useful in two circumstances. First, if a transient arrhythmia is noted on the oscilloscope but there is insufficient time to activate the direct write-out device, the arrhythmia can be recaptured and recorded by using the memory system. Second, if an observer is not near the monitor when an alarm is triggered, the memory mechanism will replay the events that preceded the triggering event. Hold or "freeze" devices stop the movement of the ECG across the oscilloscope screen, keeping a particular pattern in place until it can be interpreted. These devices do not print out an ECG (from which precise measurements can be made), and for this reason they may be less useful than direct write-out or memory mechanisms.

THE OPERATION OF CARDIAC MONITORS

Four steps are involved in cardiac monitoring: (1) attaching electrodes to the patient's chest wall; (2) connecting the wires from the electrodes to the monitor (by way of a patient cable); (3) adjusting the monitor to obtain an effective ECG; and (4) setting the high-rate and low-rate alarm system at desired levels. Each of these aspects will be discussed separately.

Electrodes and Their Attachment

The electrodes used in cardiac monitoring serve to pick up the heart's electrical signals at the skin surface. It is apparent that unless the signals are detected accurately, the remaining phases of cardiac monitoring will have little meaning. Therefore the electrodes themselves and the manner in which they are applied to the skin is of critical importance.

The electrodes are disks that are deliberately separated (or "floated") from the skin by a built-in "spacer" (Figure 3–2). A conductive gel is placed in

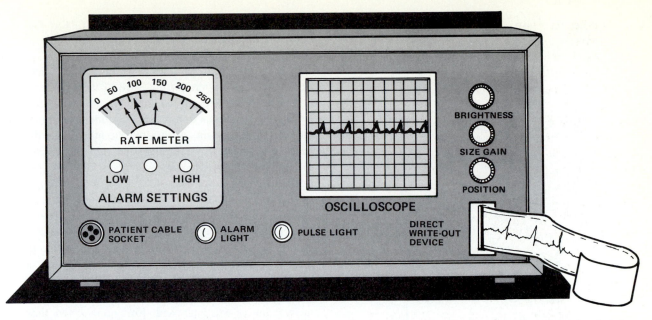

Figure 3–1. Basic cardiac monitor with oscilloscope, alarm settings, and adjustment settings for brightness, size (gain), and position.

the spacer, and the electrode is then attached to the skin by means of a surrounding ring of adhesive material. The main purpose of separating the electrode from the skin is to reduce local electrical interference at the skin surface, thus improving the quality of the ECG. In addition, disk electrodes do not have to be changed more than once a day, since the electrode gel remains moist in the spacer. Furthermore, the electrodes are lightweight, simple to apply, and seldom annoy the patient.

At present, nearly all CCUs use a modified version of the basic disk electrode. These electrodes are prepackaged, pregelled, and disposable. Their principal advantage is that they greatly reduce the time needed for electrode placement and permit cardiac monitoring to be instituted without delay. Peeling off a paper backing from a porous adhesive pad renders the gel-filled electrode immediately ready for use. Moreover, the electrodes can often remain in place for several days, since the gel does not dehydrate and seldom produces skin irritation. Equally important is the reduced likelihood of poor ECG signals resulting from too much or too little gel.

Location of Electrodes

In positioning the electrodes on the chest wall, the object is to select locations that will provide the clearest ECG wave forms, permitting arrhythmias to be identified readily. Electrode position depends on

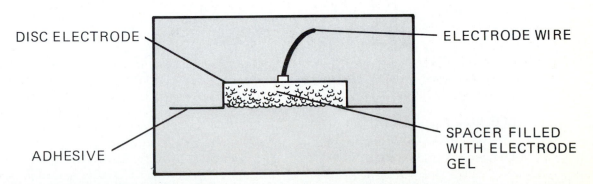

Figure 3–2. Disk-type or "floating" electrode.

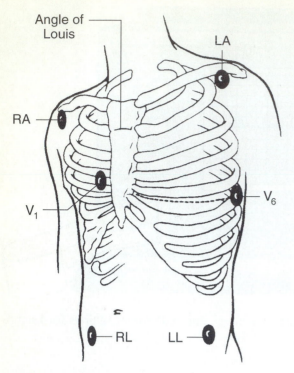

Figure 3–3. Lead placement for Leads V_1 and II using a five-wire patient cable. The location of the electrode for V_6 is also shown.

which of the 12 ECG leads are chosen (these are described in Chapter 8). The placement and number of electrodes also depend on the monitoring capability of the cardiac monitor being used. Patient cables can have three, four, or five lead wires, and the number and position of the electrodes therefore depends on the number of lead wires that the patient cable can hold and on whether the monitor provides dual- or single-channel monitoring.

With older cardiac monitors, only three electrodes are used for monitoring. Two of these serve to detect the heart's electrical activity; the third is a ground electrode that carries off ("grounds") extraneous electrical currents from sources other than the heart. With newer monitoring equipment, five electrodes may be used; the purpose of the additional electrodes is to permit multiple ECG views of the heart.

A true unipolar lead on the chest (ie, a V lead) can be obtained only with five electrode wires. Therefore, if there is a choice in monitoring equipment, a system with five lead wires is optimal. A system with three or four lead wires allows the monitoring only of a modified chest lead (eg, MCL_1 or MCL_5). Research has shown that when MCL_1 is used, supraventricular tachycardia is misdiagnosed 40% more often than when a true V1 lead is used.

If five lead wires are available on a dual-lead monitor, the nurse can monitor two leads simultaneously. The optimal first lead for monitoring is lead V1. The choice of the second lead depends on the patient's status and the goal of treatment. If detection of arrhythmia is a priority, lead II is the optimal second lead. Lead II is particularly helpful in identifying atrial activation and therefore in diagnosing atrial fibrillation/flutter. If monitoring of the ST-segment of the ECG is a priority, then leads III or AVF are optimal. Lead placement using leads V1 and II is shown in Figure 3–3.

The two most common positions in a three-lead system are lead II and a modified chest lead position (usually MCL_1). With lead II (Figure 3–4), the right

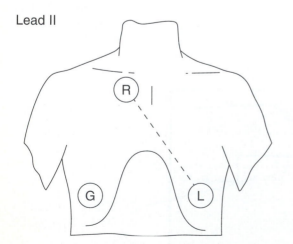
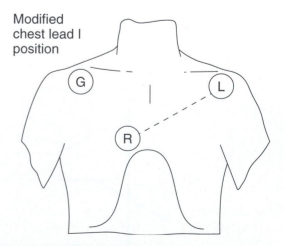

Figure 3–4. Lead placement for lead II and MCL_1 for use in a three-wire patient cable. Either lead can be chosen for display, depending on its placement in the cable receptacle.

TABLE 3–1. RECOMMENDED LEADS FOR ACCURATE CARDIAC MONITORING

System Characteristics	Patient Characteristics

Monitors with five-lead-wire patient cables and dual-lead capability
  First choice: V1 and appropriate limb lead
  Second choice: V6 and appropriate limb lead
Monitors with five-lead-wire patient cables and single lead capability
  First choice: V1
  Second choice: V6
Monitors with 3 lead-wire patient cables
  First choice: MCL_1
  Second choice: MCL_6
	Atrial fibrillation/flutter: II, III, or aVF
	Following angioplasty: III or aVF (the one with the tallest R wave)
	Inferior myocardial infarction: II, III, or aVF
	Anterior myocardial infarction: Lead with maximum ST deviation on 12-lead ECG
	Arrhythmia detection: V1 and V6
	Axis deviation: I and aVF

(R) electrode is placed on the right side of the sternum below the clavicle and medial to the pectoral muscles. The left (L) electrode is situated at the level of the lowest palpable rib on the left side of the chest in the anterior axillary line. The ground (G) electrode is placed at the area of the lower right rib cage, opposite the L electrode. With the electrodes in these positions the monitor records the electrical activity between the R and L electrodes. This particular path (or lead) normally produces the tallest atrial and ventricular complexes (P waves and R waves), and is chosen primarily for this reason.

The modified chest leads (particularly MCL_1) are optimal monitoring leads for patients with acute myocardial infarction because they are sensitive to bundle branch block, which is an important complication of acute myocardial infarction. In a three-wire patient cable, one opening is marked either R (right) or RA (right arm). The second opening is designated L (left) or LA (left arm). The third opening is identified as G (ground) or RL (right leg). To record a modified chest lead (MCL_1) position, the right (R) electrode is placed in the fourth interspace at the right border of the sternum. The left (L) electrode is located near the left shoulder, just under the outer portion of the clavicle. The ground (G) electrode is situated in the area of the right shoulder. Because the electrical path between the R and L electrodes in this position is different than that with the conventional chest lead, the resultant electrocardiographic pattern is also different (as will be explained in Chapter 8). The nurse should select the position that provides the clearest and most informative ECG for each individual patient (see Table 3–1).

Attachment of Electrode to Skin

Proper attachment of the electrodes to the skin is undoubtedly the single most important preliminary step in effective cardiac monitoring. Unless there is excellent contact between the skin and the electrodes, the electrocardiographic wave form will be distorted and artifacts will appear. In addition, the electrodes must be anchored firmly to prevent their movement or displacement. The procedure for attaching electrodes is as follows:

1. Prepare the skin areas designated for electrode placement.
   a. If necessary, chest hair should be shaved in 4-inch areas around the intended electrode sites.
   b. The area is cleansed with alcohol to remove skin oils and tissue debris, and then rubbed dry with a towel or gauze sponge. With some electrodes, mild abrasion of the skin is recommended in order to reduce skin-to-electrode impedance. The abrasion may be done with an abrasive pad or, simply, with a gauze sponge.
   c. If the chest wall is damp or wet with sweat, the electrode sites should be dried thoroughly so the adhesive pad will adhere to the skin. (If sweating continues and the area cannot be kept dry, an antiperspirant spray can be used and a thin coat of tincture of benzoin applied to the peripheral area.)
2. Prepare the electrodes for use, connect to the lead wires, and apply the electrodes to the skin. (It is advisable to attach the connecting wires to the electrodes before electrode placement: this avoids applying pressure to the positioned electrode, which could squeeze gel onto the adhesive area as well as cause discomfort to the patient).
   a. When pregelled, disposable electrodes are used, the package in which each electrode is sealed is opened just before the electrode is applied. (If the foil package remains open for too long, the conductive gel may dry.)
   b. The protective paper covering is peeled from the electrode, exposing the adhesive backing and the gel-covered disk. Contact with the adhesive surface should be avoided as completely as possible.

c. The electrode is attached by simply pressing the adhesive foam pad firmly onto the skin surface. The gelled portion of the electrode should not be pressed, since the gel may be squeezed out and interfere with adhesion.

d. If the electrodes are not pregelled, conductive gel is placed in the spacer before electrode application. Excessive amounts of gel should be avoided because the conductive medium may spread and interfere with the adhesion of the electrode.

3. Change electrodes as necessary. Pregelled disposable electrodes may remain in place for several days. However, if the electrocardiographic pattern becomes less distinct (from drying of the electrode gel), if the patient is diaphoretic, or if skin irritation develops, the electrode must be changed and reapplied.

Connecting the Wires from the Electrodes to the Monitor

The signals detected by the electrodes are transmitted to the monitor through an electrical cable known as the patient cable (in contrast to the monitor cable, which goes to a wall socket for electrical power). The electrodes are connected to the patient cable by means of thin wires 12 to 18 inches in length. These connecting wires, called lead wires, snap onto or clamp onto the electrodes; the other ends of the wires plug into a receptacle on the patient cable. The receptacle has designated openings for the respective electrode wires.

The following steps are involved in connecting the electrodes to the patient cable and then to the monitor:

1. After the electrodes are firmly attached to the skin, the connecting wires are snapped into place on the electrodes.

2. When the conventional electrode position is used for monitoring, the wires from the right (R), left (L), and ground (G) electrodes are inserted into the corresponding R, L, and G terminals of the cable receptacle.

3. In contrast, when the modified chest lead position is used, the electrode wire from the right (R) electrode is inserted in the L opening, and the wire from the left (L) electrode into the R opening. In other words, the R and L electrode wires are placed in a reversed position in the receptacle. The ground (G) electrode is placed in the G terminal.

4. After verifying that all connections are secure, position the connecting wires and the patient cable so that there is no tension on the electrode wires. The patient-cable receptacle is then pinned to the patient's gown.

5. The monitor end of the patient cable is then inserted into the cable socket of the monitor.

Adjusting the Monitor

If the electrodes have been applied properly and all wires connected securely, the ECG pattern appearing on the oscilloscope screen should be clear and distinct. Failure to obtain clear signals is due, in most instances, to faulty technique during the first two steps of the monitoring procedure, or to external electrical interference (as described in the following pages).

Even with flawless technique, three monitor adjustments may be necessary: brightening (or darkening) of the display, centering of the pattern on the screen, and adjusting the height of the wave forms, particularly for the waves of ventricular activation (R waves). The amplitude of the ventricular complexes is of great importance, because if these waves are too small, the rate meter will not recognize and count them and therefore the heart rate will appear falsely low. In this circumstance the height (gain) control dial is adjusted to increase the amplitude of the wave forms. If the height of the waves cannot be increased sufficiently by adjusting the dial, they should be monitored with a different lead.

Setting the Alarm System

As noted previously, the high- and low-rate alarms are integrated with the rate meter and are triggered when the heart rate displayed on the meter falls below or exceeds predetermined levels. The alarm limits should be set according to the patient's prevailing heart rate. If the patient's heart rate is between 60 and 100 per minute, it is customary to set the low alarm at 50 per minute and the high alarm at 140 per minute. However, if the heart rate is either very slow or very fast, the range for the alarm settings should be narrowed. For instance, if the patient's rate is 50 per minute, the low-rate alarm should be set at 40 and the high-rate alarm at about 80 per minute. In this way the observer will be alerted to even slight rate changes, which may be very significant.

Because of false alarms (described in the following paragraphs), there may be a temptation to set the alarm limits widely apart (eg, 40 and 180 per minute) or worse, to turn off the alarm mechanism entirely. This practice defeats the purpose of the alarm system and should *never* be adopted.

PROBLEMS WITH CARDIAC MONITORING

Many different problems may be encountered during cardiac monitoring; some are due to limitations of the monitoring system itself, but the great majority are the result of improper technique. The most common difficulties are discussed here.

False High-Rate Alarms

The alarm system depends on the accuracy of the rate meter. In principle, the meter is meant to count the average number of heartbeats (ventricular complexes) per minute; but most meters are not this specific and actually count all high deflections on the ECG, assuming that these are ventricular waves. Unfortunately, contraction of skeletal muscles also produces tall waves (called muscle potentials), which the rate meter cannot distinguish from ventricular complexes. Consequently, turning in bed, sudden movements of the extremities, brushing of the teeth, and shivering may all produce rapid, tall muscle potentials which the rate meter will misinterpret as heartbeats, causing a false high-rate alarm (Figure 3–5).

Attempts have been made to control this problem by equipping rate meters with electronic filters to "absorb" muscle potentials and by programming rate meters to count only waves of a particular configuration rather than all tall spikes. Despite these measures, false high-rate alarms are still common occurrences in cardiac monitoring.

One simple method for reducing interference from muscle potentials is to place the electrodes used in monitoring in positions that are not directly over large muscle masses (eg, not over the pectoral or shoulder muscles).

False Low-Rate Alarms

Any disturbance in the transmission of electrical signals between the skin surface and the monitor can produce a false low-rate alarm. This problem is caused most often by ineffective skin-to-electrode contact resulting from separation of an electrode from the skin, profuse sweating, or drying of the conductive gel. Disconnection of an electrode wire (or the patient cable) is another common source of false low-rate alarms. In all of these situations no electrical activity will be transmitted to the rate meter and oscilloscope, and it might appear at first glance that the heartbeat has stopped (Figure 3–6). The danger of mistaking this technical error for ventricular standstill is obvious and of serious consequence. To prevent this particular problem, specific alarms have been incorporated in some monitoring systems to distinguish "lead failure" from lethal arrhythmias.

False low-rate alarms can also occur if the ventricular waves are not tall enough to activate the rate meter. For example, if an arrhythmia develops in which every other ventricular complex is oriented in a direction opposite to the normal beats (R waves), and is of reduced amplitude (Figure 3–7), the rate meter may not be able to detect the smaller complexes. In the ECG in Figure 3–6, for example, the actual heart rate is 64 per minute; however, if the rate meter detected only the taller upright waves, only 32 beats per minute would be counted. This would create a false low-rate alarm. This problem can be corrected either by increasing the amplitude of the complexes or by changing the lead position.

Electrical Interference

Electrical current from external sources, such as power lines or other electronic equipment, may create

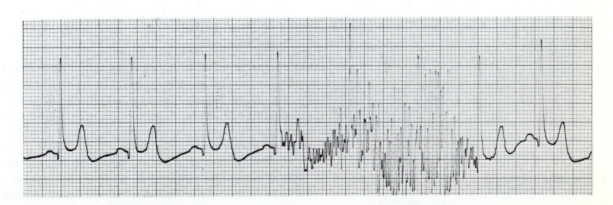

Figure 3–5. False high-rate alarm caused by muscle potentials.

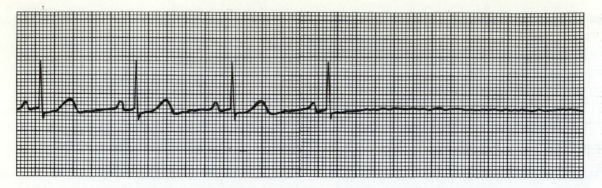

Figure 3–6. False low-rate alarm caused by one or more leads becoming disconnected from the patient cable or electrode(s).

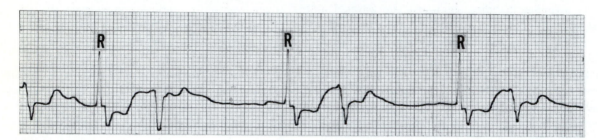

Figure 3–7. False low-rate alarm caused by some ventricular waves being not tall enough to activate the rate meter.

interference with the monitor signal. This form of interference appears on the oscilloscope screen as a series of fine, rapid spikes (at a rate of 60 per second because alternating current has a frequency of 60 cycles per second) that distort the baseline of the ECG. The effect of electrical interference is shown in Figure 3–8A. Note the difference in clarity of the pattern when the interference from an external voltage source was eliminated (Figure 3–8B). Electrical interference may arise from improper grounding of equipment or from loose connections.

When electrical interference occurs, the first step is to determine whether electrode contact with the patient's skin is secure and whether all connecting wires are firmly in place. Failure of these measures to eliminate interference suggests improper grounding of other electrical equipment being used. Frequent or persistent electrical interference may indicate a defect in the wiring system in the CCU. (An electrical engineer should be consulted in this circumstance, particularly since the problem may represent an electrical hazard to the patient.)

Wandering Baseline

At times the ECG pattern displayed on the oscilloscope may wander up and down on the screen (Figure 3–9). This movement, called a wandering baseline, makes it difficult to identify arrhythmias, particularly when part of the pattern moves completely off the screen. These excursions are generally produced by motion of the patient (eg, turning in bed) or simply by respiration. When the problem is caused by body movement, the fluctuation is transient and can be corrected by adjusting the "position" dial of the monitor to center the ECG. A wandering baseline caused by respiratory motion usually has a cyclic pattern related to inspiration and expiration. In such cases the electrodes should be repositioned away from the lowest ribs to minimize the effect of chest-wall movement.

Skin Irritation

Because monitoring electrodes must remain attached to the skin for several days, inflammatory reactions may occur at the sites of their attachment. These irritations may develop from the adhesive that secures the electrodes or from the conductive gel. Manufacturers now generally use adhesive material that is hypoallergenic and less irritating gels, but some patients may have particularly sensitive skin. If inflammation does develop at the electrode site, the area should be treated with an emollient or anesthetic cream and the electrode repositioned a few inches away. Regardless

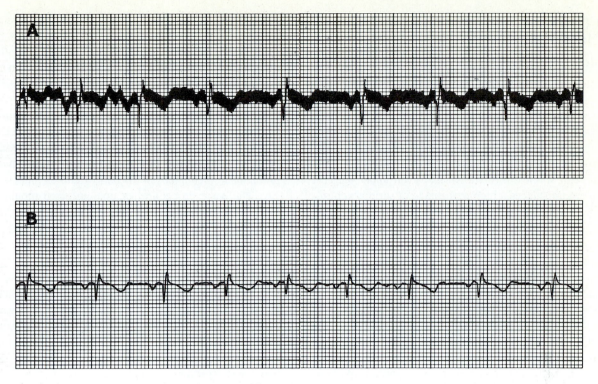

Figure 3–8. A. Electrical interference from an external source such as a power line. **B.** Pattern is clear after interference is eliminated.

of the brand of electrode used, it is important to examine the sites of electrode attachment at regular intervals to determine whether skin irritation is present.

Electrical Hazards

Until recently there were no uniform safety standards for electronic equipment, and some monitors (particularly older models) may therefore expose patients to electrical hazards. The main threat is from leakage currents that may pass from the monitor to the pa-

tient, particularly when more than one piece of equipment is being used. For example, if a temporary transvenous pacemaker has been positioned in the heart, leakage current from the monitor may travel down the pacing catheter to the heart and induce ventricular fibrillation. It is mandatory that all electrical equipment used in the CCU be designed in a way that avoids electrical hazards of this kind. Moreover, the grounding system within the CCU must be wholly effective in its purpose.

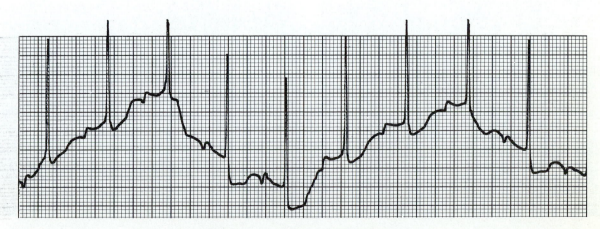

Figure 3–9. Wandering baseline.

COMPUTERIZED ARRHYTHMIA MONITORING

Computerized monitoring for arrhythmias is used in many CCUs to support nurses in the detection, analysis, and recording of arrhythmias. The main advantage of such monitoring is its ability to identify warning arrhythmias more accurately than can conventional cardiac monitoring, thus allowing preventive treatment to be undertaken as soon as possible. Several studies have shown that even under the best of circumstances a high percentage of serious ventricular warning arrhythmias go unnoticed in CCUs. This is not surprising, since the detection of warning arrhythmias with customary cardiac monitoring depends largely on nurse surveillance of the electrocardiographic patterns of several patients on multiple screens; also, most warning arrhythmias are transient and do not trigger high- or low-rate alarms. Because nurses have scores of other responsibilities in the CCU and cannot (and should not) spend their time in constantly observing cardiac monitors, many significant arrhythmic events are never recognized, particularly those that last for only a few beats. Even if cardiac monitoring is accomplished by having a nurse or specially trained technician sit in front of a bank of monitors (as is the case in some CCUs), the rate at which warning arrhythmias are missed may still be substantial because of human fatigue and the monotony of this practice. In addition to this fundamental flaw in the detection of warning arrhythmias, conventional electrocardiographic monitoring represents a time-consuming, arduous, and repetitive nursing task, especially in large CCUs, and in this sense detracts from direct patient care. In principle, computerized arrhythmia monitoring can alleviate these problems to the benefit of the patient and the nurse.

The basic procedure for computerized monitoring is essentially the same as for customary cardiac monitoring. The electrocardiographic signals picked up by electrodes on the patient's skin are displayed on monitor screens and relayed to a computer system. Through a sophisticated computer algorithm, the ventricular complexes on the monitor are classified and labeled. The algorithm filters the electrical signal from the patient's heart and detects and classifies each complex as normal or a particular arrhythmia. The computer program is designed to identify and tabulate several different types and classes of arrhythmias, and depicts these findings (along with the heart rate) on a separate screen in the form of an ongoing status report for each patient (Figure 3–10). The com-

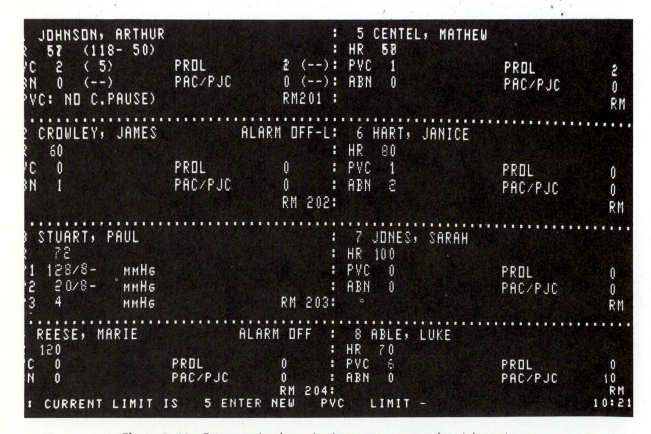

Figure 3–10. Computerized monitoring: status reports for eight patients.

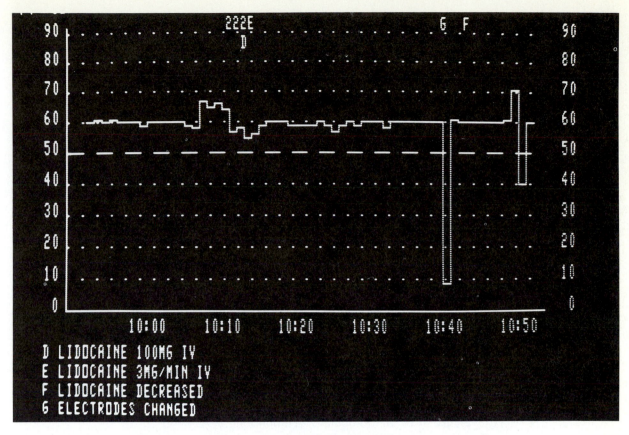

Figure 3–11. A. Computerized monitoring: Heart rate trend.

puter system stores this information and presents it graphically as an hourly trend (Figure 3–11 A and B).

The most significant feature of a computerized monitoring system is its alarm mechanism. Unlike ordinary cardiac monitors, whose alarm systems are triggered only by high or low heart rates, computerized arrhythmia monitors are programmed to deliver visual and audible alarms for many other disturbances as well, especially warning arrhythmias. The alarm limits for each type of arrhythmia are set individually. If any of these limits are surpassed, the respective alarm is activated and a rhythm strip documenting the event is produced. Printed across the top border of the ECG strip are the patient's name, room number, time of the event, and reason for the alarm (Figure 3–12). This added information simplifies and expedites the charting of arrhythmic events.

Despite the apparent advantages of computerized cardiac monitoring, some CCUs continue to use standard cardiac monitoring equipment. The reasons for this decision are several. First, computerized monitoring systems are far more expensive than customary monitors and are usually designed to monitor eight (or more) patients. Thus, for smaller CCUs automated monitoring is often a luxury. Second, conventional monitors are just as effective as computerized monitors in detecting *lethal* arrhythmias (eg, ventricular fibrillation) or, for that matter, any other fast- or slow-rate arrhythmias that trigger the alarm system. Third, computerized monitors are neither entirely accurate nor foolproof. Much of this problem stems from the rigid mathematical criteria by which computers analyze arrhythmias; because of this, even slight variations in the configuration or timing of the ventricular (QRS) complexes (which are of no clinical significance) may be misinterpreted as constituting an arrhythmia. It is also difficult (and sometimes impossible) for a computerized monitoring system to distinguish between various rhythms. For example, a large atrial (P) wave will be read as a ventricular (R) wave and the monitor will record the heart rate as being twice

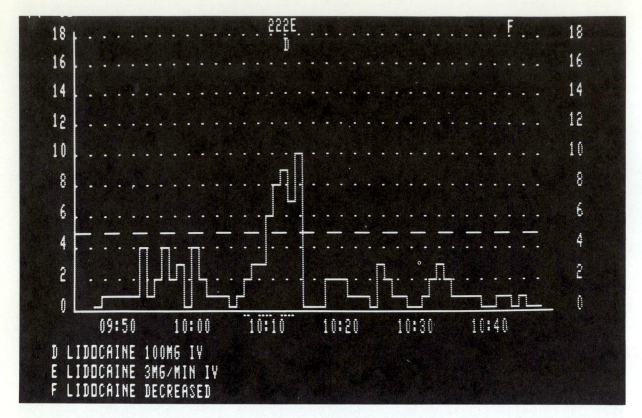

Figure 3–11. B. Computerized monitoring: PVC trend.

what it is. Accordingly, false alarms are relatively common with most computerized arrhythmia detection systems. Also, the computer programs used in these systems often experience difficulty in analyzing complicated arrhythmias, particularly if the shape of the waves varies greatly. Furthermore, since P waves are not analyzed, there is no way to distinguish atrial arrhythmias.

Nevertheless, computerized monitoring holds great promise. As its technology improves and its costs are controlled, this form of continuous surveillance will play an increasingly important role in the CCU.

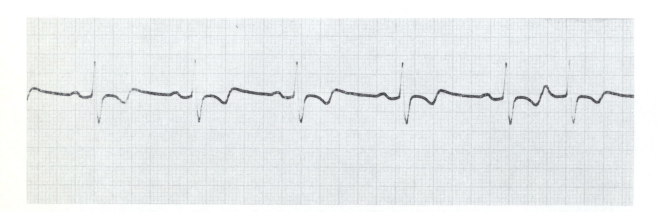

Figure 3–12. Rhythm strip produced by computerized monitoring system.

COMPUTERIZED ST-SEGMENT MONITORING

As discussed in Chapter 14, changes from baseline (either elevation or depression) in the ST-segment of the ECG can indicate myocardial ischemia. Ischemia can be assessed with a 12-lead ECG. Some bedside cardiac monitoring systems have incorporated ST-segment monitoring, using multichannel recorders. ST-segment monitoring may be especially helpful in patients receiving thrombolytic therapy or following percutaneous transluminal angioplasty (PTCA). ST-segment monitoring can be helpful in identifying successful reperfusion, and may reveal patients in whom further treatment can prevent angina or a myocardial infarction. Although ST-segment monitoring is highly accurate, it may falsely identify artifactual changes in the ST segment as being ischemic.

The lead with the tallest R wave is the best lead with which to assess changes in the ST-segment, since the amplitude of the ST-segment parallels that of the QRS complex. Leads III or AVF are usually the most accurate in monitoring ST-segment changes. The lead that is used for monitoring ST-segment changes is designated as the second lead in a dual-channel monitoring system.

TELEMETRY

The heart's electrical activity can be recorded without direct wiring from the patient to the monitor. This method, called *telemetric* monitoring or telemetry, can be utilized with conventional or computerized monitoring systems. It works as follows: the eletrode wires are connected to a small, battery-operated radio (FM) transmitter, about the size of a cigarette package, which is pinned on the patient's gown or worn about the neck. The transmitter sends the electrical signals to a receiver by means of a radio beam. The receiver then feeds the signals into the monitoring system. Among the advantages of telemetry are that the patient is not restricted by wires and can sit in a chair or use the bathroom without the risk of disconnecting the monitoring system. More important is that monitoring can be accomplished even though the patient is no longer in the CCU; in fact, the patient can be on a different floor in the hospital, hundreds of feet away from the monitor.

Many institutions use telemetric cardiac monitoring for patients who have been transferred from the CCU, particularly those who have experienced serious arrhythmias during the acute phase of their illness and may be at high risk of developing recurrent problems. In this situation telemetry may be a suitable alternative to intermediate (stepdown) CCUs. The main disadvantage of telemetric monitoring is that the electrocardiographic signals it transmits are usually not of as high a quality as those recorded with direct wiring. Radio transmission is often distorted by steel beams, elevator shafts, and other structures within the hospital.

ECGs can also be transmitted by telephone, enabling cardiac monitoring to be accomplished from hundreds of miles away if necessary. The telephone number of the monitor in the CCU (or emergency department) is dialed, and a special transmitter sends the patient's ECG signals through the telephone line to the monitor. Rescue squads sometimes use telephonic monitoring when they need assistance or advice from hospital personnel. Patients may also check their pacemaker function or heart rhythm by using a transmitter at home and dialing a monitor located in the CCU.

INVASIVE HEMODYNAMIC MONITORING

Hemodynamic monitoring is the second most common form of physiologic monitoring in a CCU. It provides an assessment of a patient's condition and response to treatment that is related to pressure changes within the systemic arteries, central veins, pulmonary artery, and heart.

Hemodynamic monitoring depends on a pressure transducer (a transducer is a device that converts an analog or physical signal into a digital or electronic signal). The transducer is connected to an indwelling catheter (eg, an arterial line or a pulmonary artery catheter) by high-pressure tubing. To prevent errors caused by the dampening of pressure impulses, the high-pressure tubing must be quite short, and never longer than 48 inches.

The transducer used in hemodynamic monitoring creates an electrical signal from pressure impulses or waves that are conducted from the catheter through a fluid-filled system. The nurse must prime the system with a heparin flush solution and then provide a continuous flush solution (usually at the rate of 3 to 5 mL every hour) to keep the system patent (Figure 3–13).

The transducer must be level with the patient's right atrium, a reference point found at the phlebostatic axis. In a patient lying supine, the phlebostatic axis is at the intersection of the midaxillary line and fourth intercostal space. Research has shown that patients may be elevated from 0 to 60 degrees without altering the accuracy of hemodynamic measurements. However, the transducer must always be leveled at the phlebostatic axis. When patients move to the lateral (particularly the left lateral) position, hemodynamic measurements are no longer reliable. The transducer

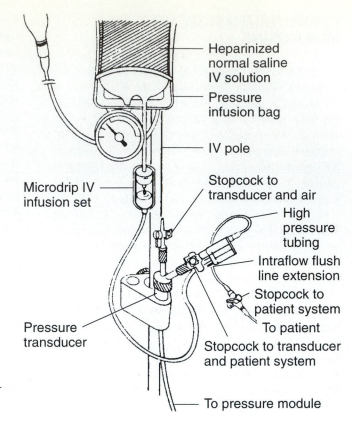

Heparinized
normal saline
IV solution

Pressure
infusion bag

IV pole

Stopcock to
transducer and air

High
pressure
tubing

Intraflow flush
line extension

Stopcock to
patient system

To patient

Stopcock to transducer
and patient system

To pressure module

Microdrip IV
infusion set

Pressure
transducer

Figure 3–13. Hemodynamic monitoring set-up with transducer flush system.

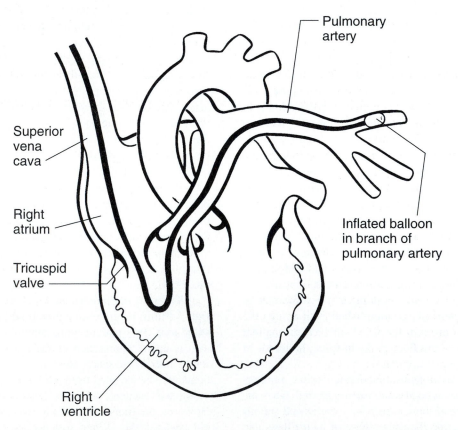

Pulmonary
artery

Superior
vena
cava

Right
atrium

Tricuspid
valve

Right
ventricle

Inflated balloon
in branch of
pulmonary artery

Figure 3–14. Course of a pulmonary artery catheter through the heart into the pulmonary artery.

and phlebostatic axis should be checked whenever the nurse is examining the catheter for problems.

There exist a variety of pulmonary artery catheters. The simplest is the double-lumen catheter. The larger lumen of this catheter measures the pressure in the pulmonary artery, while the smaller lumen leads to a small balloon just proximal to the tip of the catheter. When inflated, the balloon serves to guide the catheter through the right atrium and right ventricle, and into proper position in the pulmonary artery. The catheter is inserted through an arm (antecubital) vein and advanced to the superior vena cava. After the catheter enters the vena cava, the balloon is fully inflated with air and allowed to float through the right atrium and right ventricle into the pulmonary artery. The balloon finally wedges in a small branch of the pulmonary artery; this is called the *pulmonary capillary wedge position.*

The course traversed by the double-lumen catheter in reaching the wedge position is illustrated in Figure 3–14. Continuous pressure recordings are made during passage of the catheter, in order to verify its location. As shown in Figure 3–15 the pressure waves recorded with the catheter are distinctly different in the right ventricle, pulmonary artery, and pulmonary wedge position.

The pulmonary capillary wedge pressure (PCWP) represents the pressure in the pulmonary capillary bed, which reflects left ventricular end-diastolic pressure (in the absence of mitral-valve disease). The PCWP cannot be measured continuously because the inflated balloon of the pulmonary artery catheter obstructs the flow of blood through a segment of the lung and can cause pulmonary embolism. Consequently, as soon as the PCWP is determined, the balloon is deflated. Deflation of the balloon (with the catheter still in the wedge position) permits pulmonary artery systolic and diastolic pressures to be read continuously. Figure 3–16 demonstrates the characteristic pattern change from the pulmonary artery wave form as the catheter is moved into the pulmonary capillary wedge position.

The most common type of pulmonary artery catheter used in the CCU is the thermodilution catheter, because it allows the measurement of cardiac output (see Figure 3–17). A proximal lumen of the catheter is inserted into the right atrium and provides an assessment of right atrial pressure (similarly to a central venous pressure catheter). A venous infusion port, situated close to the proximal port in the right atrium, provides access to the venous system for fluid administration. A distal lumen is located at the end of the catheter and provides an assessment of pulmonary artery pressure. A thermistor wire is embedded in the exterior wall of the catheter. The thermistor wire ends 4 cm from the tip of the catheter and measures temperature changes

when fluid is injected into the proximal port of the catheter in the right atrium. An extra port is provided for inflation of the balloon located 1 mm from the tip of the catheter in order to obtain the PCWP.

The thermodilution catheter has the capacity to measure both the core body temperature and cardiac output. Cardiac output measurements are obtained by taking the average of three cardiac output readings (obtained with 10 mL injections of normal saline at room temperature or 10 mL injections of iced normal saline in patients with less than 3 L/minute). A cardiac output computer calculates the cardiac output from the changes in temperature between the proximal and distal ports of the catheter that occur with each 10 mL infusion.

Systemic and pulmonary vascular resistance can be derived with a pulmonary artery thermodilution catheter. Both resistances are helpful in assessing the amount of resistance experienced by the left and right ventricles during contraction. The following formulas are used to calculate resistance:

$$\text{Systemic vascular resistance (measured as dynes-sec-cm}^{-3}) = \frac{\left(\begin{array}{c}\text{mean} \\ \text{arterial} \\ \text{pressure}\end{array}\right) - \left(\begin{array}{c}\text{right} \\ \text{atrial} \\ \text{pressure}\end{array}\right)}{\text{cardiac output}} \times 80$$

$$\text{Pulmonary vascular resistance} = \frac{\left(\begin{array}{c}\text{pulmonary} \\ \text{artery} \\ \text{mean} \\ \text{pressure}\end{array}\right) - \left(\begin{array}{c}\text{pulmonary} \\ \text{artery} \\ \text{wedge} \\ \text{pressure}\end{array}\right)}{\text{cardiac output (L/min)}}$$

Normal hemodynamic values are summarized in Table 3–2.

Troubleshooting

When problems arise with hemodynamic monitoring, the nurse must examine all components of the system (the monitor, cable, transducer, pressure bag, flush device and flush solution, high-pressure tubing and connectors, and the pulmonary artery catheter itself). The most common problems are reflected in a damping of the pressure wave form or difficulty with the wedge. The latter includes both the inability to obtain a wedge pattern despite inflation of the balloon with the requisite 1 mL of air, or obtaining a continuous wedge pressure despite releasing the balloon.

Wave forms are damped when something prevents transmission of the blood-pressure wave. Damping may occur if the catheter is resting against the wall of the pulmonary artery (requiring that the balloon be inflated and "floated" a short distance distally). It also occurs when air bubbles appear

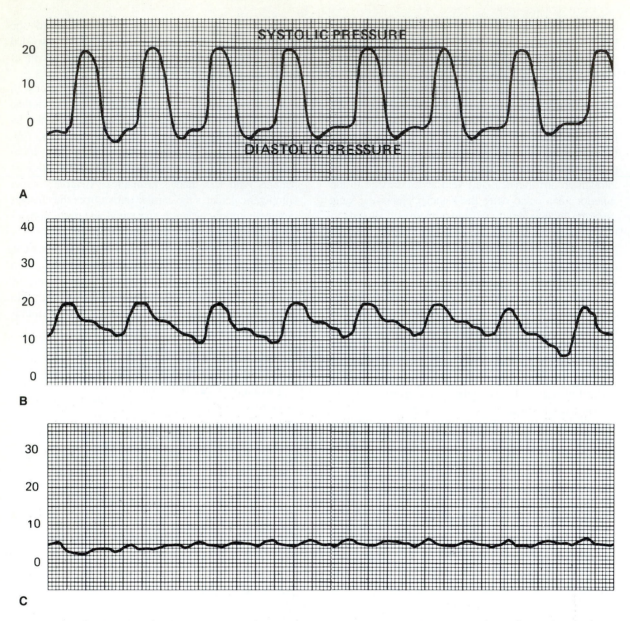

Figure 3–15. Pressure tracing, moving from right ventricle **(A)** to pulmonary artery **(B)** to pulmonary capillary wedge pressure (PCWP) **(C).** In tracing **(A)** the catheter tip is in the right ventricle. The normal pressure in the right ventricle is 20 mm Hg systolic and 5 mm diastolic (20/5). In this example the pressure is 20/0 mm Hg. In tracing **(B)** the catheter tip is in the pulmonary artery. The normal pulmonary artery pressure is 25/10 mm Hg. In this case the systolic pressure is 20 mm Hg and the diastolic pressure is between 10 and 12 mm Hg. The diastolic pulmonary artery pressure is used to assess left ventricular function if a pulmonary artery wedge pressure cannot be obtained; the pressure rises above 12 mm Hg when the left ventricle begins to fail. In tracing **(C)**, the catheter tip (with the balloon inflated) is in a small branch of the pulmonary artery. A PCWP of 5 to 12 mm Hg is considered normal. Levels above 12 mm Hg indicate reduced left ventricular emptying and high filling pressures (preload). The PCWP in this instance is about 5 mm Hg, indicating normal preload.

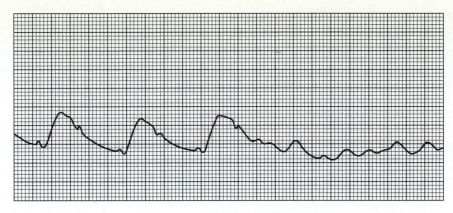

Figure 3–16. Characteristic pattern change from pulmonary artery pressure wave form to pulmonary capillary wedge pressure wave form.

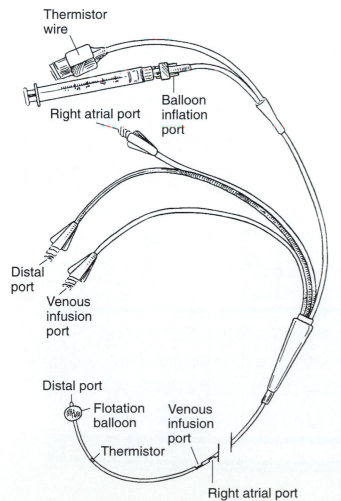

Figure 3–17. Thermodilution pulmonary artery catheter.

TABLE 3–2. NORMAL RANGES OF HEMODYNAMIC PARAMETERS

Right atrial pressure	Mean:	2–6 mm Hg
Right ventricular pressure	Systolic:	20–30 mm Hg
	Diastolic:	0–2 mm Hg
	End-diastolic:	2–6 mm Hg
Left atrial pressure	Mean:	4–12 mm Hg
Pulmonary artery pressure	Systolic:	15–30 mm Hg
	Diastolic:	8–12 mm Hg
	Mean:	10–20 mm Hg
Pulmonary capillary wedge pressure	Mean:	4–12 mm Hg
Arterial pressure	Systolic:	100–140 mm Hg
	Diastolic:	60–80 mm Hg
	Mean:	70–90 mm Hg
Cardiac output	4–8 L/minute	
Cardiac index	2.5–4 L/minute/m^2	
Mixed venous oxygen saturation (S$\bar{v}$O$_2$)	60–80%	
	60-80%	
Systemic vascular resistance	800–1200 dynes/sec/cm^{-5}	
Pulmonary vascular resistance	37–250 dynes/sec/cm^{-5}	
Stroke volume	60–100 mL/contraction	

in the tubing or transducer dome, or when small blood clots form on the distal tip of the catheter. Solutions to these problems involve inspecting the system for air bubbles and flushing the system with several short infusions of 1 second each. *The nurse should avoid a long flush, which can dislodge a blood clot at the distal tip of the catheter and carry it into the pulmonary capillary bed at a pressure of 300 mm Hg, resulting in a pulmonary embolism.*

If a wedge wave form cannot be obtained when the balloon is injected with 1 mL of air, the tip of the catheter may be misplaced. Sometimes the

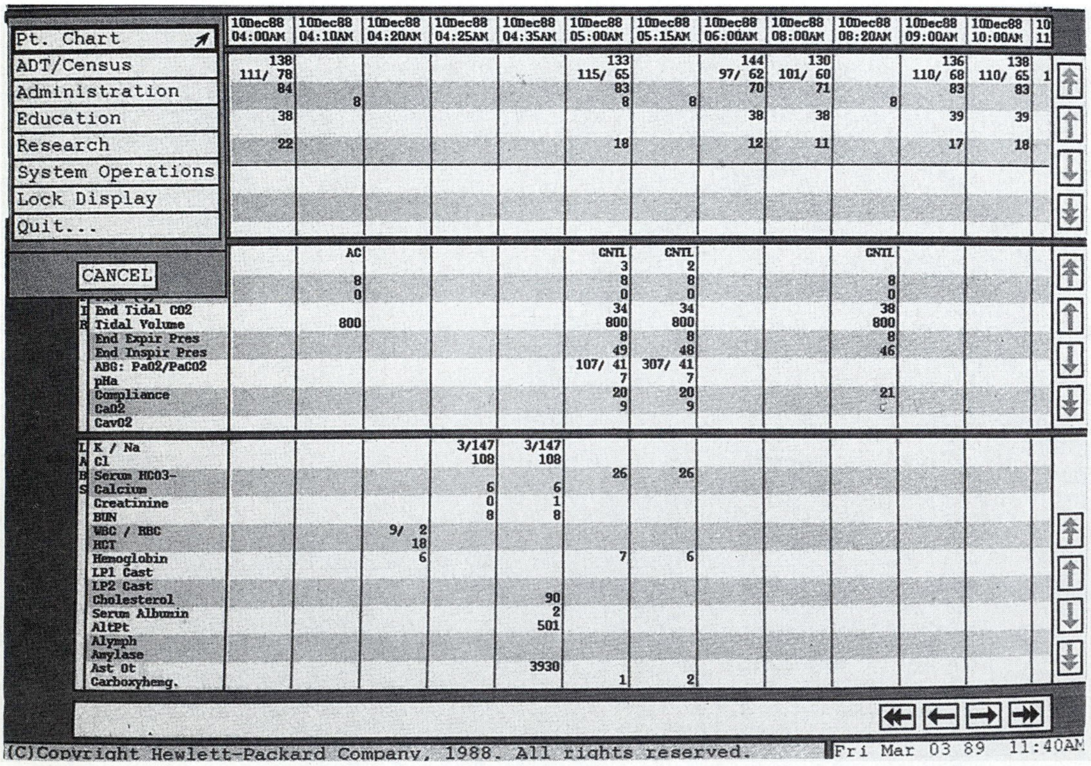

Figure 3–18. Flow-sheet screen. (Reproduced with permission from Hewlett-Packard Co, 1988.)

catheter tip has floated back into the large branch of the pulmonary artery or right ventricular outflow tract, and the catheter must be advanced again into a terminal branch of the pulmonary artery. If the monitor reflects a permanent wedge pattern, the cause is usually forward migration of the catheter tip, which becomes trapped in an arteriole and must be pulled back.

CLINICAL INFORMATION SYSTEMS

Clinical information systems (also called patient-data management systems) are systems of microcomputers used at patients' bedsides to collect, process, retrieve, and display information related to patient care. Such systems are basically extensions of the monitoring systems already used in the CCU, and represent an automation of flow sheets (Figure 3–18). Flow sheets were developed by critical-care nurses, who increasingly had the ability to monitor multiple patient parameters simultaneously. They represent a type of shorthand charting and are used by many CCU nurses to record changes in a patient's physiologic status and identify medications and intravenous fluids that the patient has received.

Some CCUs are now moving to "paperless" patient charts, for which the bedside nurse, physician, and all other personnel enter all information about the

TABLE 3–3. ALERT PARAMETERS AVAILABLE IN SOME CLINICAL INFORMATION SYSTEMS

Arterial Blood Gases	Hematology
pH	Hemoglobin
PO_2	Hematocrit
PCO_2	White blood count
Cardiac Enzymes	Partial thromboplastin time
Creatinine kinase (CK)	Prothrombin time, % activity
CK-MB	
Serum Chemistries	**Drug Levels**
Sodium	Lidocaine
Potassium	Quinidine
Chloride	Procainamide
Bicarbonate	Thiocyanate
Calcium	Digoxin
	Gentamicin
	Tobramycin

patient into a computer. Some systems also provide decision-support tools for use in making treatment decisions relating to antibiotic therapy, nutritional management, and management of mechanical ventilation. Others provide alarms (similar to the heart rate alarm on the cardiac monitor) that automatically alert the nurse when a significant change occurs in the patient's status or when incompatible or contraindicated drugs are ordered. A list of possible "alert" parameters is presented in Table 3–3.

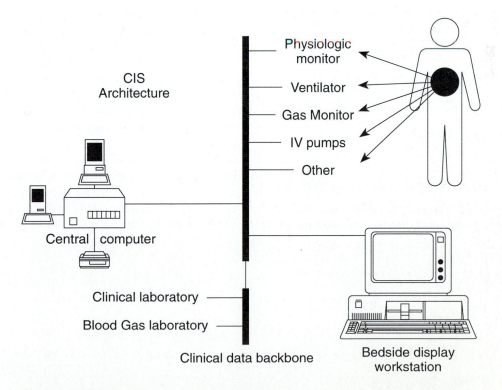

Figure 3–19. Architecture of a clinical information system. (Redrawn with permission from Williams D, Brown DL. Automation at the point of car. *Nursing Management.* 1994; 25:33.)

TABLE 3–4. FEATURES OF AN IDEAL CLINICAL INFORMATION SYSTEM FOR THE CCU

Departmental Interface	**Charting**	**Planning**
Admissions	Flow sheet	Physician and nurse orders
Clinical laboratories	Fluid intake and output	Automated care plans based on problem-oriented charting
Pharmacy (for drug orders and billing)	Medications	Individualized care plans
Accounting and billing	Physical assessment	Reference library and on-line help
CCU Interface	Nursing and physician progress notes	**Review and Analysis**
Monitors	**Task Management**	Quality assurance
Ventilators	Task lists for each shift	Severity of illness score
Intravenous drug pumps	Medication schedule and management	Graphic displays of data over time
	Diagnostic test schedule	

The Ideal Clinical Information System

The "minimal" ideal clinical information system is depicted in Figure 3–19. It is integrated with the clinical and blood-gas laboratories and also provides computerized management of mechanical ventilation and intravenous infusions. All CCU personnel use the system for documentating the patient's status as well as recording physician and nurse orders. The system incorporates the flow sheet, fluid intake and output, medications, physical examination results, nutritional status, progress notes, and laboratory results. It provides automated care plans based on problem-oriented charting, and gives a patient-specific task list for each shift, as well as a medication schedule.

However, many clinical information systems have the capability of doing much more than this minimum. A more extensive system can handle the tasks listed in Table 3–4. The goals with any system are to automatically collect source data whenever possible, in order to reduce duplication of charting and provide all pertinent data to caregivers in a central location (at the computer itself).

Problems with Clinical Information Systems

A major problem with current patient-data management systems is that many do not yet interface with hospital departments outside the CCU (clinical and diagnostic laboratories, radiology departments, operating rooms, outpatient clinics, and the pharmacy). If a truly integrated system can be achieved, the interface must ensure the accurate and timely acquisition and processing of patient data from all relevant sources.

A second problem relates to support for clinical decisions. Numerous guidelines have been developed over the past two decades to help nurses and physicians make clinical decisions based on controlled clinical trials. Unfortunately, computers still seem a long way from incorporating these guidelines into algorithms that can assist the nurse at the bedside. Despite recent advances, a system that can appropriately support the clinical decisions of nurses and physicians working in the CCU seems a distant prospect.

A final problem stems from the lack of research on the results of computerizing CCUs. Given the high cost of computerization, hospital administrations need to be convinced that the use of computers will result in cost-effective care. Researchers have shown that computer systems reduce the number of errors in charting and improve the quality, accuracy, and timely capture of patient data. However, they have not shown that such systems reduce the number of nursing hours required for charting or improve the quality of patient care.

Chapter 4

Coronary Heart Disease

When the incredible complexity of the human system is considered along with the vast number of possible sources of illness and death, it seems incongruous that the lives of so many persons depend finally on the health of two small arteries; but the fact is undeniable. Disease of the coronary arteries has become the single greatest threat to life in industrialized countries throughout the world. In the United States and Canada, for example, more than 1 million persons die of myocardial infarction, cardiac dysrhythmias, and heart failure annually. All are sequelae of coronary artery disease (CAD). The resulting economic cost is over $100 billion each year.

As the sole conduits of blood supply to the musculature of the heart (myocardium), the coronary arteries assume extreme importance. Any significant interference with blood flow through these vessels can impair the entire function of the myocardium, with dire consequences including sudden death. Before describing the clinical aspects of coronary artery disease, it is pertinent first to consider the coronary arteries and the most common disease process that affects them.

THE CORONARY ARTERIES

The two coronary arteries, the left and right, arise from the aorta just above the aortic valve. The left coronary artery then divides into two large branches: the left anterior descending artery and the left circumflex artery. The relationship of these three arteries is shown in Figure 4–1.

Each artery supplies a different area of the heart. Briefly, the left anterior descending artery supplies most of the anterior wall of the left ventricle, the anterior portion of the interventricular septum, and the anterior wall of the right ventricle. The left circumflex artery supplies the lateral aspect of the left ventricle and the left atrium. The right coronary artery supplies the right atrium and the right ventricle, along with the posterior portions of the left ventricle and interventricular septum. The arteries lie on the outer surfaces of the ventricles and give off numerous branches that penetrate all parts of the heart. The terminal branches of the arteries have many interconnections, forming an extensive vascular network throughout the myocardium.

The function of the coronary arteries is to bring oxygen-carrying blood to the myocardium, oxygen being an essential ingredient in producing the energy the heart requires to contract. As a pump that works incessantly (contracting more than 100,000 times a day), the myocardium has very great oxygen needs. This constant demand can be met only by an adequate coronary blood flow. Indeed, 250 mL of blood per minute, or 360,000 mL per day, pass through the coronary arteries to oxygenate the myocardium under normal conditions. The oxygen demands of the myocardium increase greatly with exercise or emotional stress. Since the heart utilizes nearly all of its available oxygen supply even with normal activity, and has a very limited oxygen reserve, these additional needs can be satisfied only by an increase in coronary blood flow (supply).

CORONARY ATHEROSCLEROSIS

The primary disease affecting the coronary arteries is atherosclerosis, a process in which fatty substances (particularly cholesterol) deposit as plaques along the

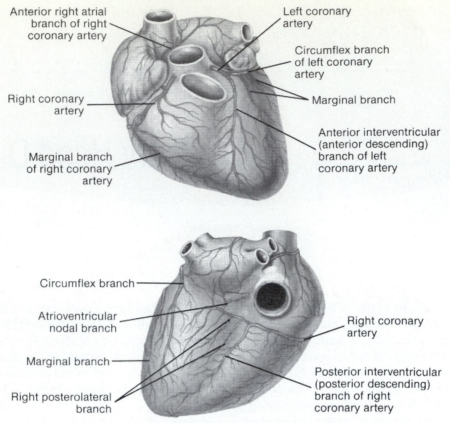

Figure 4–1. Anatomy of the coronary circulation.

inner lining of the vessels, narrowing the passageways for blood. The beginning of atherosclerosis may be the shear stress caused by blood flow at certain vascular sites (eg, bifurcations of vessels and bending points). This may produce a chronic minimal injury in the arterial endothelium, which can be aggravated by various cardiac risk factors, such as cigarette smoking and hyperlipidemia. Even a minimal injury can lead to the accumulation of lipids and macrophages, ultimately damaging the intimal surface and leading to the aggregation of platelets in the area. Both macrophages and platelets release growth factors that prompt smooth-muscle cells to multiply and form a "fibrointimal lesion." These plaques easily rupture, resulting in thrombus formation (Figure 4–2).

Coronary atherosclerosis usually develops gradually over a period of years. However, the process begins at an early age, so that by middle adulthood most men (and women, to a lesser degree) have some evidence of atherosclerosis in their coronary arteries. Autopsy studies have shown, for example, that among young American soldiers (average age, 22 years) killed in action during the Korean war, nearly 80% had definite signs of coronary atherosclerosis. It is essential to realize, however, that the critical deter-

minant of CAD is not the mere presence of atherosclerosis but rather the extent of arterial narrowing and reduction in blood flow resulting from atherosclerotic lesions.

Coronary atherosclerosis can be categorized into four grades according to the degree of arterial obstruction it causes. Grade 1 atherosclerosis indicates that the diameter (lumen) of the artery is reduced by no more than 25%; grade 2 atherosclerosis represents a 50% reduction, grade 3 a 75% reduction, and grade 4 complete (100%) obstruction of the vessel. An obstruction of at least 75% is necessary to significantly reduce coronary blood flow; lesser degrees of narrowing can usually be tolerated without affecting myocardial function or causing pain. Obstruction may occur in any (or all) of the coronary arteries, but involvement of the left anterior descending artery is particularly dangerous. This vessel supplies a much larger portion of the total myocardial mass than the right coronary or left circumflex arteries, and therefore carries a greater blood flow than either of these other vessels. Even more serious is obstruction of the left main coronary artery. Significant narrowing of this short (2 cm) vessel causes a reduction in blood flow through *both* the left anterior descending and

A. Stable angina pectoris

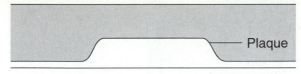

Plaque

B₁.

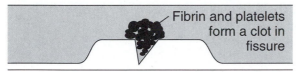

Fissure

B₂. Unstable angina

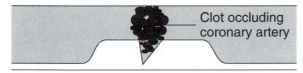

Fibrin and platelets form a clot in fissure

C. Acute myocardial infarction

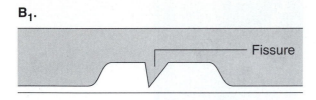

Clot occluding coronary artery

Figure 4–2. Comparison of partial and complete obstruction of the coronary artery.

left circumflex arteries, and therefore compromises the blood supply to nearly all of the left ventricle. Fortunately, obstruction of the left main coronary artery is the least common lesion of the coronary circulation, occurring in only 5% to 10% of patients with symptoms of CAD.

The site and extent of narrowing in a coronary artery can be determined by *coronary angiography,* a technique that permits the arteries to be visualized with X-rays. The procedure involves the insertion of a catheter into the root of the aorta (by way of a peripheral artery) and the injection of a radiopaque dye into the left and right coronary arteries through their openings (ostia). As the dye is being injected, a rapid series of X-ray films or photographs (cineangiograms) are made to outline the entire arterial tree; significant lesions can readily be detected in this way. Figure 4–3 compares a normal coronary artery with one that has a 90% obstruction.

Myocardial ischemia may be caused by obstructive coronary atherosclerosis, coronary embolism, or anomalies of the coronary arteries. It may also be caused by severe aortic valve stenosis, severe aortic regurgitation, hypertension, or cardiomyopathy. However, by far the most common cause of myocardial ischemia is coronary atherosclerosis.

CAUSES OF CORONARY ATHEROSCLEROSIS

Coronary atherosclerotic heart disease is a multifactorial disease. Over the past 50 years, researchers have identified the various factors that put individuals at risk for developing atherosclerosis. Some of these factors are nonmodifiable while others are subject to modification. Nonmodifiable risk factors are sex, age, and family history. Modifiable factors are smoking, hypertension, hyperlipidemia, diabetes, obesity, a sedentary life style, and psychosocial factors (see Table 4–1).

Nonmodifiable Risk Factors

Sex and Age. Before the age of 50, CAD is distinctly more prevalent in men than in women. Symptomatic CAD may occur in men as young as 30 years of age (or even younger), while during the childbearing years women are seemingly protected from CAD unless they have other risk factors for it (eg, hypertension and diabetes). After the menopause, however, the incidence of CAD in females rises rapidly and exceeds the rate in males. The mean age of men with a first myocardial infarction is 55 years, while that of women is 65 years. This sex–age discrepancy, combined with data showing a reduction in heart disease with estrogen replacement therapy, suggests that hormonal influences may be important in the disease process.

The incidence of CAD increases greatly with age in both sexes. The risk of myocardial infarction or sudden cardiac death doubles with each decade of age. For example, a man in his fifties has four times as great a risk of having a heart attack as a man in his thirties. The fact that young persons may develop CAD, however, makes it clear that coronary atherosclerosis is not simply a disease of aging.

Heart disease is often incorrectly associated with male sex. However, heart disease is the number one killer of women in the United States, with approximately 500,000 women dying of it each year. This far exceeds the mortality rate for all types of cancer deaths combined.

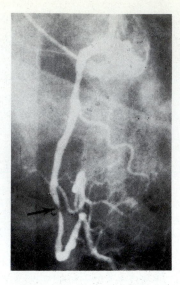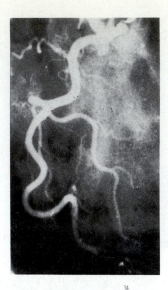

Figure 4–3. Arteriograms comparing a normal right coronary artery (*right*) with one that has a 90% obstruction (*left*).

Numerous studies have been conducted over the past decade to identify sex differences in the incidence, treatment, and prognosis of heart disease. Although women over the age of 55 have a higher incidence of heart disease than do men, they are less likely to be examined and diagnosed as having heart disease. Fewer angiograms are ordered for women than for men, and women are less likely to receive thrombolysis if they present to an emergency department with symptoms of acute myocardial infarction (AMI). Unfortunately women with documented heart disease also have a poorer prognosis than do men.

TABLE 4–1. RISK FACTORS FOR CORONARY ATHEROSCLEROTIC HEART DISEASE

Age
  Males >45 years
  Females >55 years or premature menopause without
    estrogen replacement therapy
Positive family history
Current cigarette smoking (pack-years[a])
Hypertension
  >140/90 mm Hg or on antihypertensive medication
Low HDL cholesterol
  <35mg/dL
Diabetes mellitus
Obesity
Sedentary lifestyle
Emotional stress/behavioral patterns

[a] Pack-years, number of packs of cigarettes smoked per day multiplied by the number of years of smoking.

Modifiable Risk Factors

Heredity. A familial pattern of CAD has long been recognized as an important nonmodifiable risk factor for the disease. The risk is significantly greater if either of the individual's parents have experienced myocardial infarction before the age of 55 years. Having a sibling with CAD doubles an individual's risk. When CAD occurs during the fourth or fifth decade of life, it is common to find that an individual's father, grandfather, and brothers developed CAD at about the same age. It has been postulated (but not proven) that the physical structure of the coronary arteries and the rate of atherosclerosis may be genetically determined.

The relative risk of a family history of CAD may be partially mediated through other risk factors, such as inherited abnormalities of cholesterol and lipoprotein metabolism. Because dietary patterns, personality structures, and smoking habits may also be influenced by heredity, the influence of genetics in CAD is difficult to isolate.

Diet, Cholesterol, and Lipoproteins. Many epidemiologic studies have shown that the incidence of CAD is positively correlated with the average population consumption of both dietary cholesterol and dietary saturated fat. Both dietary cholesterol and saturated fat intake are directly correlated with blood total cholesterol levels. In those countries in which animal fats (eg, eggs, butter, cream, milk, and fatty meats) constitute a large percentage of the total diet, the frequency of CAD is very high, while in countries in which animal fat intake is much lower, the incidence of the disease is low. The gross disparity in the amount of animal fat eaten in different parts of the world is believed to account for the fact that "normal" serum cholesterol levels in the United States may be 200 to 240 mg/dL, whereas in those countries in which CAD is uncommon the comparable levels are only 100 to 120 mg/dL.

More specific information about the danger of high serum cholesterol levels has been obtained from the Framingham Heart Study. In this study more than 5,000 men and women in the town of Framingham, Massachusetts, have been examined at regular intervals for more than 35 years to identify factors that contribute to the development of CAD. The results indicate that the risk of a heart attack is at least three times greater in men with serum cholesterol levels exceeding 240 mg/dL than in men with levels below this. On the basis of this and other research, the National Cholesterol Education Program identified serum cholesterol levels below 200 mg/dL as optimal for reducing cardiac risk.

Although serum cholesterol has received the greatest attention among lipid risk factors for CAD, other serum lipids (eg, triglycerides) and substances that transport lipids in the blood (lipoproteins) are important risk factors in their own right. For example, an elevated serum triglyceride level (above 200 mg%) is associated with an increased incidence of CAD even though the serum cholesterol level may be normal or only slightly elevated. In other words, cholesterol and triglyceride levels are not necessarily related, and a high concentration of either lipid may indicate an increased risk of CAD. Elevated triglyceride levels, unlike elevated cholesterol levels, are usually induced by the ingestion of carbohydrates (rather than saturated fats), and are commonly associated with diabetes or abnormal glucose tolerance.

Cholesterol and triglycerides, as lipids, are insoluble in plasma and are carried in the blood in combination with a group of soluble proteins called *lipoproteins*. Lipoproteins can be separated into three main classes: low-density lipoproteins (LDLs), very low-density lipoproteins (VLDLs), and high-density lipoproteins (HDLs). About two-thirds of the cholesterol in the blood is carried by LDLs, while HDLs carry less than one-third. (VLDLs are primarily involved in the transport of triglycerides, and carry only small amounts of cholesterol.) Epidemiologic studies have revealed that the concentration of LDL cholesterol is directly related to the risk of CAD. On the other hand, there is an inverse association between HDL cholesterol and the incidence of CAD.

TABLE 4–2. NORMAL VALUES FOR SERUM LIPIDS

Lipid	Normal Range	Goal
Serum cholesterol	100–240 mg/dL	<200 mg/dL
HDL cholesterol	35–45 mg/dL	>40 mg/dL
Triglycerides	0–150 mg/dL	<150 mg/dL
LDL cholesterol	50–160 mg/dL	<130 mg/dL

This means that the higher the percentage of HDL cholesterol (as a component of the total serum cholesterol), the lower the risk of CAD. HDL cholesterol seems to *protect* against CAD. Consequently, prediction of the risk of CAD can be substantially enhanced by measuring HDL and LDL cholesterol in conjunction with the total serum cholesterol level. For example, a total serum cholesterol of 160 mg/dL and HDL cholesterol of 80 mg/dL (normal HDL cholesterol range: 35 to 45 mg/dL) gives a total cholesterol/HDL cholesterol ratio of 1.8, which is half normal. LDL cholesterol can be calculated with the following equation:

LDL cholesterol = total cholesterol
        − (HDL cholesterol + triglyceride level/5)

HDL cholesterol levels may be increased by aerobic exercise, weight reduction, and discontinuing cigarette smoking. LDL cholesterol levels may be decreased by reducing dietary fat intake (especially saturated fats found in animal and vegetable products, such as coconut and palm oil) and increasing the intake of complex carbohydrates, such as whole grains and beans. See Table 4–2 for normal values of the serum lipids.

Hypertension. High blood pressure, or hypertension, is thought to predispose to CAD by accelerating the rate of atherosclerosis and increasing the oxygen demands of the myocardium. In the Framingham Heart Study it was observed that blood pressures in excess of 160/95 mm Hg were associated with a five-fold increase in the incidence of CAD over its incidence with normal pressures. Thus, from a statistical standpoint, hypertension appears to be one of the most serious risk factors for CAD. The currently accepted definition of hypertension is a diastolic blood pressure above 90 mm Hg and a systolic blood pressure above 140 mm Hg.

Hypertension can be reduced by weight reduction, physical exercise, salt restriction, a reduction in alcohol intake, and relaxation techniques (eg, biofeedback and meditation). It has been estimated that approximately half of all persons with high blood pressure respond to reductions in dietary sodium. Unfortunately, it is impossible to tell, before instituting a reduced-salt diet, whether an individual patient will benefit from a reduced sodium intake.

Antihypertensive medications are indicated for persons who remain hypertensive despite nonpharmacologic treatment. The most commonly used medications fall into four classes: diuretics, vasodilators, sympatholytics (alpha blockers, beta blockers, and central alpha agonists), and angiotensin-converting-enzyme inhibitors. Many of the available agents are described in Appendix A.

Cigarette Smoking. There is firm statistical evidence that cigarette smokers have a higher incidence of CAD than nonsmokers. In the Framingham Study the risk of a heart attack was nearly twice as great among cigarette smokers as among nonsmokers. In other studies, men who smoked were more than twice as likely to have a heart attack or die from cardiac causes than men who did not smoke. Women who smoked were at even greater risk. Cigarette smoking is one of the most potent cardiac risk factors, and every effort should be expended in helping patients to stop smoking. The manner in which cigarette smoking affects the coronary arteries is not understood. The suggestion that nicotine may sufficiently constrict the arteries as to reduce coronary blood flow has not been confirmed. On the other hand, nicotine increases the work of the heart (by increasing the heart rate and blood pressure) and could produce a relative oxygen deficiency. Moreover, cigarette smoking is associated with elevated carbon monoxide levels in the blood, which may also interfere with myocardial oxygenation.

Regardless of its mechanism of action, cigarette smoking is generally considered among the most serious risk factors for premature CAD. The risk of CAD is linearly proportional to the number of cigarettes smoked per day. A patient who continues to smoke after a myocardial infarction has twice the risk of having another myocardial infarction as a patient who stops smoking. Continued smoking also increases the risk of obstruction of coronary artery bypass grafts and restenosis of arteries after angioplasty. However, the risk of heart disease among persons who stop smoking falls within 2 to 3 years to the same level as that for nonsmokers.

Diabetes. The diagnosis of diabetes mellitus doubles the risk of CAD. CAD develops more frequently and at an earlier age among diabetic patients than among nondiabetics. Even when diabetes is mild or well controlled the risk of CAD remains substantially greater in diabetic persons. These facts, along with data indicating that other metabolic diseases (eg, gout) are associated with a high incidence of CAD, suggest that a biochemical disturbance may be central to the underlying disease process.

Sedentary Life Style

Persons who engage in regular aerobic activity (usually defined as lasting 30 minutes three times a week) have CAD incidence rates that are one-half those of sedentary individuals. This observation has been documented in both men and women. Because people who exercise are also more likely to be nonsmokers, less obese, and less hypertensive, it has been difficult to identify the specific contribution of exercise to reducing CAD risk. Vigorous physical activity also decreases blood glucose and increases HDL cholesterol concentrations. However, in recent studies, researchers have taken into account other cardiac risk factors and have still found a sedentary life style to be an important risk factor for CAD.

Obesity

Insurance company statistics suggest that obesity predisposes to fatal CAD, but the issue is by no means settled. In fact, in the Framingham Study, moderate obesity by itself was not associated with an increased incidence of CAD. However, overweight persons are especially prone to hypertension, diabetes, and elevated lipid levels, and it may be that the risk of obesity in CAD lies with these secondary effects. In any case obesity is classified as a risk factor even though its mechanism of action is uncertain.

Emotional Stress

Epidemiologic studies have consistently shown a markedly higher rate of CAD in industrialized countries than in less industrialized, less demanding societies. Many believe that this gross disparity either reflects or results directly from emotional stress imposed by fast-paced, demanding life styles. For this reason some persons consider CAD to be a disease of "overcivilization." According to this theory, humans in industrialized societies have developed chronic anxiety in attempting to cope with rapidly changing socioeconomic and sociocultural forces, and this tension in some way promotes atherosclerosis. In principle, this is an attractive concept, since it has been shown that anxiety is often accompanied by a distinct increase in serum cholesterol, which could favor the development of atherosclerotic plaques. Moreover, stress is known to accelerate blood coagulation, allowing small clots to form within the coronary arteries. Nevertheless, the relationship between emotional stress and CAD has been difficult to prove, particularly since there are no available methods for tangibly measuring degrees of stress. Intriguing studies have documented that persons who perceive their jobs to be highly demanding but to provide low autonomy and support (eg, clerical workers) have higher rates of CAD. Further study will be needed to determine the significance of emotional stress as a risk factor for the disease.

Interpersonal relationships may mitigate the negative consequences of emotional stress. In contrast, a lack of social support seems to put people at risk for CAD. For example, in some studies recently widowed men were six times more likely to die of CAD within 6 months of the death of their spouse than were age-adjusted controls.

Behavioral Patterns

Attempts have been made to correlate CAD with certain personality traits and behavioral patterns. The heart attack-prone person (called a *type A personality*) is said to be one who is hostile, aggressive, ambitious, highly competitive, and possessed with a profound sense of time urgency. Persons with this type of behavior pattern reportedly have significantly higher cholesterol levels and a greater incidence of CAD than their counterparts (type B personalities) in whom these particular characteristics are not as apparent. This interesting observation requires confirmation in non-Western cultures, but many now accept the type A behavior pattern as a distinct risk factor for CAD.

Summary of Risk Factors

It is essential to point to the lack of definite evidence that any of the risk factors just described actually *cause* CAD. All that can be said is that individuals with multiple risk factors are high-risk candidates for CAD; conversely, the absence of these factors predicts little likelihood of developing the disease. Thus, for example, a man with hypertension and a high serum cholesterol level who is a heavy cigarette smoker may have a 10 times greater risk of sustaining a heart attack than a person with none of these factors. In other terms, there is a statistical association between risk factors and CAD, but no proof that these risk factors in themselves are the direct cause of coronary atherosclerosis.

THE CLINICAL SPECTRUM OF CORONARY ATHEROSCLEROSIS

Asymptomatic Coronary Atherosclerosis

If the degree of arterial obstruction caused by coronary atherosclerosis is moderate and does not signifi-

cantly reduce the blood supply to the myocardium, the disease may never be suspected by the patient or the health-care practitioner. Results of autopsy studies among persons dying of other causes indicate that this is a common situation. In fact, practically all men in the United States have evidence of coronary atherosclerosis by age 50; it is only the degree of involvement that varies.

Even if the coronary arteries are grossly narrowed by intimal plaques, it still does not follow that the disease will be clinically evident or produce symptoms. This paradox can be partly explained by the frequent accompaniment of coronary arterial narrowing by the enlargement of small branches of these vessels or the formation of new branches in order to bring more blood to the myocardium. This additional blood supply, called a *collateral circulation,* is of great importance in determining the clinical effects of coronary atherosclerosis, since it is often sufficient to sustain portions of the myocardium despite the existence of advanced atherosclerosis in a major vessel. It is the *total* blood supply to the myocardium, rather than the state of the main coronary arteries, that determines whether the disease will be symptomatic.

It is important to realize there is no definite correlation between the extent of CAD and symptoms. In fact, about 30% of patients who die of CAD experience no symptoms of the disease before the fatal event. Stated in another way, sudden death is the first symptom in 30% of patients who die from coronary atherosclerotic heart disease.

Symptomatic Coronary Disease

By definition, CAD implies that the myocardium is affected by inadequate coronary blood flow. The symptoms of CAD are due to myocardial oxygen deprivation and are manifested in a progressive order of severity by three main clinical patterns: angina pectoris, unstable angina, and acute myocardial infarction. Each of these syndromes is described separately in the following pages.

Angina Pectoris

The classic indication of impaired circulation to the myocardium is a distinctive type of chest pain called *angina pectoris*. The pain signifies insufficient oxygenation (*ischemia*) of the myocardium; it occurs when the oxygen demands of the myocardium exceed the capacity of the coronary circulation to supply oxygen to the heart. In other words, angina represents a signal from the heart that the myocardium is not receiving sufficient oxygen to meet its immediate needs. Because angina pectoris is usually the key to the diagnosis of CAD, it is essential to understand its clinical features.

Site of Pain.
The pain of myocardial ischemia is located most often directly under the center of the breastbone. It may radiate from this substernal location to both sides of the chest, the left or right arm, the neck, the jaws, or the shoulders and upper back. In some instances the pain occurs only at these latter sites without a substernal component; this pattern, however, is much less common than central chest pain.

Quality of Pain.
The discomfort in angina pectoris is usually described as pressure, tightness, or constriction within the chest. Some patients place a clenched fist against the sternum in attempting to characterize the tight, constricting nature of the sensation. Although angina generally lasts for only a few minutes (as described below), the pain is steady and is not influenced by breathing, breath-holding, or changes in body position. This constancy of the pain is a characteristic aspect of angina and is often more significant than other descriptive qualities of the condition (eg, burning, pressure, or " indigestion").

Occurrence of Pain.
Any situation that increases the myocardial demand for oxygen is capable of producing angina. In general, this oxygen demand is determined by the amount of work the heart performs. As would be anticipated on this basis, the pain of angina is usually brought on by physical effort that increases the heart rate and cardiac workload, in turn increasing myocardial oxygen requirements. Certain activities are especially prone to precipitate angina, including walking uphill or against the wind, hurrying after eating a meal, and unaccustomed exercise. Conversely, angina is relieved by rest. As soon as physical activity stops the oxygen demand of the myocardium promptly declines, and as a consequence the pain subsides. The relationship of activity with pain, and rest with the disappearance of pain is typical of transient myocardial ischemia, and distinguishes angina of effort from other, nonischemic causes of chest pain in which this pattern does not occur. In addition to physical exertion, sudden emotional stress (e.g., anger, fear, or even the excitement of watching a football game) may induce an anginal episode. The mechanism in such cases is the same as with angina of effort: the workload of the heart is transiently increased beyond the ability of the coronary circulation to satisfy the additional oxygen demands of the myocardium. In summary, any physical or emotional stress that produces a sudden increase in the heart rate or elevation in blood pressure may induce angina.

Duration of Pain.
Angina is characteristically of brief duration, lasting usually from 1 to 5 minutes before abating with rest. Occasionally the pain may last for more than 5 minutes, particularly if the stimulus for the attack persists. The cessation of pain indicates that the myocardial demand for oxygen has been met and that the oxygen deficit was only transient and not destructive to the myocardium. If the pain does not subside within minutes after the beginning of rest, myocardial damage should be suspected.

Relief of Pain.
A distinctive feature of anginal pain is its prompt relief by nitroglycerin. The failure of sublingual nitroglycerin to terminate anginal pain is unusual, and a cause for suspicion that the attack is not due to angina of effort. Anginal attacks are precipitated by exercise, emotion (stress), elimination (the Valsalva maneuver), and extremes in temperature. Nitroglycerin acts by dilating the venous capacitance vessels, thus decreasing the return of blood to the heart. This decreases the cardiac workload and myocardial oxygen consumption. Nitroglycerin also acts directly on the coronary arteries by dilating them to increase the myocardial oxygen supply.

Diagnosis of Angina Pectoris

The most important diagnostic evidence of angina pectoris is the patient's history. If chest pain is centrally located, of brief duration, oppressive in quality, and related to effort, the diagnosis of angina pectoris is virtually assured and no further confirmation is necessary. Physical examination and ECGs at rest are normal in most patients with angina and seldom contribute directly to the diagnosis. When the chest-pain pattern is suspicious but not entirely characteristic of angina, several diagnostic tests may be performed to determine whether the pain is ischemic in origin.

Exercise (Stress) Testing.
The simplest and most widely used method for diagnosing angina is the exercise, or stress, test. It consists of recording an ECG during progressively strenuous exercise, when the oxygen demands of the myocardium increase greatly and signs of myocardial ischemia are most likely to appear in an ECG. The exercise is performed by riding a stationary bicycle or walking on a treadmill while the heart rate, blood pressure, and ECG are monitored continuously. The test starts with low-level exercise which is increased in stages until a target heart rate (based on the patient's age) is achieved. In patients with significant obstructive disease of the coronary arteries, the exercise test soon leads to a point at which myocardial oxygen demand exceeds oxygen supply and signs of myocardial ischemia ap-

pear in the ECG. Although chest pain may develop during exercise, a positive stress test is defined only on the basis of electrocardiographic changes characteristic of ischemia (as described in Chapter 15), and not by the presence or absence of angina. One of the main limitations of stress testing is that many elderly sedentary patients are unable to exercise sufficiently to achieve the target heart rate; the test must often be terminated prematurely in this group because of fatigue, leg weakness, or shortness of breath.

Radionuclide Studies. In recent years, various nuclear scanning techniques have assumed an increasingly useful role in the diagnosis and assessment of CAD. One of these methods, *radionuclide angiography,* provides indirect information about myocardial blood flow and is used in combination with exercise testing to confirm the diagnosis of angina pectoris. Use of this technique is based on the fact that myocardial ischemia, besides producing typical electrocardiographic signs, also causes abnormalities in contraction of segments (regions) of the left ventricle. These transient, regional abnormalities in ventricular wall motion with exercise can be detected by nuclear scanning of the heart. The procedure involves the intravenous injection of a radioactive isotope during the period of peak exercise followed by sequential recording of the motion of the ventricular wall with a nuclear camera. With significant CAD, blood flow is reduced in the region supplied by the involved vessel, as reflected by an abnormal contractile pattern of that portion of the ventricle. Radionuclide angiography has greater diagnostic accuracy than customary stress testing, but is much more costly. (Radionuclide scanning is also described in Chapter 5.)

Coronary Arteriography. The most definitive method for the diagnosis of CAD is *coronary arteriography.* In fact it serves as the standard of accuracy for the comparison of all other tests used in the diagnosis of CAD. As mentioned previously, coronary arteriography permits visualization of the coronary arteries (with a radiopaque dye), and thereby defines the precise number of arteries involved by CAD, the extent of narrowing in each vessel, and the degree of collateral circulation. This anatomic description of the disease process is particularly important in evaluating patients for coronary bypass surgery.

In addition to coronary arteriography, cardiac catheterization and ventriculography are also performed as part of a complete study of the heart and its arteries. *Cardiac catheterization* involves the introduction of catheters into the cardiac chambers and great vessels in order to measure pressures and oxygen concentrations in each of these sites. These data are essential for patients in whom cardiovascular surgery is contemplated. *Ventriculography* is used to assess the pumping function of the ventricles and to detect regional abnormalities in the motion of their walls. The technique consists of injecting a radiopaque dye through a catheter introduced into the left ventricle and recording motion pictures of ventricular motion. This latter information is similar to, but more precise than that obtained in radionuclide studies. The main disadvantage of coronary arteriography (and its procedural components) is that catheterization of the heart is an expensive, invasive procedure that is not entirely without risk.

Stable and Variant Angina Pectoris

Classic angina pectoris, as described above, behaves in a predictable and reproducible manner: it is brought on by physical activity or emotional stress that increases the myocardial oxygen demand, and is relieved promptly by rest, which decreases the oxygen requirement of the heart. This classic form of angina, with its established pattern of pain, is called *stable* angina pectoris. It is associated with fixed narrowing of the coronary arteries and results from advanced atherosclerosis. Coronary angiograms usually show at least 75% narrowing of one or more of the arteries; most often, two or three vessels are involved.

Angina pectoris may also result from coronary artery spasm. The arterial spasm reduces coronary blood flow sufficiently to produce myocardial ischemia. Coronary artery spasm may be manifested clinically in several ways, but its most typical form is described as *variant* or Prinzmetal's angina. The pattern of pain in variant angina differs greatly from that in stable angina; indeed, it contrasts almost directly with the latter in many of its characteristics. The main feature of variant angina is that pain occurs with *rest* rather than with activity. In fact, patients with variant angina do not develop chest pain or characteristic electrocardiographic signs of ischemia even during exercise testing. The pain also has an unusual cyclic pattern, often awakening the patient each night at about the same time. Furthermore, the electrocardiographic changes that accompany variant angina are entirely different from those associated with stable angina (see Chapter 14). The cause of coronary artery spasm is still unknown, but the condition is related somehow to abnormal contraction of the smooth muscles in the walls of arteries.

Although variant angina is less common than stable angina, it has commanded increasing attention in recent years. Part of the interest in it can be attributed to the *calcium antagonists* or calcium blocking agents (diltiazem hydrochloride, nifedipine, and verapamil hydrochloride), which have proven very effective in preventing and interrupting coronary artery spasm and relieving variant angina. Much more important is that these drugs also seem to benefit certain patients with fixed coronary artery obstruction. This implies that coronary artery spasm may contribute to the classic anginal syndrome even when the dominant cause of ischemia is advanced coronary atherosclerosis.

Unstable Angina

The term *unstable angina* has been used to characterize a clinical state that lies between stable angina pectoris and acute myocardial infarction. The syndrome has several different patterns, thus accounting for the variety of names given to it in the past. Among the older (but still used) terms are impending myocardial infarction, preinfarction angina, crescendo angina, accelerated angina, and acute coronary insufficiency. At present the preferred term is unstable angina, connoting that the common feature of the syndrome is its clinical instability.

Unstable angina may occur as the initial symptom of CAD or, more often, as a sudden worsening of stable angina. The chest pain, instead of lasting briefly as with stable angina, usually persists for 10 to 20 minutes or longer. It develops with increasing frequency and is provoked by less effort, often occurring during rest. Nitroglycerin provides incomplete or no relief in most cases of unstable angina. Electrocardiographic signs of ischemia are common but without definite evidence of acute myocardial infarction.

The mechanism of unstable angina is not entirely clear, but progressive narrowing of the coronary arteries probably plays a major role in this condition, especially in patients with previously stable angina. In any case, unstable angina is more serious than stable angina, since it is often an immediate forerunner of acute myocardial infarction. Approximately 750,000 patients are hospitalized each year in the United States with the diagnosis of unstable angina. From this number, 70,000 go on to have an acute myocardial infarction and 30,000 die while hospitalized.

The diagnosis of unstable angina theoretically implies that despite prolonged ischemia adequate oxygenation was restored to the heart before myocardial destruction occurred. From a clinical standpoint, however, it is often difficult to rule out the possibility that small areas of the myocardium have been injured or destroyed by episodes of ischemia. For this reason, and because of the changing and unpredictable course of the condition, patients with unstable angina are ad-

mitted to a CCU at least until the diagnosis of acute myocardial infarction has been excluded.

Acute Myocardial Infarction

When a portion of the myocardium experiences profound and sustained ischemia, the cells deprived of oxygen cannot survive, and tissue in the involved area dies (undergoes *necrosis*). This destructive process is termed *acute myocardial infarction.* The event that produces this irreversible tissue damage (infarction) is often called a coronary thrombosis, a coronary occlusion, a "coronary," or a heart attack. These latter terms are used synonymously in clinical practice to describe what properly should be designated as an acute myocardial infarction (AMI).

With few exceptions, AMI results from advanced atherosclerosis of the coronary arteries. This final consequence of progressive coronary atherosclerosis usually occurs when one of the main coronary arteries or its branches becomes occluded. Although the process by which this occurs is gradual, the obstruction occurs suddenly in most instances. Exactly why a coronary artery becomes blocked at a certain moment is not fully understood, but three main factors have been incriminated: 1) a clot may develop on the roughened surface of an atherosclerotic plaque and occlude the lumen of the artery; 2) an atherosclerotic lesion in the artery may irritate the underlying arterial wall, causing bleeding beneath the plaque (subintimal hemorrhage) that dislodges the plaque and obstructs the artery; 3) a piece of a large plaque may break off and block a small distal artery. Although all of these mechanisms offer a logical explanation for the suddenness of a myocardial infarction, it is now clear that none of them can account for all infarctions. Autopsy studies have shown, for instance, that AMI can occur even though the coronary arteries have no clots and are not completely obstructed. In these latter instances it is presumed that at a particular moment the heart is faced with an enormous oxygen demand (eg, during intense physical activity, such as shoveling snow) that cannot be met by the available blood supply through partially narrowed arteries. In effect, even though the coronary arteries are not completely obstructed, the persistent myocardial demand for oxygen simply overwhelms the limited supply, and tissue necrosis develops because of this relative oxygen deprivation. Another possibility in the occurrence of myocardial infarction is that coronary artery spasm is superimposed on existing CAD, causing a partially narrowed vessel to close completely during the transient spasm.

The site of an infarction depends fundamentally

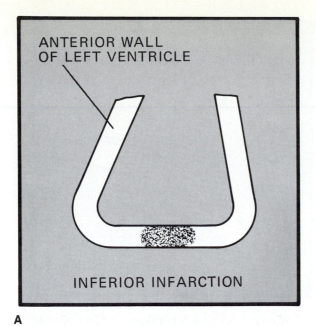

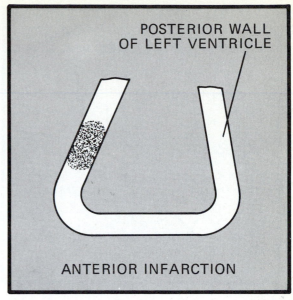

A   **B**

Figure 4–4. Side view of the left ventricle showing the respective locations of an inferior (**A**) and anterior (**B**) infarction. Because the inferior surface of the left ventricle faces the diaphragm, inferior infarctions are also called diaphragmatic infarctions. Anterolateral infarctions involve both the anterior and lateral (side) wall of the left ventricle.

on which coronary artery (or arteries) is blocked. When the left coronary artery or its branches are occluded, the infarction primarily involves the anterior wall of the left ventricle, and is called an *anterior infarction*. Occlusion of the right coronary artery results in infarction of the inferior (diaphragmatic) wall of the left ventricle, which is designated an *inferior infarction* (Figure 4–4). Very often the ischemic process damages more than one area of the left ventricle; in these cases more specific terms are used to describe the location of an infarct. For example, an infarction that involves both the anterior and lateral walls of the left ventricle is termed an *anterolateral infarction*. Similarly, an infarction that damages both the anterior wall of the left ventricle and the interventricular septum is called an *anteroseptal infarction*.

Myocardial infarction involving the *right* ventricle alone is very rare because this chamber is supplied with a relatively greater proportion of blood for its (smaller) muscle mass than is the left ventricle, and also has lower oxygen requirements. However, right ventricular infarction is not uncommon in conjunction with inferior myocardial infarction. This relationship is understandable, since the right ventricle and the inferior wall of the left ventricle share a common blood supply through the right coronary artery. Nevertheless, the frequency of such combined infarc-

tions was not appreciated until the recent introduction of radionuclide techniques for the diagnosis of AMI (as described in the Chapter 5). With these (and other) means it has been shown that at least 25% of patients with acute inferior myocardial infarction also have some evidence of right ventricular damage.

The extent of an infarction is determined first by the size of the vessel obstructed and second by the capacity of the collateral circulation to bring additional blood to the oxygen-deprived areas of the heart. Until the 1980s the terms *subendocardial* and *transmural* infarctions were used to categorize myocardial infarctions. Transmural infarctions were defined by widespread myocardial necrosis extending through the entire ventricular wall (from the endocardium to the pericardium). Subendocardial infarctions were defined as involving less severe damage that did not extend through the full thickness of the ventricular wall (Figure 4–5) Other descriptive terms for subendocardial infarctions were *intramural* and *nontransmural*.

Numerous studies of autopsy findings have since shown that myocardial infarctions are more accurately categorized by their size, as reflected in Q-wave changes on the ECG (discussed in Chapter 14). *Q-wave myocardial infarctions* (formerly called transmural infarctions) are medium to large in terms of the weight of myocardial tissue they in-

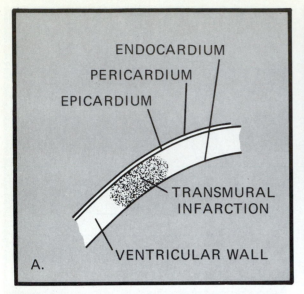

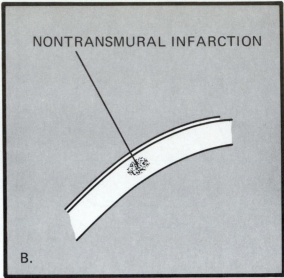

Figure 4–5. Comparison of transmural and subendocardial myocardial infarctions. **A.** The necrotic area extends all the way through the ventricular wall from the endocardium, through the myocardium, and to the pericardium. **B.** With a nontransmural infarction the damage is less extensive, involving only a portion of the ventricular wall.

volve, whereas *non-Q-wave myocardial infarctions* (formerly called subendocardial infarctions) are smaller. A non-Q-wave infarction may involve only the myocardium, or may extend from the subendocardium through the myocardium to the epicardial area.

Consequently, the presence or absence of a Q-wave on the ECG does not reveal whether or not an infarction involves all three layers of the ventricle, and is not necessarily reflected in different symptoms. However, it does have clinical and prognostic implications. Patients with non-Q-wave infarctions will have smaller changes in cardiac enzyme concentrations, will be more likely to extend their infarction (usually about 10 days after the initial event), and will have fewer in-hospital complications than patients with Q-wave infarctions. Although the in-hospital mortality rate is lower among patients with non-Q-wave infarction than those with Q-wave infarction (5% versus 15%), the 2-year mortality rate is the same for both conditions (27%-28%). These differences are summarized in Table 4–3.

Q-wave infarctions comprise about 60% of all myocardial infarctions, while non-Q-wave infarctions constitute about 30%. The remaining 10% of infarctions cannot be identified because of left bundle branch block or pacemaker dependent rhythms.

In the early stages of AMI there are, at least in concept, three zones of tissue damage. The first zone consists of necrotic myocardial tissue that has been irreversibly destroyed by prolonged oxygen deprivation. Surrounding this dead tissue is a second zone (the zone of injury) in which the myocardial cells, although injured and jeopardized, may still survive if adequate circulation is restored to the area. Zone 3, called the zone of ischemia, represents cells that have not received adequate oxygen but can be expected to recover unless the ischemic process worsens. In effect, the ultimate size of an infarction may depend on the fate of the zones of injury and ischemia. (These latter zones are not actually distinct or separate areas, as the foregoing description suggests. Instead, they appear histologically as a combined outer zone surrounding the central zone of necrosis. This outer zone is diffuse and consists of patchy areas of necrotic, in-

TABLE 4–3. COMPARISON OF Q-WAVE AND NON-Q-WAVE MYOCARDIAL INFARCTIONS

	Q-Wave Infarction	Non-Q-Wave Infarction
Incidence	55–60%	35–40%
Coronary artery	Total occlusion	Partial occlusion
ECG	Q waves, ST elevation and T wave inversion	Nonspecific ST-T Changes or ST elevation
Hospital mortality	15–20%	5–8%
Two-year mortality	25–30%	25–30%

jured, and ischemic tissues merging with normal myocardium. Because of its intermediate location and status, this peripheral zone is usually described as the *border* zone).

Once the coronary circulation is interrupted and a myocardial infarction occurs, there follows a series of events that put life in the balance. This book is concerned with these events, and describes a concept of specialized care, known as *intensive coronary care,* that is designed to reduce the death rate from CAD, particularly from acute myocardial infarction and its sequelae.

Chapter 5

Acute Myocardial Infarction

THE ONSET OF THE ATTACK

Most patients with acute myocardial infarction (AMI) seek medical assistance because of *chest pain.* The pain is usually quite distinctive; it occurs suddenly and is of severe, crushing quality. It is more intense than the pain of angina and may be unlike any sensation the patient has experienced previously. Typically the pain is concentrated directly beneath the sternum, but it frequently radiates across the chest or to the arms and neck. Patients commonly describe the pain as a heavy weight or pressure or a knot in the chest. Unlike angina, the pain does not necessarily occur with exertion; in fact, it may even occur during sleep. Its occurrence after eating explains why many patients interpret the pain of a myocardial infarction as indigestion. The chest pain is continuous and is not relieved by changes in body position, breath-holding, or home remedies (eg, bicarbonate). It usually persists for 30 minutes or more, and may not subside until morphine is administered. Nitroglycerin seldom influences the duration or severity of the pain. Drenching perspiration usually begins soon after the onset of the substernal pain, and nausea and vomiting often occur at the same time. Fear and apprehension are usual, and most patients sense that a catastrophe has happened. Within minutes, many patients are aware of dyspnea and marked weakness. This symptom complex of substernal pain, sweating, nausea, and vomiting along with dyspnea and sudden weakness can be considered the typical history of AMI.

Not all patients, of course, present such typical histories, and there are many variations to patients descriptions of an infarction. Sometimes the pain is centered not in the chest but, as with angina, in the arms, neck, or shoulders. Sweating, nausea, vomiting,

and dyspnea are not constant features of the attack and may not appear at all. The severity and duration of chest pain can vary greatly, and it is often difficult to distinguish angina pectoris, unstable angina, and AMI on the basis of the quality of pain alone. Typical signs and symptoms of a myocardial infarction are listed in Table 5–1.

Some patients experience acute infarction apparently without any chest pain or other clear-cut symptoms. The diagnosis becomes evident when signs of an old infarction are found on a routine ECG while the patient denies having had any symptoms. Such infarctions are called *silent* infarctions. It is estimated that at least 20% of all infarctions fall into this category.

At the other end of the spectrum are patients who develop a serious or fatal complication of AMI immediately with or after the onset of the attack. In these cases the complication itself (eg, pulmonary edema or a fatal arrhythmia) suggests that an acute infarction has occurred. Each year approximately 1.2 million Americans experience an AMI, and 500,000 die before reaching the hospital.

CHANGES IN THE HEART

An AMI usually occurs when plaque ruptures inside a coronary artery and a clot (thrombus) forms at the site of the rupture. With this, blood can no longer flow through the artery, and the portion of the myocardium that depends on the artery for the delivery of oxygen and removal of waste products becomes cyanotic. Active myocardial contractions stop within 1 minute, and cell death (necrosis) begins within 20 to 40 minutes after coronary artery occlusion, begin-

TABLE 5–1. SIGNS AND SYMPTOMS OF ACUTE MYOCARDIAL INFARCTION

Pain
  Substernal chest pain radiating to the left arm, both arms, or neck
  A feeling of heaviness or oppression

Autonomic Stimulation
  Parasympathetic: nausea, vomiting, weakness
  Sympathetic: diaphoresis, cold and clammy skin

Inflammatory Response
  Mild fever and increased heart rate

Cardiac Findings
  S_3 (if heart failure) and S_4
  Systolic murmur (if mitral regurgitation or ventricular septal defect)
  Pericardial friction rub (if pericarditis)

Other
  Jugular venous distension (if right ventricle involved)
  Pulmonary rales (if heart failure)

ning at the subendocardial surface and spreading outward through the myocardium to the epicardium (transmural). Unless blood flow to the affected portion of myocardium can be restored within minutes, it becomes irreversibly damaged. Myocardial necrosis occurs within 8 to 12 hours. Leukocytes begin to infiltrate the area, and removal of necrotic tissue occurs within 4 to 7 days. Scar-tissue formation begins in the second and third week after the infarction and is complete by 2 months.

The subendocardial surface is normally the last area of the heart to be perfused and the first to experience ischemia when blood flow is interrupted, since its blood supply comes from the epicardial surface of the heart. The terminal branches of the coronary artery bring blood to the subendocardial surface, putting this layer of the heart at greatest risk for necrosis.

THE CLINICAL COURSE IMMEDIATELY AFTER INFARCTION

It is apparent from the foregoing description of the onset of a myocardial infarction that the heart may respond in several ways to the interruption of its blood supply. Some patients develop serious or lethal complications almost instantly while others never experience any difficulties at all. The factors that influence the heart's behavior in the immediate postinfarction period are not known with certainty. There is good reason to believe, however, that the size of an infarction is the most critical determinant of the patient's clinical course. In general, if a main coronary artery is occluded and produces extensive myocardial dam-

age, the course and prognosis are much poorer than when a branch artery is blocked and the resultant injury is small. This relationship, however, is not always constant, and patients with modest areas of tissue destruction can develop serious complications. Because of this disparity it is evident that other factors contribute to the initial and subsequent outcome of an infarction.

Collateral blood supply is one of several important factors in determining the clinical course after a myocardial infarction. If sufficient blood can be diverted immediately to the border zone surrounding the necrotic area of myocardium, the jeopardized tissues may be preserved, thus limiting the size of the infarction. Conversely, if the collateral blood supply is poor, widespread myocardial destruction may result, since tissue oxygenation cannot be enhanced. By this same token, the extent of an infarction is probably influenced by the specific oxygen demands of the myocardium immediately after the attack. A rapid heart rate and high blood pressure, for example, greatly increase the oxygen requirements of the myocardium; this prevents the jeopardized zone of ischemic tissue from surviving, causing the infarction to enlarge.

Regardless of the mechanisms underlying the different responses to an obstruction of coronary blood flow, the immediate clinical course of an AMI can be generally categorized according to the following order of severity:

1. If the infarcted area is of limited size and enough blood is diverted to it by collateral channels, the myocardium may continue to function quite normally. The heart's pumping action may not be affected, and its rate and rhythm will not necessarily be disturbed. In such instances the pain gradually subsides in these instances, and the patient appears in no distress at the time of admission.

2. When the involved area is larger and has only trivial collateral assistance, the myocardium may become sufficiently damaged to impair its function. This may be manifested by signs of a decreased pumping action of the heart (heart failure) or by disturbances in the heart rate and rhythm (arrhythmias). The degree of impairment may vary greatly; some patients have only mild shortness of breath and minor arrhythmias, while others are critically ill, with marked dyspnea, pulmonary edema, and life-threatening arrhythmias.

3. If the pumping action of the heart is grossly reduced by extensive structural damage to the myocardium, the left ventricle is simply unable to pump sufficient blood throughout the body to sustain circulation to the vital organs. Accordingly, the blood pressure falls, the heart rate increases, the urinary output decreases, and the skin becomes cold and clammy. This state is called *cardiogenic shock;* it is a life-threatening state and without appropriate treatment is fatal to most patients.

4. For some patients death occurs almost instantly after an interruption of coronary blood flow. These sudden deaths are almost always due to lethal arrhythmias resulting from extraordinary changes in the electrical activity of the heart, which are probably induced by myocardial ischemia. By far the most common arrhythmic mechanism of sudden death is ventricular fibrillation, a condition in which the ventricles are stimulated so incessantly that they lose their normal contractile pattern and merely quiver without propelling blood into the aorta. There is no clear relationship between the size of an infarction and the occurrence of sudden arrhythmic death. It is estimated that 50% of all deaths from AMI occur within the first few hours after the attack as a result of arrhythmias.

Because of these different possibilities it can be appreciated that some patients admitted to the hospital with AMI have no pain by the time they arrive and are not in distress, whereas others are near death from cardiogenic shock or pulmonary edema. The ultimate clinical course is largely but certainly not entirely related to the clinical picture on admission and extent of myocardium affected by a coronary artery occlusion. *Complications may occur at any time*

THE DIAGNOSIS OF ACUTE MYOCARDIAL INFARCTION

The diagnosis of AMI is made essentially in three steps: the patient's history, the ECG, and enzyme studies. In the event that this does not lead to a definite conclusion, radionuclide imaging may be needed to confirm the diagnosis.

The Patient's History

In many ways the patient's own story of illness is the prime factor in reaching the diagnosis of AMI. This history is the basis for suspecting a diagnosis of acute infarction and admitting the patient to the hospital. The development of severe, substernal pain associated with nausea, sweating, and the other features of an infarction is often so distinctive that the emergency department or CCU team can be fairly confident that this diagnosis will be confirmed by ECG and enzyme studies. Despite this, the history, regardless of how typical it may be, is not diagnostic in its own right, and other steps must be taken to prove that an acute infarction has actually occurred.

The Electrocardiogram

The diagnosis of AMI can be made definitively only by electrocardiography. When injury and local death (infarction) of myocardial tissue occur, characteristic findings reflecting these changes are found in the electrocardiographic tracing. On many occasions the initial diagnostic (12-lead) ECG fails to show specific evidence of an infarction, and additional (serial) tracings must be obtained over the next several days until definite electrocardiographic proof of infarction has evolved. The diagnosis of acute infarction cannot and should not be made unless characteristic electrocardiographic changes are finally demonstrated. It is important to realize that the ECG does not show the actual extent of the damage incurred by an infarction, and by itself is not a true index of the seriousness of the attack. (The electrocardiographic signs of acute myocardial infarction are described in Chapter 14.)

Enzyme Studies

In some cases patients may give an impressive history suggesting AMI, whereas ECG's show equivocal (rather than definite) changes. In these cases other studies are necessary to verify the diagnosis. The most important studies are laboratory measurements of certain enzymes in the blood. The basis for these tests is that several enzymes are normally present in myocardial cells. When the myocardium is injured, these enzymes escape into the bloodstream, where they can be detected and measured. Thus, a characteristic increase in the concentration of these enzymes in the serum is to be expected after acute infarction. The three enzyme studies most frequently used to confirm the diagnosis of AMI are creatine phosphokinase (CK), aspartate aminotransferase and serum glutamic oxaloacetic transaminase (AST/SGOT), and lactic dehydrogenase (LDH).

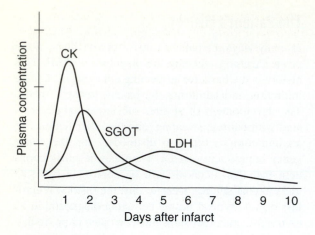

Figure 5–1. Pattern of serum enzyme changes in acute myocardial infarction. The level of CK rises several hours after the acute infarction and peaks at 25 hours; SGOT peaks at 48 to 72 hours. Serum levels of LDH rise more gradually and peak at 3 to 5 days.

Creatine Phosphokinase (CK).

CK is the first enzyme whose blood levels show an increase after myocardial infarction, and elevated levels of this enzyme can be detected within 2 to 6 hours after an infarction. The peak level is usually reached during the first 24 hours. After 2 to 3 days the CK level generally returns to normal (Figure 5–1). Accordingly, CK levels should be measured at the time of admission, 24 hours later, and at the end of the second and third days of hospitalization. Unfortunately, CK is not only a myocardial enzyme, but is also produced by the brain and skeletal muscles. Therefore, elevated CK levels may be noted after brain damage (eg, stroke) or with various muscle diseases or injuries. Even an intramuscular injection may cause a significant increase in the serum CK level. (For this reason it is wise, when possible, not to give any intramuscular injections to patients suspected of having had an AMI.)

CK has three isoenzymes: MM in skeletal and cardiac muscle, BB in brain, and MB in myocardium. Of the CK in the myocardium, 15% to 20% is CK-MB. To exclude the possibility that elevated CK levels are due to causes other than AMI, most laboratories measure the CK-MB isoenzyme as well as CK itself. This particular isoenzyme is found only in the myocardium and is therefore a very sensitive index of myocardial necrosis. CK-MB levels become abnormal from 2 to 3 hours and peak at 12 hours after an infarction; they then decrease rapidly and may return to normal within 24 hours. If the CK-MB isoenzyme concentration exceeds 5% of the total CK level, the diagnosis of AMI is nearly certain.

AST/SGOT.

AST/SGOT levels rise less rapidly than do those of CK after myocardial infarction. Although minor increases in AST/SGOT may be detected after 8 hours, their peak levels do not occur until 24 to 48 hours have elapsed. The levels usually return to normal after 4 to 6 days. AST/SGOT is a nonspecific marker of myocardial infarction because it also rises in other diseases (eg, liver disease, skeletal muscle injury, and, to a lesser degree, in heart failure). Given its nonspecificity it should only be used in those hospitals that lack facilities for the accurate measurement of CK-MB.

Lactic Dehydrogenase (LDH).

Serum levels of LDH increase after infarction at a slower rate than those of either CK or AST/SGOT. Peak concentrations of this enzyme do not usually occur until the third day or fourth postinfarction day, and return to normal on about the sixth or seventh day. The laboratory determination of LDH should therefore be performed on days 3, 4, and 5, but only if CK and SGOT levels have not already confirmed the diagnosis. The measurement of LDH is useful in patients who have delayed coming to the hospital beyond 2 or 3 days after a possible infarction, because by that time the CK-MB has returned to normal.

As with CK and SGOT, LDH levels may increase from causes other than AMI. Elevations occur with pulmonary, renal, and skeletal muscle diseases. These latter causes can be excluded by measuring the isoenzymes of LDH. It has been shown that the ratio of two LDH isoenzymes, LDH1/LDH2, is a far more specific indicator of AMI than is the total LDH level. An LDH1/LDH2 ratio that exceeds 1.0 is indicative of myocardial necrosis.

Significance of Enzyme Studies.

Although the degree of serum enzyme elevation cannot be correlated precisely with the size or severity of myocardial infarction, serum enzyme levels do provide a general indication of the extent of tissue destruction. Markedly increased serum enzyme levels, especially of CK-MB, appearing promptly after infarction and remaining elevated longer than anticipated, usually suggest an extensive myocardial infarction.

Despite the sensitivity of isoenzyme determinations, the diagnosis of AMI should not be made solely on the basis of elevated enzyme levels; the value of these tests is only supplemental. Conversely, negative results of enzyme studies should not be grounds to abandon the diagnosis of acute infarction.

Radionuclide Imaging

Occasionally the diagnosis of AMI cannot be definitely confirmed either electrocardiographically or by enzyme studies. Characteristic electrocardiographic signs of an acute infarction may, for example, be obscured by preexisting abnormalities, such as an old infarction. Even CK-MB, the isoenzyme most sensitive to infarction can be misleading if the patient has delayed coming to the hospital. If, for instance, the test is delayed more than 12 hours after a small infarction, the diagnosis may be missed because the CK-MB peak has passed and levels of the enzyme may be returning toward normal. A more common diagnostic problem is AMI occurring during or after open heart surgery. In this circumstance there is no way to tell whether elevated postoperative enzyme levels are due to a heart attack or to myocardial injury from the surgical procedure itself. These (and other) diagnostic dilemmas can in many instances be resolved by means of radionuclide imaging.

Radionuclide imaging can be used in two basic ways to diagnose AMI: "hot spot" imaging and "cold spot" imaging. Hot spot imaging involves the intravenous injection of a radionuclide-containing substance, most often technetium-99m pyrophosphate, that accumulates selectively in areas of myocardial necrosis. The uptake of the radionuclide in the infarcted area can be visualized in emission images made with a specialized nuclear camera. Acute myocardial infarction appears in these images as an area of increased uptake of the radionuclide (greater radioactivity), called a hot spot. By contrast, normal myocardial tissue demonstrates no visible uptake of the radionuclide. The technique therefore demarcates the zone of necrosis from normal myocardium, which in effect defines the size and location of an acute infarction. An example of AMI as determined by hot spot imaging is shown in Figure 5–2. Images reflecting acute infarction become evident about 10 to 12 hours after the attack and peak at 24 to 72 hours; they may remain positive for 7 to 10 days. Although very attractive as a diagnostic concept, hot spot imaging has several associated pitfalls, including varying results with different types of infarction and different timings of the test. At present it is estimated that the sensitivity of technetium-99m pyrophosphate for the diagnosis of AMI is about 80% to 90% for transmural infarctions and 50% for small, nontransmural infarctions.

Cold spot imaging is based on a different principle than hot spot imaging. It has been demonstrated that certain radionuclides, especially thallium-201, are taken up by the myocardium in direct relation to coronary blood flow (myocardial perfusion). If myocardial perfusion is normal, radionuclide imaging following the intravenous injection of thallium-201 reveals an even, homogenous distribution of radioactivity throughout the myocardium, mostly within the left ventricle. The images show a horseshoe or doughnut appearance reflecting the configuration of the left ventricle (Figure 5–3). On the other hand, if an area of the myocardium is infarcted, there is no uptake in this nonperfused segment, and a void or cold spot is seen on the myocardial images. In other words, myocardial infarction is revealed by a cold

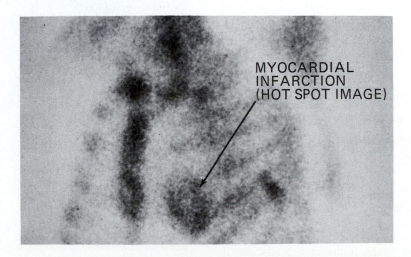

MYOCARDIAL INFARCTION (HOT SPOT IMAGE)

Figure 5–2. Technetium scan showing a large myocardial infarction as a "hot spot" (arrow). A smaller, old infarction is also apparent.

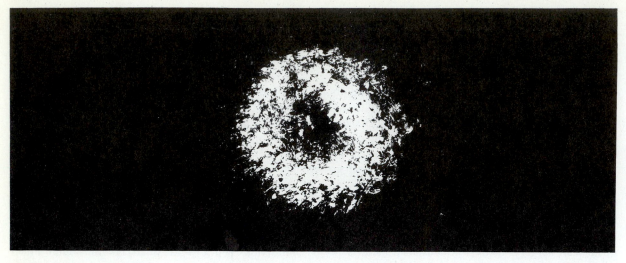

Figure 5–3. Normal thallium scan showing homogenous uptake of radioactive isotope by the left ventricle.

spot with thallium-201 perfusion and by a hot spot with technetium-99m pyrophosphate. The relative accuracy of these two tests is still undetermined, but one drawback of the thallium-201 study is that an area of old infarction will also produce a cold spot, preventing an acute infarction from being distinguished from an old one.

As noted in the Chapter 4, thallium-201 studies are also used to confirm the diagnosis of angina pectoris and unstable angina; in fact, the greatest usefulness of the test is for these latter purposes. Since the thallium-201 study reflects myocardial perfusion, ischemia of the myocardium is manifested by abnormalities in the perfusion pattern of this radionuclide, particularly in the form of transient cold spots. Thallium-201 imaging is especially useful in conjunction with exercise testing designed to induce temporary ischemia. In normal myocardium there is a brisk uptake of thallium-201 after exercise, but the ischemic area shows scant or no uptake. As the ischemia subsides, however, the cold spot gradually assumes a normal appearance because of redistribution of the isotope. A positive thallium-201 exercise test is considered strong evidence for CHD and is probably more reliable than exercise testing alone (as described in Chapter 4).

Cardiac Radiography

The chest radiograph (X-ray) is generally used to evaluate the sizes of the heart chambers and status of the pulmonary system. Both frontal and lateral images are made. The frontal image should be a posterior-to-anterior (PA) view to avoid the magnification of anatomic structures on the X-ray plate. Unfortunately, many patients in the CCU are too sick either at the time of admission to the emergency department or during their stay in the CCU to tolerate standing in front of an X-ray machine. These patients can have portable chest X-rays, which are always taken with the X-ray film behind the patient. This anterior-

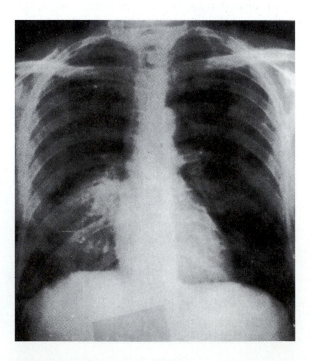

Figure 5–4. Normal chest X-ray with cardiothoracic ratio of less than 50%.

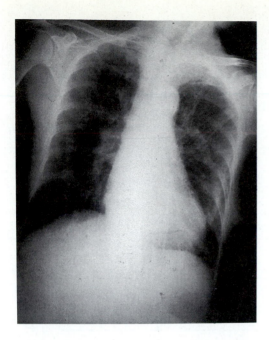

Figure 5–5. Chest X-ray demonstrating pulmonary congestion.

to-posterior (AP) view tends to exaggerate the size of the heart chambers. Nonetheless, the chest AP plate does provide important information about the heart.

In the frontal view, an adult's heart shadow should occupy 50% or less of the maximal width of the thorax (Figure 5–4). This relationship of the width of the heart to the total width of the thorax is called the cardio/thoracic ratio. The ratio becomes larger when the patient has heart failure, valvular lesions, intracardiac shunts, or certain pulmonary diseases. The patient with an enlarged heart is said to have *cardiomegaly.*

The X-ray is also useful for identifying pulmonary congestion (Figure 5–5), which can result from AMI. Pulmonary vascular congestion, which occurs in left heart failure, is seen in the form of increased vascular markings, redistribution of blood flow from the bases to the apices of the lungs, pulmonary edema, septal lines (showing fluid between the lobes of the lungs), and pleural effusions.

THE ACUTE PHASE OF MYOCARDIAL INFARCTION

In general, the clinical course after myocardial infarction can be considered in two phases: the *acute* phase, which usually involves the first few days fol-

lowing the attack, and the *recovery* phase, which concerns the remaining period of hospitalization. During the acute phase patients are treated in a CCU. For a patient with an uncomplicated infarction this may cover only 2 or 3 days, while patients who experience cardiogenic shock may be in the CCU for a much longer period (eg, several weeks).

The most characteristic aspect of the acute phase of myocardial infarction is its uncertainty; there is no typical course. The variation in course is quite remarkable, but three broad patterns can be described.

Some patients' clinical course is truly uncomplicated. They show no evidence of cardiogenic shock, acute left ventricular failure, arrhythmias, or other major problems during the acute phase of the illness. Most of these patients make uneventful recoveries regardless of the type of treatment employed.

Other patients' illness appears benign at the time of admission, but is then suddenly marked by major complications. These complications account for nearly all deaths from myocardial infarction, and it is the unpredictability of these catastrophes that makes infarction such a lethal condition. The concept of intensive coronary care is based on preventing or immediately detecting and treating life-threatening complications of heart disease. The system of intensive coronary care has made its greatest contribution in its ability to prevent sudden, unexpected death in patients, who are in the acute phase of myocardial infarction.

When serious complications already exist at the time of admission, the clinical course is usually hectic and the prognosis becomes extremely poor. For example, if shock exists when the patient is admitted, there is more than a 70% likelihood that the patient will die within the next 48 hours. If acute heart failure is evident on admission, the mortality rate may be as high as 50%. Consequently, the original clinical picture is very important in determining the ultimate course of an infarction, and an uncomplicated picture at the time of admission should not lead to a false sense of security.

That AMI may have such widely divergent courses explains why the death rate may be as high as 90% at one extreme and as low as 0% to 5% at the other. Probably no other disease behaves in this unpredictable fashion.

THE COMPLICATIONS OF ACUTE MYOCARDIAL INFARCTION

Four major complications threaten life after myocardial infarction (see Figure 5–6). The two most common are heart failure and arrhythmias. Both will be

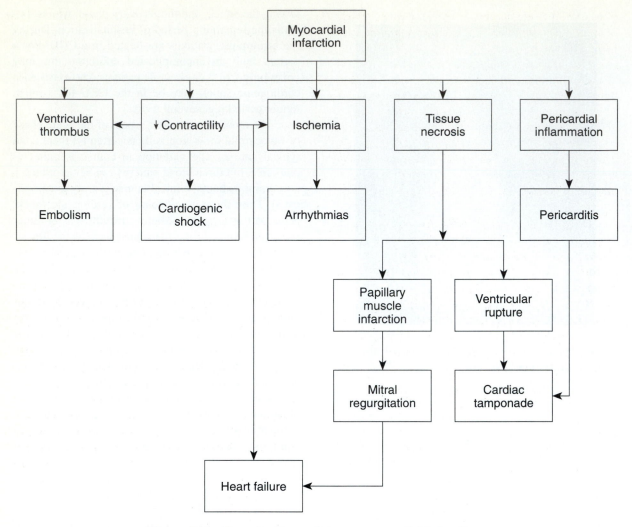

Figure 5–6. Complications of acute myocardial infarction.

discussed only briefly here because they are considered in detail in Chapters 7 and 8. The other two complications are thromboembolism and cardiac tamponade. Although quite rare, each alters the clinical course of infarction in a significant manner, and each is life-threatening. Two of the primary objectives of coronary-care nursing are to prevent the development of these complications whenever possible and to treat them rapidly and effectively when they do occur.

Arrhythmias

Disturbances in the cardiac rate or rhythm (arrhythmias) are the most common complications of AMI. At least 90% of patients with acute infarction develop some form of arrhythmia during the acute phase of the illness. Arrhythmias pose two serious threats: they may reduce the pumping efficiency of the heart, precipitating acute heart failure; and more seriously, they may produce *sudden death*. Although not all dis-

orders of rate and rhythm are life-threatening, the critical fact is that *fatal arrhythmias, particularly ventricular fibrillation, can occur at any time in someone who has had an infarction.*

Conduction blocks are also frequent in AMI. They may result from ischemia or necrosis of conduction tracts in the heart, or from increased vagal tone. The increased vagal activity is the result of stimulation by the inflamed myocardium (affecting the afferent fibers of the vagus nerve), or of stimulation of the autonomic nervous system by pain.

Heart Failure

The contractile ability of the myocardium is inevitably reduced after infarction, often causing the heart to fail as a pumping system. Such failure can occur suddenly, resulting in acute pulmonary edema, or gradually (if the ventricle recovers from the original ischemia but subsequently falters). Clinical signs of heart failure are observed in about 60% of patients with infarction, but the degree of this pumping deficit varies considerably.

Heart failure usually results from a compromise in the contractility of the heart secondary to infarction and myocardial necrosis. However, it may also result from ischemia or infarction of the papillary muscles, which anchor the valve leaflets during systole. If any of these muscles rupture, the valve leaflet becomes incompetent. Blood flows backward into the left atrium during systole, and left ventricular filling pressures rise dramatically, thereby precipitating heart failure.

Heart failure may also result from rupture of the ventricular septum. This is extremely rare but usually occurs when an infarction involves the septum. The outcome is not necessarily immediately fatal, but the prognosis is very poor. In this situation blood from the left ventricle is forced into the right ventricle (because the left ventricle has a higher pressure than the right ventricle) and produces an abrupt overload of the right ventricular and, in turn, severe right heart failure. The patient goes into heart failure because of the high volume of blood forced into the pulmonary capillaries.

The diagnosis of a perforated interventricular septum can often be suspected from the sudden appearance of a loud systolic murmur that was not present previously. This finding, coupled with the abrupt development of right heart failure (from the opening between the left and right ventricles), strongly suggests septal rupture. The diagnosis can be confirmed with pulmonary artery catheterization, which reveals a marked increase in oxygen saturation in the right heart (reflecting the passage of oxygenated blood from the left ventricle into the right ventricle).

The most advanced form of left ventricular pump failure is described as *cardiogenic shock*. It occurs when the heart is unable to sustain the circulation and provide adequate oxygen to the vital organs and tissues. Cardiogenic shock is an extremely serious complication of myocardial infarction, and despite all present forms of treatment for it, has a mortality of greater than 70%. Although cardiogenic shock develops most often during the first 12 hours after the infarction, it can occur several days later.

Thromboembolism

There is a propensity for blood to clot on the inner wall of the injured left ventricle. Poor left ventricular contraction at the site of infarcted tissue leads to blood stasis and turbulence, both of which enhance thrombus formation. It is unusual for a thrombus to occur in an inferior myocardial infarction, but it can be seen during the period of recovery in up to 30% of patients with anterior infarctions, especially those that involve the left ventricular apex or when an aneurysm has formed. The thrombus may break loose and leave the heart (as an embolism) that blocks the arterial blood supply to peripheral organs (eg, the brain or kidneys).

The majority of thrombi, however, arise in the deep veins of the lower extremities (peripheral thrombi). These thrombi develop as a result of the venous stasis of blood and muscular inactivity (related to bed-rest), as well as from certain blood factors that induce abnormal coagulation (hypercoagulability). It is estimated that approximately 40% of all patients with AMI develop clots in their calf veins during the period of hospitalization. However, in only a small percentage of cases do these thrombi produce symptoms or affect the clinical course of myocardial infarction. When a deep-vein thrombus breaks loose it travels to the lung, with potentially devastating results. The incidence of peripheral thrombosis is highest in elderly patients and those with heart failure.

Embolic phenomena, from either the left ventricle or the leg veins, can produce sudden death, but this complication is uncommon and accounts for a relatively small percentage of deaths after infarction. When a peripheral or mural thrombus breaks loose from its site of origin it migrates through the circulatory system as an embolus. Depending on where they ultimately lodge, emboli are classified as pulmonary, cerebral, or peripheral. These three types of embolization are discussed separately.

Pulmonary Embolism. Pulmonary emboli nearly always originate in the deep veins of the legs. A thrombus that is dislodged from one of these veins travels through the inferior vena cava, right atrium, and right ventricle, and finally occludes a branch of the pulmonary artery. There is little chance of mural thrombi causing pulmonary embolism, since such thrombi are confined almost exclusively to the *left* heart and consequently remain in the systemic rather than the pulmonary circulation.

Of the three kinds of thromboembolic complication of infarction, pulmonary embolism is by far the most common. Autopsy studies indicate that pulmonary embolism occurs in about 25% of patients with AMI. These embolic episodes are, however, seldom fatal; the total mortality from pulmonary embolism in patients with acute myocardial infarction is about 1% to 2% at most. With a massive pulmonary embolus (obstructing more than 50% of the main pulmonary artery), hypotension and circulatory collapse develop, and in this circumstance death is usually rapid.

Clinical Manifestations of Pulmonary Embolism.
The clinical response to pulmonary embolism depends

on the size of the embolus and the degree of obstruction it produces in the pulmonary circulation. Most pulmonary emboli are small and do not produce distinct signs or symptoms; indeed, the majority of embolic episodes go unnoticed. A large pulmonary embolus that occludes a major branch of the pulmonary artery usually produces clinically recognizable findings. These typically consist of sudden chest pain, dyspnea, cough (sometimes with hemoptysis), tachycardia, and marked anxiety. The chest pain, often described as crushing or oppressive, may be located substernally or in the right or left side of the chest. The pattern of pain frequently resembles that in AMI, but differs from the latter in that it ordinarily does not radiate to the arms or jaws and is usually increased by inspiration (pleuritic pain). Rapid respiration and tachycardia are observed in nearly all cases of pulmonary embolism soon after its onset. Physical examination of the chest may reveal wheezing or rales, but these findings are inconsistent.

Because pulmonary embolism often resembles AMI, the nurse must consider that recurrent chest pain may be due to a complication of embolism rather than to infarction. Whenever pulmonary embolism is suspected, the nurse should record a 12-lead ECG and prepare the patient for arterial blood-gas studies. Routine inspection of the legs for signs of thrombophlebitis (warmth, tenderness, or swelling) is important, particularly in high-risk patients.

Several diagnostic tests are used to identify pulmonary embolism. X-ray examination of the chest, which is probably the most common method of identifying an embolism, is of minimal diagnostic value immediately after an embolic episode because the characteristic findings of the condition rarely appear at once. A normal chest X-ray offers no assurance that embolization has not occurred. A more reliable diagnostic procedure is the lung scan. Injecting a radioactive isotope intravenously and scanning the lung fields, reveals at an early stage the segment of the lung deprived of oxygen by an embolism. Figure 5–7 shows comparison of a normal lung scan with one demonstrating a large pulmonary embolism. The diagnosis of pulmonary embolism can sometimes be suspected from acute changes in the ECG that indicate a strain on the right heart (which develops from resistance in the pulmonary circulation created by the embolus). Arterial blood-gas determinations may also be useful in establishing the diagnosis. Nearly all patients with large pulmonary emboli exhibit hypoxia.

The onset of pulmonary embolism is by no means constant or predictable; however, its sudden occurrence after straining during defecation or when the patient first gets out of bed after prolonged inactivity is common enough to merit special precautions against its occurrence in these circumstances.

Cerebral Embolism. Cerebral emboli, unlike pulmonary emboli, originate as *mural* thrombi in patients with myocardial infarction. Clots from the injured wall of the left ventricle travel through the aorta

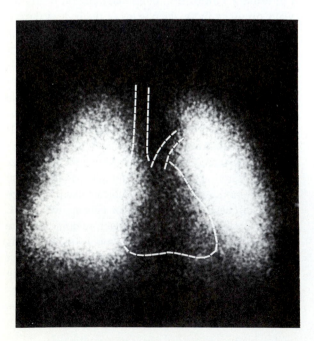 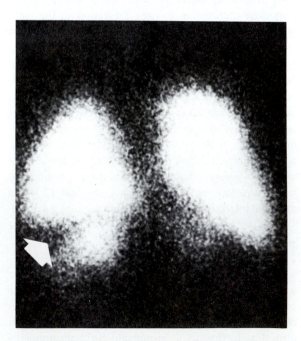

Figure 5–7. Lung scans: **A.** Normal. **B.** Large pulmonary embolism (*arrow*).

and occlude arteries in the brain, producing cerebral infarction. In some instances the embolic episode occurs very soon after acute infarction, making it not uncommon for patients to be admitted to a hospital with typical findings of a stroke when the underlying problem is in fact an AMI. In this situation the effects of the stroke usually dominate the clinical picture and obscure cardiac symptoms. (For this reason it is a wise practice to record an ECG routinely in all patients with sudden cerebrovascular events.)

Clinical Manifestations of Cerebral Embolism.
The most characteristic feature of cerebral embolism is the *sudden* onset of stroke. In contrast to customary (nonembolic) strokes, there are no premonitory warnings, and the neurologic findings appear abruptly. Therefore, if a patient with an AMI suddenly develops signs of a stroke (eg, motor weakness, paralysis, or a speech disturbance), it can be assumed that cerebral embolism has developed as a complication of the infarction.

Diagnostic studies are seldom necessary to confirm the presence of a cerebral embolism, but if uncertainty exists, computerized axial tomography (CAT scan) may be utilized. The combination of an acute myocardial infarction and a stroke is usually overwhelming, particularly in elderly patients.

The clinical course after an embolic stroke depends on the location of the cerebral infarction and the extent of the neurologic deficit it produces. Although death does not generally occur suddenly, the prognosis is extremely poor.

Peripheral Embolism.
Like cerebral emboli, peripheral emboli arise from mural clots that form within the left heart. Although these mural thrombi may lodge anywhere in the systemic arterial system, the most frequent sites of peripheral embolism are the femoral or iliac arteries supplying the lower extremities. The outcome of peripheral embolism depends on the artery involved and whether the embolus can be removed surgically (embolectomy).

Clinical Manifestations of Peripheral Embolism.
Embolic occlusion of the major arteries to the lower extremities produces a distinctive clinical picture. There is a sudden onset of pallor, coldness, and numbness of the involved extremity. Within minutes, the patient develops pain in the leg along with decreased sensation. Physical examination reveals an absence of arterial pulsations in conjunction with a cold, pale extremity. In some instances both extremities are involved simultaneously, indicating that the embolus is at the bifurcation of the aorta. Unless embolectomy can be performed promptly, gangrene develops.

Treatment of Thromboembolism.
Because emboli originate as thrombi, the ideal treatment for all forms of embolism is to prevent thrombus formation. This can often be accomplished by means of anticoagulant therapy. Low-dose subcutaneous heparin is routinely administered to bedridden patients to prevent deep venous thrombosis. Full-dose intravenous heparin is administered: (1) after thrombolytic therapy, to maintain vessel patency; (2) to prevent reinfarction if recurrent unstable angina/ischemia follows AMI; or (3) to prevent thrombus formation when large regions (usually the anterior wall) of the left ventricle have infarcted. If the latter occurs, or if a mural thrombus is viewed by echocardiography, long-term therapy with oral anticoagulants (warfarin) is continued.

A second method of reducing the incidence of thrombus formation is to avoid venous stasis whenever possible. This can be achieved by exercising the extremities, changing the body position frequently, and minimizing the duration of complete bed rest. Elastic stockings may be applied to the legs to prevent venous pooling. If support stockings are used it is important to verify that they remain in proper position and do not produce a tourniquet effect. Placing pillows (or elevating the gatch of the bed) under the knees must be avoided, since this can obstruct venous flow in the extremities. The nurse should caution the patient about straining at defecation, and should provide stool softeners or laxatives if needed.

If the patient is not receiving anticoagulants and develops a thrombus, intravenous heparin is started immediately. In this situation the purpose of anticoagulants is not to prevent embolism but to prevent further clot formation at the site of the original clot, which will reduce the risk of embolism. Also, anticoagulant therapy may inhibit extension of the embolus.

A continuous intravenous drip containing 20,000 units of heparin in 500 mL of dextrose solution is administered at a rate (usually 500 to 750 units per hour) that will achieve and maintain the activated partial thromboplastin time (aPTT) at 2 to 2.5 the normal control value. The aPTT level should be checked at 4 to 6 hours after heparin therapy is begun and once a day thereafter. Intravenous heparin may also be administered intermittently by way of a heparin lock positioned in a peripheral vein. The usual dosage with this method is 5,000 to 10,000 units every 4 to 6 hours, depending on the aPTT. Heparin is continued for 5 to 7 days, after which oral anticoagulating agents are used.

During the course of anticoagulant therapy the nurse must observe the patient carefully for signs of bleeding. Excessive doses of anticoagulant drugs can cause hemorrhage anywhere in the body, but the most common bleeding sites are the skin, kidneys, and gastrointestinal tract. Careful examination of the body surface should be made during routine nursing care to detect evidence of ecchymosis. The urine and stools must be observed on each occasion. Any evidence of bleeding should be reported to the physician promptly. Anticoagulant therapy may have to be discontinued or anticoagulant antagonists (protamine sulfate or vitamin K) administered.

Cardiac Tamponade

Myocardial infarctions often extend to the epicardial surface of the heart and produce inflammation of the overlying pericardium. In most cases the pericardial reaction (pericarditis) is confined to the area over the infarction, but in 10% to 15% of patients, diffuse pericarditis develops within a few days of the infarction, probably from inflammation at the surface of the infarction site caused by the death of myocardial cells. Patients with pericarditis secondary to AMI usually experience chest pain, which is often increased by deep breathing or changes in body position, and fever. The characteristic physical finding in pericarditis is a pericardial friction rub—a grating sound occurring each time the heart beats. A transient friction rub can be detected in nearly 50% of patients with AMI. The pericarditis usually disappears spontaneously within a few days and seldom causes serious problems.

Signs and Symptoms of Pericarditis

1. Pericardial friction rub
2. Fever
3. Pain of inspiration
4. Pain relieved by leaning forward
5. ST-segment elevation in all 12 leads of ECG

When there is extensive damage to the ventricular wall, the necrotic area may weaken, leading to rupture. This catastrophe is life-threatening. When the wall of the ventricle ruptures, blood from the ventricle instantly fills the surrounding pericardial sac and causes compression of the heart (cardiac tamponade). Death usually occurs within minutes.

Rupture of the ventricular wall rupture may occur at any time during hospitalization for myocardial infarction, but the highest incidence is within the first 5 to 7 days. The rupture is nearly always associated with extensive transmural infarction involving myo-

cardial necrosis extending completely through the wall of the heart. Consequently, these patients are not candidates for early discharge. The perforation, which develops suddenly, occurs in the center of the necrotic area (or at the junction of the infarcted area with healthy tissue), apparently from softening and weakening of the muscle fibers. It is more likely to occur in women, in patients over 50 years of age, and in patients who have been hypertensive prior to the onset of their myocardial infarction. Luckily, ventricular rupture is a relatively rare occurrence, causing less than 5% of the total mortality from AMI.

For many years it was believed that physical activity during the early period after infarction was a major factor in causing ventricular rupture. It now appears that this concept is incorrect, since many ruptures occur despite complete bed rest. Moreover, about one-third of cardiac ruptures develop within the first 2 days after hospitalization for infarction. Sustained hypertension and the use of anticoagulant therapy have also been incriminated as possible causes of ventricular rupture, but there is little evidence to substantiate this in either case. Perhaps the most significant factor in the development of ventricular rupture is the size and extent of the infarction and the degree of collateral circulation to the involved area. Curiously, ventricular rupture occurs more often in women than in men, and is the only complication of AMI with a female preponderance; the reason for this is uncertain. The highest incidence of ventricular rupture is in the seventh decade of life.

The extravasation of blood into the closed pericardium that follows rupture of the outer ventricular wall causes cardiac tamponade and prevents ventricular filling. Death usually occurs within minutes. Occasionally the patient may complain of recurrent chest pain just before the event, and a sudden decrease in blood pressure and abrupt slowing of the heart rate accompany the rupture. Clinically the picture is that of an arrhythmic death. Although the mechanical (pumping) action of the heart ceases immediately after cardiac rupture, the heart's electrical activity may persist for many minutes or longer (because electrical impulses continue to be generated even though the ventricles cannot contract). Because of this, electrical activity may be noted on the cardiac monitor during resuscitation attempts even though the patient is dead.

In cases of apparent sudden death, the nurse must make certain that the catastrophe is not in fact due to a treatable and reversible cause, such as ventricular fibrillation or standstill, rather than ventricular rupture. Cardiopulmonary resuscitation should be attempted immediately and continued until it is definitely ascertained that an arrhythmia is not responsible for the fatal event.

OTHER ASPECTS OF THE ACUTE PHASE OF MYOCARDIAL INFARCTION

In addition to major complications, many other problems may develop during the acute phase of myocardial infarction. Some of these problems represent natural responses to tissue damage, whereas others can be considered to be complications.

Fever

Most patients with AMI develop temperature elevations during the acute phase of the illness. Typically, the body temperature rises after the first 24 hours of the attack to 38°C (or more), and remains elevated for 2 to 3 days before gradually declining. By the fifth day the temperature has usually returned to normal. It is thought that this febrile pattern reflects the local death of myocardial tissue. (The white blood cell count and erythrocyte sedimentation rate also increase during this period, for the same reason.) Fever is therefore an anticipated finding and ordinarily does not indicate an infectious process in patients with acute infarction. However, if the fever is prolonged, excessively high, or develops after the first few days, the possibility of pneumonia, thrombophlebitis, or other systemic infection must be considered.

Recurrent Chest Pain

Some patients develop additional episodes of ischemic chest pain during the acute phase of myocardial infarction. This pain may represent angina pectoris or, worse, an extension of the original infarction. (The possibility of the pain being caused by pericarditis must also be considered.) Recurrent ischemic pain generally indicates that the acute process accompanying infarction has not stabilized and that further damage may occur. Serial ECGs and enzyme studies should be done after any significant episode of chest pain. It is also critical that patients have their pain promptly relieved (usually with morphine sulfate).

Emotional Disturbances

Profound emotional reactions are frequent among patients with AMI during the period of intensive coronary care (as discussed in Chapter 2). In the majority of cases these emotional reactions are not related to the severity of the infarction. The basis of such reactions can be readily appreciated: the abrupt interruption of normal life, the fear of death, and the possibility of permanent invalidism are powerful psychological threats. Because numerous factors inherent in the patient's personality influence the response to this stress, the spectrum of reactions is very wide.

Treatment During the Acute Phase

During the past decade, the treatment of AMI has undergone a complete revision. In the early days of intensive coronary care, both medical and nursing care were focused on reducing myocardial oxygen demand. The rationale was that if oxygen demand could be reduced, the heart would be more likely to heal without further complication and without an extension of the infarction. Given this philosophy, all efforts were oriented to reducing physical and emotional exertion. Patients were put on bed-rest and given tranquilizers. The care unit was designed to provide optimal rest and quiet.

Recent developments in revascularization techniques have translated to important changes in patient care in the CCU. Although efforts are still made to reduce myocardial oxygen demand (by asking patients to minimize their physical exertion and giving them beta blockers), treatment is also oriented to increasing myocardial oxygen supply. Whenever possible, drugs are given to dissolve (lyse) the arterial blood clot (thrombus) that causes myocardial necrosis. If such thrombolysis is contraindicated, then revascularization is attempted with percutaneous coronary angioplasty. Given the important role of the CCU nurse in these treatments, they will be discussed in detail in Chapter 6.

THE RECOVERY PHASE OF MYOCARDIAL INFARCTION

The overall incidence of complications declines greatly after the first 2 to 3 days in myocardial infarction, and for this reason patients are usually transferred from the CCU at this time, assuming that their clinical condition is stable. During the recovery phase, while the infarction is healing, the main objective is to observe the clinical course carefully, focusing on the prevention of new complications. At the same time it is important to prepare patients for hospital discharge and the resumption of activities by instructing and counseling them about their illness and starting a planned program of physical rehabilitation.

In general, physical activity is restricted during the recovery from infarction in order to limit the work of the heart as its heals. However, complete bed-rest is contraindicated because of the high risk of complications related to physical deconditioning. It is customary to allow patients to sit in arm chairs and walk to the bathroom and in the hallways (usually with telemetry monitors). The objective of such early ambulation is to prevent the deleterious physiologic and psychologic effects of cardiovascular deconditioning, skeletal muscle wasting, and anxiety or depression. This is accomplished by a program of progressive physical activity starting with low-intensity exercise and gradually building the degree of exercise to a level that will prevent the patient from returning home as an invalid. In many hospitals, staff from the cardiac rehabilitation program evaluate the patient in the CCU (usually on the third day of hospitalization) or immediately upon discharge to the stepdown unit, and prescribe an activity regimen during the patient's stay in the hospital.

The hospital course for patients who develop complications during the acute phase of myocardial infarction varies with the nature of the problem and the response to treatment. Understandably, the basic program of care just described must be adapted according to the clinical picture.

Although the recovery phase of infarction is undoubtedly less hazardous than the acute phase, substantial evidence indicates that the period after transfer from the CCU is by no means without danger. *Indeed, complications, especially sudden death from arrhythmias, may develop at any time during the hospital stay.* For this reason, many hospitals use specially designated coronary progressive units (variously known as telemetry units, intermediate coronary care units, or stepdown units) to ensure careful observation and continued cardiac monitoring for several days after transfer from the CCU in a less intensive but nonetheless prepared setting.

CRITICAL PATH FOR ACUTE MYOCARDIAL INFARCTION

Patients' progress through the acute and recovery stages of myocardial infarction has been standardized in a critical path for Diagnostic Related Grouping (DRG) #122, under the Medicare system, with an anticipated stay of 7 days. The government reimburses hospitals for expenses incurred by all patients on Medicare. Reimbursement is based on the patient's diagnosis and Diagnosis Related Grouping or DRG. Although the path may vary slightly from one hospital to another its general elements are similar. Each element addresses standard diagnostic tests to be performed, diet and activity recommendations, medications, treatments, and educational topics to be discussed. An example is provided in Table 5–2.

The goals of using critical paths are to decrease

fragmentation of care, enhance collaboration among disciplines, provide a database for quality assurance, and decrease patient length of stay (when appropriate). The increase in managed-care contracts in United States hospitals has provided a strong impetus for the development of critical paths and for the role of a case manager who is responsible for overseeing the patient's progress in relation to a particular critical path.

HOSPITAL DISCHARGE

The usual duration of hospitalization for most patients with AMI is about 7 to 10 days, including the period in the CCU. However, with continuing pressure on practitioners to reduce hospital stays because of health-care reform, periods of hospitalization are continuing to decrease. In the Minnesota Heart Survey, a comparison was made between the lengths of hospitalization for more than 3,000 patients who experienced AMIs between 1985 and 1990. In 1985 male patients were discharged after an average length-of-stay of 9.8 days and female patients after 10.4 days. In 1990 that average had dropped to 8.0 and 9.0, respectively. The difference in average duration of stay by sex is undoubtedly related to the generally older and sicker status of female patients with AMI as compared with their male counterparts.

Patients who experience no significant complications of infarction are sometimes discharged even earlier than the 7- to 10-day average. In one large clinical trial, patients with uncomplicated acute infarctions were randomly assigned to an early-discharge group (discharged after 3 days) or to customary care. No significant differences were found in the two groups' morbidity or mortality, suggesting that early discharge of selected patients is safe and not associated with a higher subsequent mortality.

In keeping with the trend toward early mobilization, of patients with myocardial infarction, many physicians now request that a patient perform a *low-level treadmill exercise test* before hospital discharge. Unlike the maximal (or submaximal) stress test used for the diagnosis of angina pectoris, the exercise level in this test is of low intensity and designed to increase the heart rate only moderately. The primary purpose of the procedure is to assess the patient's clinical and ECG response to exercise as a means of determining the type and amount of activity that the patient can safely tolerate at home and subsequently at work. In addition, exercise testing soon after AMI provides prognostic information about the future course of the patient's illness. The risk of angina pectoris, recurrent myocardial infarction, and sudden death occurring in the first year or two after infarction may be predicted from the results of low-level exercise testing.

Myocardial perfusion imaging performed in conjection with exercise testing has been shown to be more accurate than exercise testing alone in distinguishing high- and low-risk survivors of uncomplicated infarction. In such imaging thallium-201 is injected prior to the exercise test. Following exercise, the degree of redistribution of the thallium within the zone of infarction, and the ratio of heart/lung uptake of thallium, are measured by scintigraphy.

Predischarge exercise testing is reserved for patients whose hospital course is uncomplicated; it is not performed in those with arrhythmias, heart failure, or angina. Nevertheless, the procedure is not without potential risk, and always carries the possibility of provoking serious myocardial ischemia or dangerous arrhythmias.

DISCHARGE TEACHING

The topics that need to be covered prior to a patient's discharge are summarized in Table 5–3. It is important that patients and their families have all their questions answered before discharge, and that they feel a sense of partnership with the nurses and physicians caring for them. A partnership philosophy is an important aspect of achieving patient compliance with treatment protocols.

Patients who have had an infarction must reduce any and all cardiac risk factors (eg, smoking, hypertension, or hypercholesterolemia). Much of patient and family education is oriented to achieving compliance in reducing these risk factors. Written educational materials prepared by the American Heart Association or other associations can be useful adjuncts to verbal instruction of the patient and family. Interactive video programs and videotapes (used while the patient is still hospitalized) also serve to reinforce this important aspect of discharge teaching.

Patients and their families should be taught what to do in case cardiac symptoms occur after they return home. They should be instructed about those symptoms that indicate a possible AMI and who to call in an emergency. Research shows that the median delay time between the onset of symptoms of acute infarction and arrival at a hospital is 4 hours. Surprisingly, patients who have already experienced an AMI also show a median delay of 4 hours. Previous experience does not reduce the time to hospitalization. Patients need to be taught the value of coming to the hospital early in the case of possible infarction (so that thrombolysis can be given, thereby saving heart muscle). They need to be told to take three nitroglyc-

erin tablets sublingually over a 10 minute period (3 minutes apart) upon experiencing pain, and to then call 911 or their seven-digit emergency access code if the pain does not abate. Nitroglycerin tablets must be kept in a cool, dark place if they are to retain their potency. *Patients should be instructed to not call their physician if they experience the symptoms of AMI.* In all research done to date, calling one's physician prolongs the time to treatment.

Patients and their families should review the patient's activity instructions. Patients with uncomplicated AMIs can begin a walking program (5 minutes twice a day, on a flat surface) as soon as they return home. Discussion about activity should also include information about returning to sexual activity and to work. In the case of an uncomplicated myocardial infarction, patients can resume sexual activity within 2 to 3 weeks of their discharge from the hospital.

Standard therapy for all infarct patients being discharged from the hospital without specific contraindications includes low-dose aspirin (to reduce the incidence of reinfarction) and beta-blocker therapy (to reduce mortality). Patients need to understand the rationale for these drugs and learn how to monitor their side effects. They must also review any other medications that they will be taking at home, and clearly understand the purpose and action of each one, as well as all untoward side effects. Many CCUs use individual "drug sheets" that provide this information in a one-page description.

CONVALESCENCE AFTER ACUTE MYOCARDIAL INFARCTION

After discharge from the hospital, it is customary for patients who have had a myocardial infarction to remain at home on a limited activity program until the infarction has healed. As a general rule, necrotic areas of the myocardium heal within 6 weeks after infarction. Thus, if a patient were hospitalized for 1 week, the period of convalescence at home would be an additional 5 weeks. The duration of convalescence depends on several factors, the most important of which are the functional capacity of the heart and the patient's age.

Physical activity is increased gradually during the convalescent phase of infarction. Patients who are enrolled in an outpatient cardiac rehabilitation program are interviewed by one or more of the program personnel and given an exercise prescription to follow at home until they begin their thrice-weekly visits to the program. The exercise prescription is based on the patient's discharge exercise stress test and medical history. It usually involves increasing levels

TABLE 5–2. CRITICAL PATHWAY FOR ACUTE MYOCARDIAL INFARCTION

Level of Care	Day 1 (CCU)	Day 2 (CCU)	Day 3 (CCU)	Day 4 (PCU)	Day 5 (PCU)	Day 6 (PCU)	Goals/Outcomes
Diagnostic Tests	ECG CK total stat and q. 8 h. ¥2 CK-MB CBC Chemistry panel PTT Urinalysis Chest X-ray	ECG PTT if on heparin Cardiac enzymes	ECG PTT if on heparin Cardiac enzymes as ordered	PTT if on heparin PTT if on oral anticoagulants	PT if on oral anticoagulants Treadmill as ordered Cardiac catheterization as ordered	Discharge home Exercise stress test	1. Ischemic ECG changes will be resolved. 2. Laboratory values will remain within normal limits.
Fluids/intake and output	Heparin lock/IV access intake and output	Heparin lock intake and output	Heparin lock intake and	Heparin lock		Discharge home	Patient will maintain a normal fluid balance
Treatments	Continuous oxygen VS per protocol Cardiac monitor in lead of suspected infarct	Continue oxygen VS per protocol Cardiac monitor Echocardiogram	Oxygen PRN VS per protocol Cardiac monitor → telemetry	O₂ PRN VS per protocol → Telemetry	Same as day 4	Discharge home	Patient will have a positive response to treatment as by: Vital signs within normal limits Control of cardiac arrhythmias
Medications	Beta blocker ASA Antiarrhythmic Heparin IV Nitrates	Same as day 1	Reassess medication needs Oral anticoagulants Reevaluate IV heparin order	Reassess medication needs Oral anticoagulants as ordered Reevaluate IV heparin order	Reassess medication needs Oral anticoagulant as ordered Discontinue heparin as ordered	Discharge home	1. Adequate cardiac peformance will be maintained with absence of arrhythmias, ischemia 2. Patient's anxiety will be controlled 3. Patient's comfort level will be maintained
	PRN: Pain meds Antiemetic Sedative Stool softener						

	Day 1	Day 2	Day 3	Day 4	Day 5	Discharge	Outcomes
Diet	Low fat, low cholesterol 3 g sodium	Same as day 1 Diet teaching	Same as day 1 Reinforce dietary instructions	Same as day 1	Same as day 1	Discharge home	Patient's nutritional needs will be met with restriction of fat/cholesterol/sodium
Activity	Bedrest except to commode	Up in chair as tolerated	Ambulate as tolerated	Ambulate as tolerated	Ambulate as tolerated	Discharge home	Patient will return to pre-hospital level of activity
Education/discharge planning	Explain procedures/treatment plan to patient and family Inform patient to report sex immediately Teach bleeding precautions if on heparin Instruct patient on action/rationale for medications	Assess knowledge of disease process Identify patient risk factors Begin teaching	Continue/reinforce teaching Identify lifestyle changes with written instructions	Review/reinforce day 3 Identify discharge Medications with written instructions	Continue review/reinforcement	Discharge with written information about heart disease Written instructions for follow-up care Written instructions for cardiac symptoms	1. Patient/family understands disease process and rationale for treatment pain 2. Patient is able to identify cardiac risk factors and appropriate interventions 3. Patient/family understand discharge instructions including diet/exercise instructions
Consults	Cardiologist	Cardiologist Dietary	Cardiologist Cardiac rehabilitation	Cardiologist	Cardiologist	Instruct on when to see cardiologist	

TABLE 5–3. SUGGESTED TOPICS FOR PATIENT AND FAMILY EDUCATION AND COUNSELING FOLLOWING ACUTE MYOCARDIAL INFARCTION

General Counseling

Explanation of coronary atherosclerotic heart disease and acute myocardial infarction

Cardiac risk factors

Symptoms of angina and acute myocardial infarction

What to do if symptoms occur

Explanation of treatment plan

Clarification of patient's responsibilities

Role of family members in treatment plan

Importance of cessation of tobacco use

Availability and value of qualified local support group and/or outpatient cardiac rehabilitation program

Prognosis

Life expectancy

Advice for family members in the event of a cardiac emergency

Activity Recommendations

Recreation, leisure, and return to work

Exercise

Sexual activity

Dietary Recommendations

Low cholesterol

Low sodium

Medications

Review of all medication actions

Potential side effects and what to do if they occur

Dosing

Coping mechanisms for complicated medical regimens

Availability of lower cost medications or financial assistance

Importance of Compliance with Cardiac Risk Factor Reduction and Treatment Plan

of walking. Walking is considered to be one of the most sensible and effective forms of exercise and should be encouraged in all patients, with the distance (and then the pace) being increased daily. In addition to its helpful effect on the heart and circulation, physical activity at this stage of the illness is of great value in combating the weakness and fatigue that are so common after myocardial infarction. These symptoms, resulting mostly from disuse of the skeletal muscles during the period of hospitalization, are usually alleviated soon after a regular walking program is instituted.

Although excessive rest during the convalescent period immediately following discharge is unnecessary, stair-climbing or heavy household chores should be minimized (unless the patient has already progressed to this stage with an early ambulation program, or predischarge exercise testing indicates that these activities can be tolerated safely). Toward the end of the healing phase, a deliberate program of progressive, monitored physical activity is often prescribed in an outpatient cardiac rehabilitation program.

Most patients, especially those without serious complications of infarction, are able to resume their customary lives and return to work about 2 months after the attack. Clearly, this schedule must be flexible and adjusted according to the patient's age, general health, and cardiac status. It has become increasingly clear that the resumption of normal activity is highly desirable after an infarction, and every effort should be made to meet this objective. There is no reason to believe that deliberate inactivity or retirement from work after a myocardial infarction is conducive to longevity; in fact, the evidence is strictly to the contrary.

The resumption of a normal, useful life after a heart attack depends not only on physical but also on emotional recovery. Approximately 25% of patients, despite an excellent physical recovery, develop profound psychological reactions to their illness. They remain depressed and incapable of returning to their former life style. Emotionally induced cardiac invalidism produces no less functional impairment than true physical invalidism. The clinical features of this distressing problem are inability to tolerate physical activity, weakness and fatigue (which are often overwhelming), and an intense awareness of and concern about any discomfort or pain.

Patients who have had an AMI must understand the serious implications of this diagnosis. They must be provided with accurate information so that they can make decisions about the changes in their lives that such a diagnosis requires. At the same time, it is important that they maintain hope for a high quality life in the future. Psychological factors may be more important to a patient's quality of life and social functioning than any degree of physiologic impairment. The teaching and counseling given by nurses in the ICU provide the groundwork for the patient's future psychological adjustment.

PROGNOSIS IN ACUTE MYOCARDIAL INFARCTION

The outcome of AMI during the period of hospitalization depends on several factors, including the size and location of the infarction, the extent of CAD, and the occurrence of complications. However, the key determinant of the outcome is the pumping ability (ventricular function) of the heart after the attack. If ventricular function is not significantly affected and there are no signs of left ventricular failure, the prognosis is usually very good, whereas if ventricular function is reduced substantially, the outcome is generally poor. The relationship between the left ventricular ejection fraction and level of mortality in myocardial infarction is an inverse one. Patients with normal ejection fractions have an annual mortality rate of 2% to 5%, while patients with low ejection fractions (below 20% of normal) and symptoms at rest have an annual mortality rate exceeding 50%. Patients who have symptoms during moderate activity have an annual mortality of 20% to 40%.

Among all patients who suffer an AMI and are discharged from the hospital, 10% will die within one year after the infarction. After the first year the mortality decreases substantially to about 5% annually. It must be emphasized that these are average mortality rates and therefore do not define the prognosis for an individual patient. Indeed, some patients survive for 15 to 20 years or more, especially those who are young and those with normal ventricular function.

Chapter 6

Medical and Surgical Treatment of Acute Myocardial Infarction

The treatment of coronary atherosclerotic heart disease has undergone a dramatic evolution over the past three decades. The development of coronary ICUs and of cardiac nursing as a specialty were fundamental to that evolution and are briefly reviewed here.

THE DEVELOPMENT OF INTENSIVE CORONARY CARE

The concept of intensive coronary care originated in 1962 when two parallel avenues of research converged. One of these avenues concerned the manner and mechanisms by which AMI causes death; the other involved new techniques of cardiac resuscitation.

It had been known for many years that death from AMI always came from complications of the attack, rather than from the occlusion of a coronary artery itself. However, the relative frequency with which the complications of AMI caused death was uncertain. In 1961 Meltzer and Kitchell answered this question by studying the mechanisms of death in 171 patients who died of AMI. On the basis of their investigation they concluded that death was attributable to the following causes:

Arrhythmias	47%
Left ventricular failure	28%
Cardiogenic shock	15%
Emboli	8%
Rupture of ventricle	2%

These findings were extremely important in pointing a way toward improving the survival rate after acute infarction. It was evident that rupture of the ventricle and embolism, the two complications that rarely can be treated successfully, were uncommon causes of death, producing only 2% and 8%, respectively of total mortality. Left ventricular failure and cardiogenic shock, representing failure of the heart to pump effectively, collectively produced 43% of deaths. *By far the most important observation was the unusually high percentage (47%) of deaths from arrhythmias.* Although sudden and unanticipated deaths resulting from electrical disturbances in the heart were not uncommon, their true incidence had previously been grossly underestimated. (Indeed, before this study, the impression existed that arrhythmic deaths were relatively uncommon.) That nearly half of all deaths from AMI resulted from arrhythmias became the cornerstone for the concept of intensive coronary care, since it was known that arrhythmic deaths were preventable.

In fact, it had been known for more than 50 years that ventricular fibrillation, the arrhythmia responsible for at least 90% of all sudden cardiac deaths, could be terminated and the life of the patient saved if a powerful electric shock was delivered to the heart immediately after the onset of the arrhythmia. At first it was believed that the electrodes used to deliver the shock had to be applied directly to the surface of the ventricles. Because this procedure required the chest to be opened (thoracotomy) in order to expose the heart, application of this life-saving measure was confined primarily to the prepared setting of operating rooms. For this reason the technique of open-chest cardiac resuscitation never became a practical method for preventing death from AMI.

In 1956 this particular problem was solved when Dr. Paul Zoll and his colleagues demonstrated that ventricular fibrillation could be terminated by means of an electric shock delivered externally through the intact chest wall, thus eliminating the need for thoracotomy. However, even this major medical advance had limited practical application until the development of the concept of coronary care, because of the extraordinarily short interval between the onset of ventricular fibrillation and irreversible death. *Usually only 1 to 2 minutes are available to stop ventricular fibrillation and restore an effective heartbeat.*

The chance of effecting such defibrillation within this very brief period is remote under ordinary circumstances. Specifically, successful defibrillation in the era before coronary care required that a physician be in attendance when the lethal arrhythmia began, and that an ECG machine (to identify the arrhythmia) and a defibrillator be brought to the bedside and an electric shock be delivered to the heart, *all within two minutes or less!* From the results of the 1961 study by Meltzer and Kitchell, in which nearly half of all deaths from AMI were due to arrhythmias, it is clearly apparent that these fortuitous circumstances rarely prevailed, even though hospitals had highly trained personnel and the necessary equipment to perform defibrillation.

Results of resuscitation from ventricular asystole—the second of the arrhythmias that cause sudden death—were equally poor. There was good evidence that if cardiac asystole occurred the normal rhythm of the heart could be reactivated under certain conditions by rhythmic electrical stimuli delivered to the myocardium from a device called a pacemaker. Again, however, although pacing techniques had been known for more than a dozen years, very few lives were ever saved with this ingenious method because of the same time limitation as in ventricular fibrillation; restoration of the heartbeat after ventricular asystole can be accomplished only if pacing is begun within seconds after the onset of the arrhythmia.

Thus, as late as 1960, and despite the availability of methods and equipment to prevent arrhythmic deaths, little headway had actually been made in decreasing mortality from AMI. The fault was readily apparent: insufficient time to permit corrective action to be taken once a lethal arrhythmia developed. Attacking this critical problem, Kouwenhoven and co-workers, at the Johns Hopkins Hospital in Baltimore, in 1960 devised a simple procedure to sustain the circulation until defibrillation or cardiac pacing could be performed. This procedure, now known as cardiopul-

monary resuscitation (CPR), involves rhythmic compression of the lower sternum (to compress the heart) and mouth-to-mouth ventilation (to supply oxygen). With this technique the circulation can be adequately supported for many minutes (or longer), thus providing additional time to terminate an arrhythmia. Although CPR was instrumental in saving the lives of many patients who would have died otherwise, its failure to reduce substantially the total number of arrhythmic deaths soon became evident. This was because most patients who died of lethal arrhythmias were unattended at the moment of the catastrophe, and death was already irreversible by the time the event was recognized.

Finally, in 1962, Day, at Bethany Hospital in Kansas City, Kansas, and Meltzer and Kitchell, at the Presbyterian-University of Pennsylvania Medical Center in Philadelphia, independently conceived a plan by which sudden arrhythmic deaths among patients hospitalized with AMI might be prevented in nearly all instances. All three investigators reasoned that if patients were kept under constant surveillance in a special unit in which their cardiac rhythm could be observed continuously and resuscitative equipment was always ready for immediate use, it would be possible to detect and terminate lethal arrhythmias the instant they occurred. In this way, sudden, unexpected deaths from arrhythmia could be avoided. *It was calculated that if this scheme were successful, the in-hospital mortality rate from AMI might be reduced by nearly 50%.*

The development of monitoring equipment that permitted constant viewing of the cardiac rate and rhythm brought the plan closer to reality. One last step had to be accomplished before intensive coronary care could be implemented: the training of personnel to assess the patient's clinical course, identify and interpret arrhythmias, and above all, to act alone if necessary in terminating lethal arrhythmias. But who would assume this demanding role? At that time it seemed that only physicians could possibly undertake the responsibility, but then research studies at the Presbyterian-University of Pennsylvania Medical Center revealed that specially educated nurses were fully capable of serving in this critical position. It was with this background that the original system of intensive coronary care was finally designed and tested.

Coronary care has come a long way since those early days of converted patient wards and rudimentary monitors. The CCU is credited for reducing the mortality rate from in-hospital AMI from 30% to 15%. The success or failure of in-hospital treatment for acute infarction (as well as for other manifestations of CAD) continues to depend on the skill and knowledge of nurses working in the field of coronary intensive care. Both the medical and surgical treatment of AMI will be reviewed in the following sections, with special emphasis on the responsibility of nurses in the provision of such treatment.

PHARMACOLOGIC TREATMENT OF ACUTE MYOCARDIAL INFARCTION

Several important advances in the medical treatment of symptomatic CAD and AMI have brought hope that drug treatment may in one way or other inhibit serious complications of CAD and promote the long-term survival of those it affects. Treatment goals for the patient with acute infarction have always been to alleviate pain and anxiety, to preserve as much myocardium as possible, and to prevent and treat complications. The most effective way to accomplish these goals is with thrombolytic therapy.

Thrombolysis

Prior to the availability of thrombolytic agents, the management of AMI was largely passive and reactive. Physicians and nurses watched and responded to complications as they occurred. There was no way to prevent myocardial damage. Clinical goals were limited to preventing or reducing serious complications. If a fatal arrhythmia did not occur, a delay in therapy in the prethrombolytic era was generally not serious. This situation has now changed. If a patient receives care soon enough, thrombolytic therapy can alter the course of AMI, limit the extent of damage and subsequent morbidity from the condition.

The modern era of thrombolytic therapy began in 1980, when DeWood and colleagues reported that occlusive coronary artery thrombi are present within 1 hour of the onset of symptoms in 90% of all patients with acute infarctions. The coagulation cascade is susceptible to intervention, and researchers began to study the biochemical events that lead to intravascular thrombosis. In the United States, three thrombolytic agents have been developed and are currently available for lysing (dissolving) thrombi: streptokinase, tissue plasminogen activator (Alteplase, also known as TPA or rt-PA), and anisoylated plasminogen-streptokinase activator complex (APSAC), which has a sustained action and similar structure and function to those of streptokinase. All three drugs work by lysing occlusive intracoronary thrombi, as well as by reducing blood viscosity (which results in better distal coronary perfusion).

Since the mid-1980s, several large-scale studies have shown that thrombolytic therapy can significantly reduce mortality from AMI. Studies with more than 10,000 patients have shown that thrombolytic therapy delivered within 6 hours of the onset of symptoms significantly affects infarct size, ejection fraction, and mortality. The benefits of thrombolytic therapy are directly related to the interval between the onset of symptoms and the administration of the thrombolytic agent. The shorter the interval, the better the outcome. When administered within 3 hours of the onset of symptoms, thrombolytic therapy reduces mortality by 23%. Mortality can be reduced by approximately 50% if thrombolytic therapy is begun within 1 hour of the onset of symptoms. After 12 hours, there is no effect. Similarly, the shorter the interval between symptom onset and treatment with a thrombolytic agent, the greater the resulting cardiac function. Because cardiac function is the best predictor of subsequent mortality and is also a good indicator of morbidity, early treatment (particularly within 60 minutes of the onset of symptoms) with a thrombolytic agent can dramatically reduce mortality and morbidity.

For the past 10 years controversy has raged over which thrombolytic agent is most effective. This debate is important from the standpoints of both patient welfare (i.e., which drug provides the best therapeutic outcome) and cost. The cost of rt-PA is approximately $2,400 per dose, while that of streptokinase is $320. In the Global Utilization of Streptokinase and t-PA for Occluded Coronary Arteries (GUSTO) trial, more than 40,000 patients with myocardial infarctions were randomly assigned to receive alteplase, streptokinase, or combination therapy with alteplase and streptokinase. Patients had to have arrived at the hospital within 6 hours of symptom onset and to have had a documented myocardial infarction (the diagnosis was later confirmed in 97% of enrolled patients). All patients also received aspirin at a dosage of 160 to 325 mg daily and a beta-blocking agent (atenolol), if no contraindications to these drugs were present.

Accelerating the dosage regimen for alteplase (by giving it over 90 minutes rather than 3 hours) produced the best outcomes. Mortality (at both 24 hours and 30 days after admission) was significantly better in the alteplase group. At 30 days there was a 14% risk reduction for the alteplase-treated patients (which translates into one life saved per 100 patients). This decrease in mortality was accompanied by a slight increase in the incidence of stroke (1.55% for the alteplase group versus 1.40% for the streptokinase and intravenous heparin groups). However, the administration of alteplase after 4 hours resulted in no significant reduction in mortality.

Given the overwhelming benefit of thrombolytic therapy, it is somewhat dismaying to discover that less than 35% of all eligible patients receive it. The primary reason for patients not receiving thrombolytic therapy is delay in coming to the hospital. The average patient delay exceeds 4 hours in most studies, and approximately one-third of all patients with acute infarctions delay coming to the hospital by more than 12 hours. Nurses working in the CCU need to exert particular effort to educate patients and their families about the need to respond to symptoms of possible infarction (as discussed in the last chapter) and underscore the potential benefit that would accrue from coming to the hospital as soon as possible.

Protocol for Thrombolytic Therapy.
Patients with acute myocardial infarction should be evaluated immediately for thrombolytic therapy, since time is critical to the benefit of such therapy. Absolute and relative contraindications to thrombolytic therapy are summarized in Table 6–1. The effectiveness of thrombolytic therapy in the elderly has been somewhat contradictory from one study to another. Many protocols have excluded patients over the age of 70 years from such therapy, but this policy is being evaluated in ongoing trials. In general, patients under the age of 75 years seem to benefit from thrombolytic therapy, but this positive result is lost when the delay to therapy exceeds 4 hours.

The following is a protocol for thrombolytic therapy with rt-PA:

1. In preparation for thrombolytic therapy, the nurse should start three intravenous infusions; two should involve large-bore catheters (14 or 16 gauge). One line is for the thrombolytic agent, another for heparin, and the third for maintenance fluids and other medications.
2. The standard dose of rt-PA is 100 mg in 100 mL sterile water. The first 15 mg is given as an IV bolus dose over a period of 3 minutes.
3. The remaining 85 mg are administered by infusion pump at a rate of 0.75 mg/kg over a period of 30 minutes (with the total dose not to exceed 50 mg), and at a rate of 0.5 mg/kg over a period of 60 minutes (with the total dose not to exceed 35 mg). The total rt-PA dose will equal 100 mg.
4. Fifty minutes after the start of the rt-PA infusion, the nurse should give a bolus of 5,000 units of heparin followed by a continuous intravenous heparin drip given at a dose that will produce an APTT of 60 to 85 seconds (usually 12,500 units of heparin in 250 mL of

TABLE 6–1. ASSESSMENT OF PATIENTS FOR THROMBOLYTIC THERAPY

Absolute Contraindications
Active internal bleeding
Known history of cerebrovascular accident
Severe, uncontrolled hypertension (>200/120 mm Hg)
Intracranial or intraspinal surgery or trauma within the past 2 months
Known coagulation disorder
Brain tumor, arteriovenous malformation, or aneurysm

Relative Contraindications
Cerebrovascular disease
Hypertension (>180/110 mm Hg)
High likelihood of left heart thrombus (eg, mitral stenosis with atrial fibrillation)
Acute pericarditis
Severe renal or hepatic disease
Pregnancy
Diabetic hemorrhagic retinopathy
Current anticoagulant therapy, such as with warfarin
Major surgery within the past 10 days
Gastrointestinal or genitourinary bleeding
History of prolonged or traumatic cardiopulmonary resuscitation.

5% dextrose in water [D_5W] at an infusion rate of 1,000 units/hour).
5. Serial coagulation times (PTT and activated clotting time) should be measured every 6 hours following the heparin bolus.
6. The heparin infusion is continued for 48 hours, and is usually tapered slowly, on the belief that its abrupt discontinuation may increase reocclusion (a belief that needs to be tested in a clinical trial).
7. Because rt-PA has a relatively short (3–7 minutes) half-life, a full dose can be readministered 6 hours after the completion of treatment if reocclusion occurs. Adjusted doses can be readministered sooner than this.

Streptokinase is used by many nurses and physicians for thrombolysis. Although it is not clot specific (as is rt-PA), numerous randomized clinical trials have found no difference in the outcomes of patients treated with streptokinase and rt-PA. The protocol for administering streptokinase is straightforward. A dose of 1.5 million units diluted in 100 mL D_5W is given over a period of 1 hour. The drug can be readministered for 5 days following the initial treatment, but should not then be readministered for 6 months.

Long-term anticoagulation following the administration of both rt-PA and streptokinase is usually managed with aspirin or oral anticoagulants (warfarin). In one study of patients treated with thrombolytic agents, secondary prevention proved better with warfarin than with aspirin in terms of the combined incidence of unstable angina, emergency bypass surgery, and death. However, the benefits of warfarin are partly offset by a higher incidence of hemorrhagic complications.

Patient Assessment. Careful patient assessment during thrombolytic therapy is critical. Pain and vital signs should be monitored every 15 minutes, with *total pain relief* always being the nurse's goal of treatment. Neurologic observations should be made to detect early signs of intracranial hemorrhage. Stools should be tested for occult blood.

Reperfusion arrhythmias may occur in patients undergoing thrombolytic therapy, but usually do not require treatment. They are caused by the gathering of metabolic wastes, oxygen-free radicals, and potassium in nonperfused areas of the myocardium. With reperfusion these substances are "washed out," and the myocardium may show some irritability. This usually resolves without treatment, but ventricular tachycardia and sinus bradycardia have been documented in some cases, and must be quickly diagnosed and treated.

Clinical signs of reperfusion

> Relief of chest pain
> Reperfusion dysrhythmias: accelerated idioventricular rhythm, ventricular ectopy, bradycardia
> Reduction of ST-segment elevation
> Cardiac isoenzyme levels (CK-MB) peak in less than 12 hours

The majority of reocclusions occur within the first few days after thrombolytic therapy, while the patient is in the CCU. A correlation between inadequate anticoagulation and reinfarction has been clearly demonstrated. The nurses and physicians following the patient must therefore keep informed of APTT results. Blood specimens for baseline APTT testing should be drawn every 12 hours while the patient is receiving a heparin drip. If any changes are made in the heparin drip, a new specimen for APTT testing should be drawn 2 to 3 hours later.

Careful monitoring of the patient who has had thrombolytic therapy requires serial ECGs and cardiac enzyme studies. ECGs should be monitored at baseline, the beginning of thrombolysis, completion of thrombolysis, every 8 hours for 24 hours, and then daily. Cardiac enzymes (CK and CK-MB) should be assayed at the time of admission, and then every hour for 3 hours, every 6 hours for 24 hours, and every morning for 2 days. Successful reperfusion is seen with normalization of the ST segment and the development of Q-waves on the ECG. CK-MB reaches peak values within 1 to 4 hours of reperfusion.

Angioplasty. In the early days of thrombolysis, patients with AMI underwent a cardiac catheterization and percutaneous transluminal coronary angioplasty prior to hospital discharge. The Thrombolysis in Myocardial Infarction (TIMI) trial compared patients who had these procedures to those who did not, and found no difference in mortality, reinfarction, or ventricular function. Other studies confirmed these findings, and the current treatment philosophy is to limit coronary angiography and angioplasty after thrombolytic therapy to patients who have spontaneous ischemia.

Nitrates

Nitrates reduce myocardial wall stress and oxygen demand by reducing the volume of blood that returns to the heart (preload) and reducing the resistance the heart experiences in ejecting blood (afterload). Additionally, nitrates increase collateral blood flow to ischemic myocardium. In several trials of patients with acute myocardial infarction, those treated with intravenous nitroglycerin had significant reductions in infarct size compared to controls. Although individual trials have had somewhat conflicting results about the benefits of nitrates to specific subgroups (patients with anterior and inferior myocardial infarctions, Q-wave infarctions, and non-Q-wave infarctions), pooled data from several trials support a significant reduction in mortality with the use of these drugs. However, early treatment is more effective than late treatment. Nitrates are clearly of benefit in AMI complicated by heart failure (see Chapter 7).

Narcotics

Pain causes a sympathetic response that dramatically increases myocardial oxygen demand. It is critical that patients with AMI have their pain relieved completely. Nitrates are helpful in this regard since they reduce oxygen demand and increase collateral blood flow to the heart. However, they are rarely adequate in eradicating the pain of infarction. Control of pain usually is accomplished with morphine sulfate, although meperidine is also used. Patients with severe pain may require large and frequently repeated doses of morphine (given by intravenous "push") for adequate analgesia. Either morphine or meperidine can be associated with vagal side effects, and atropine may have to be given to counter these effects.

Beta Blockers

Beta blockers are one class of drugs designed to interfere with the sympathetic nervous system (they can also be called *antiadrenergic drugs*). Beta-adrenergic receptors are found in heart muscle and the smooth muscle of the vascular system (both arteries and veins) and bronchial tree. Drugs that stimulate the beta receptors increase contractility and heart rate, dilate systemic blood vessels, and dilate the bronchioles. Drugs that block the beta receptors (called beta-adrenergic antagonists) have opposite effects.

The beta receptors comprise several subgroups: beta-1 receptors are found in the heart, while beta-2 receptors are found in the bronchioles and to a lesser degree in the arterioles. Drugs have been developed that have selective affinities for beta-1 and beta-2 receptors. The goal of beta-1-selective drugs (eg, esmolol, atenolol, betaxolol, and metoprolol) is to block myocardial receptors while having less of an effect on bronchial and vascular smooth muscle (ie, causing less bronchospasm and vasoconstriction, both of which are adverse effects in patients with CAD). Other beta-blocking agents, including propranolol, nadolol, timolol, and labetalol, are nonselective.

The use of beta-blocking agents in patients who had experienced a myocardial infarction was the beginning of treatment aimed at preventing anginal attacks rather than relieving them (with sublingual nitroglycerin), and of reducing infarct size rather than treating its sequelae. By blocking the effects of the sympathetic nervous system on the heart, beta-blockers reduce heart rate and contractility, thus diminishing the work of the heart and its oxygen demands. The decrease in heart rate also results in a prolongation of diastole, which improves the perfusion of ischemic myocardium (since coronary artery filling occurs during diastole). Beta blockers also appear to increase the threshold for ventricular fibrillation (a common cause of death in patients with CAD). Beta-blocking agents are generally used before the onset of AMI, in combination with long-acting nitrates such as isosorbide dinitrate; together, these drugs are highly efficacious in managing angina pectoris. They have documented efficacy in preventing myocardial ischemia and improving exercise tolerance in patients with angina.

There is impressive evidence that beta-blocking drugs prolong life in patients recovering from AMI. In a swedish study, for example, metoprolol reduced 3-month mortality in patients with acute infarction by 36%. In the First International Study of Infarct Survival (ISIS-1), atenolol reduced cardiac-related mortality at 7 days and 1 year in patients with suspected acute infarction who were treated an average of 5 hours after the onset of symptoms. Pooling of data from several large randomized trials for the purpose of examining the effects of early treatment (within 4 hours of symptom onset) with an intravenous beta-blocking agent, revealed a 20% reduction in cumulative cardiac enzyme release, preservation of R waves, and reduction in the development of Q waves. Beta blockers can be combined safely with thrombolytic agents to enhance myocardial salvage during an evolving acute infarction. They have become an important part of the early treatment of infarction.

Following acute infarction, patients are treated with long-term beta blockade with good effect. In the Beta Blocker Heart Attack Trial (BHAT), for example, propranolol was begun from 5 to 21 days after acute infarction. At 25 months, patients taking propranolol had significantly lower overall mortality and incidence of sudden cardiac death than did controls. These results are consistent across numerous research studies, and suggest that all patients with AMI who have no contraindications to taking a beta blocker (eg, severe heart failure or lung disease) should receive one. The only exception to this may be patients who have an uncomplicated myocardial infarction and preserved left ventricular function (ie, ejection fraction >60%). These patients already have a good prognosis and do not appear to benefit substantially from long-term beta-blocker therapy.

Calcium-channel Blockers

Another medical advance has been the development of the class of drugs categorized as calcium antagonists or *calcium-channel-blocking agents*. These drugs (verapamil, diltiazem, and nifedipine) have several different actions, foremost among which is their ability to increase coronary blood flow and improve myocardial oxygenation. The exact mechanism of this beneficial effect is still uncertain; however, smooth-muscle contraction depends on calcium ions, and it is believed that the calcium-channel-blocking agents reduce coronary vascular resistance by blocking the entry of calcium through cell membranes, thereby relaxing the smooth muscles within the arterial wall. In other words, these drugs inhibit smooth-muscle contraction, which in effect allows the arteries to dilate fully. Because of this antispasmodic action, calcium-channel-blocking agents were used initially to treat coronary artery spasm (variant or Prinzmetal's angina), and the results of several studies indicate that these drugs are extremely effective for this purpose. Calcium antagonists have also been employed in the treatment of stable angina, again with considerable success. In addition to preventing

TABLE 6–2. TREATMENT OF ACUTE MYOCARDIAL INFARCTION: REDUCING MYOCARDIAL OXYGEN DEMAND AND INCREASING OXYGEN SUPPLY

Decrease Myocardial Oxygen Demand	Increase Myocardial Oxygen Supply
Bed-rest	Low-flow oxygen
Pain relief: morphine sulfate and nitrates also function as venodilators and therefore diminish preload	Thrombolytic therapy: should be initiated within 1 hour of symptom onset for best results
Anxiety relief: reassurance, family support, and sedation	Anticoagulants: intravenous heparin immediately after thrombolysis to maintain vessel patency and prevent further thrombus formation
Beta blockade: decrease the sympathetic drive to the myocardium	Aspirin: decreases platelet adhesiveness
Angiotensin-converting enzyme inhibition: reduces both preload and afterload in patients with left ventricular dysfunction	PTCA: stenosis dilated with balloon to increase perfusion
Intraaortic balloon pump: balloon deflates during systole to aid in the ejection of blood from the left ventricle into the aorta	CABG surgery: increases blood supply to myocardium by providing a bypass of obstructed artery or arteries
	Intraaortic balloon pump: increases intraaortic pressure during diastole to augment blood flow through coronary arteries

myocardial ischemia, calcium-blocking agents are reported to be effective in treating resistant arrhythmias, heart failure, and hypertension.

Despite initial enthusiasm, for the use of calcium-channel blockers in treating of acute myocardial infarction, a number of clinical trials have not supported this. For example, in the Norwegian Nifedipine Multicenter Trial, there was no difference in infarct size or 6-week mortality rate among patients with AMI who were treated with nifedipine and those given placebo. Trials of verapamil and diltiazem have produced similarly disappointing results.

Angiotensin-converting-enzyme Inhibitors

Angiotensin-converting-enzyme (ACE) inhibitors (captopril, enalopril, and lisinopril) have been used to reduce infarct expansion after AMI by blocking the adverse effects of the renin-angiotensin-aldosterone system (as discussed in Chapter 7). This class of drugs seems to have important beneficial effects in patients with acute infarctions who experience left ventricular dysfunction (ie, an ejection fraction of less than 40%). The ACE inhibitors are currently underprescribed and underutilized after AMI, despite overwhelming evidence that they significantly improve survival and functional status in patients with moderate to severe heart failure. They are discussed in the Chapter 7.

SUMMARY OF PHARMACOLOGIC TREATMENT FOR MYOCARDIAL INFARCTION

The cornerstone of management of the patient with AMI is found in the CCU. Supportive measures are immediately instituted to reduce myocardial oxygen demand and prevent life-threatening arrhythmias. These measures include reassurance, effective analgesia, quiet surroundings, bed-rest, low-flow oxygen inhalation, prophylaxis against deep venous thrombosis, and treatment of arrhythmias. Attention is also directed at reducing myocardial oxygen demand and restoring blood flow to the ischemic myocardium through combination pharmacotherapy (Table 6–2). Time is of the essence in such therapy, since the greatest benefit is derived when it is begun within 1 hour of symptom onset. Administration of drugs, particularly thrombolytic agents, should begin within the initial 15 to 30 minutes of hospitalization. Thrombolytic therapy is followed by anticoagulant therapy (full dose intravenous heparin) to maintain coronary artery patency.

Other pharmacologic treatment in myocardial infarction involves the use of nitrates and morphine to relieve pain, beta-blockade to reduce myocardial oxygen consumption (thereby promoting salvage of ischemic myocardium), and the use of ACE inhibitors in patients with left ventricular dysfunction. Calcium channel blockers appear to have no role in the treatment of AMI.

CORONARY REVASCULARIZATION

Despite the significant success of thrombolytic therapy, it restores vascular patency in only 50% to 70% of patients who receive it. Moreover only 35% of patients with AMI who have no contraindications to thrombolytic therapy actually receive it. Many patients delay in seeking medical care and arrive at the emergency room beyond the 6 hour "window of opportunity" for such therapy. Therefore, other tech-

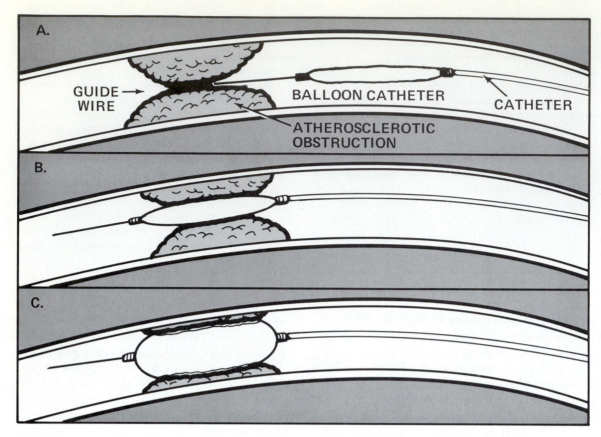

Figure 6–1. A. Guidewire of dilatation catheter (with balloon deflated) being inserted into obstructed segment. **B.** Balloon inflated within stenotic area, thereby enlarging lumen artery.

niques are used to increase blood supply to the endangered myocardium. The two most common are percutaneous transluminal coronary angioplasty (PTCA) and coronary artery bypass graft (CABG) surgery. Some patients with AMI will undergo coronary revascularization as part of their acute treatment. Many patients who have been reperfused successfully with a thrombolytic agent will eventually return to the hospital for PTCA, CABG, or both procedures because of the high incidence of restenosis after reperfusion.

Balloon Dilatation of Coronary Arteries

PTCA involves the dilatation of narrowed segments of coronary arteries by means of a small balloon catheter inserted into the obstructed vessel by way of a peripheral artery (Figure 6–1). The procedure is performed as follows: a relatively large catheter, called a guiding catheter, is introduced percutaneously through either a femoral or brachial artery and its tip positioned at the ostium of the involved vessel. The guiding catheter is used for coronary angiography so as to visualize the exact location of the obstructive lesion. A second catheter, known as a coronary dilatation catheter, is then inserted through the guiding catheter to the site of obstruction. The dilatation catheter, which has a short, flexible wire guide at its tip, is advanced until this guidewire passes through the obstruction and the deflated balloon segment of the catheter straddles the stenotic area of the affected artery. The balloon is then inflated for 3 to 5 seconds with a pressure sufficient to dilate this obstructed segment of the artery. The balloon compresses the atherosclerotic plaque and splits the intima of the artery, creating a controlled injury to the vessel. There is little evidence that emboli travel distally during PTCA, despite what logic might suggest. If the first response to inflation of the PTCA balloon is not satisfactory, the inflation cycle may be repeated several times. After the procedure the nurse must carefully monitor the patient for 6 to 8 hours.

The main advantage of PTCA, at least in principle, is that it unblocks obstructed arteries and produces an immediate increase in coronary blood flow without the need for surgery and general anesthesia. Moreover, the procedure involves a minimal hospital stay, with rapid convalescence, and is much less expensive than bypass surgery. Also, PTCA can be repeated if necessary in the event that a treated vessel again becomes obstructed. In practice, however, the technique seems to have limited application. Clinical experience suggests that PTCA is most useful in patients with CAD affecting only a single vessel that exhibits discrete lesions. Accordingly, only 5% to 10% of patients who might otherwise undergo coronary bypass surgery are considered suitable candidates for PTCA. Furthermore, this catheterization procedure is not without risk. It may cause sudden occlusion or deterioration in flow in the obstructed artery (because of dissection, thrombus or spasm), resulting in AMI or worsening of symptoms. Given its potential for producing serious complications, PTCA should be performed only in those hospitals that have a cardiac surgical team available for emergency bypass surgery. Further evaluation of the benefits, risks, and long-term effects of PTCA is continuing. Recent studies suggest that it has a success rate of 93% to 98%. The 10% to 15% in-hospital reocclusion rate following PTCA is significantly lower than that following thrombolytic therapy. However, from 25% to 50% of patients who undergo PTCA eventually need to have the procedure repeated because they develop restenosis sufficient to cause anginal symptoms.

New Developments in the Treatment of Coronary Stenosis

PTCA was first performed in 1977, when Gruentizig revolutionized cardiology by applying the technique to open narrowed or blocked arteries. Since then, new revascularization techniques have been developed in an effort to overcome the limitations of PTCA. Some of these techniques are being developed to replace PTCA, while others are envisioned as adjuncts to PTCA. Each has a unique technology, criteria for use, and complication rate. Today, patients are being treated in the catheterization laboratory with directional atherectomy, transluminal extraction/endarterectomy (TEC), rotational atherectomy, angioplastic stenting, or laser ablation. Although some of these techniques are still experimental, nurses working in CCUs are caring for increasing numbers of patients who have had one of the new procedures.

Directional Atherectomy.
Directional coronary atherectomy uses a catheter-mounted system with a rigid housing and rotating blade. The atheromatous tissue is excised and pushed into a collecting chamber (Figure 6–2). A smooth, intact arterial luminal surface is left, with a reduced tendency to form blood clots that

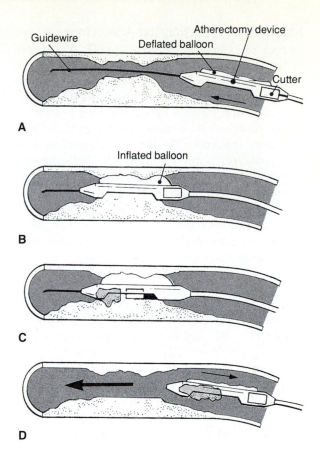

Figure 6–2. Coronary atherectomy. **A.** In coronary atherectomy procedures, a special cutting device with a device with a deflated balloon on one side and an opening on the other is pushed over a wire down the coronary artery. **B.** When the device is within a coronary artery narrowing, the balloon is inflated so that part of the atherosclerotic plaque is "squeezed" into the opening of the device. **C.** When the physician starts rotating the cutting blade, pieces of plaque are shaved off into the device. **D.** The catheter is withdrawn, leaving a larger opening for blood flow.

could reocclude the artery. The results of directional atherectomy for the treatment of CAD show a procedural success rate of 87%, complication rate of 6%, frequency of myocardial infarction of 5%, need for coronary artery bypass surgery in 1.6% of cases, and mortality rate of 1%. Restenosis rates are similar to those in PTCA, although large clinical trials need to be conducted to ascertain this. Directional atherectomy is contraindicated in heavily calcified arteries that will not bend to allow the rigid housing of the system to be threaded through the artery. The procedure appears to be a good alternative or adjunct to PTCA.

Transluminal Extraction/End-Arterectomy. Transluminal extraction/end-arterectomy (TEC) was designed to create a large lumen and smooth vascular intimal surface by excising atheroma fragments through continuous vacuum suction. It continuously removes plaque material by suction while a cutter tip rotates slowly, thus reducing the risk of distal embolization. Indications for TEC include occlusion of saphenous vein grafts, particularly in grafts that are degenerated and friable. Contraindications include proximal-vessel tortuosity and heavily calcified lesions. The complication rate is similar to that for directional atherectomy. In a recent multicenter study, the success rate of TEC was 95%, but a 6-month follow-up revealed a restenosis rate of 46%.

Rotational Atherectomy. The rotoblator used in rotational atherectomy has a diamond-coated abrasive tip that works on the principle of differential viscoelasticity. This principle holds that the microblade will push softer elastic tissue out of its way and cut more rigid atheroma and fibrotic atheromatous tissue. The tip rotates at an immense speed (up to 200,000 rpm, compared to the 2,500 rpm of the TEC device). The debris generated by the procedure is not collected but thrust into the distal coronary microcirculation. Rotational atherectomy is particularly useful for calcified lesions; long, diffuse, and distal disease; chronic total occlusions; and lesions in small tortuous vessels. A patient registry has reported a success rate of 95% with rotational atherectomy, with adjunctive PTCA performed in 44% of lesions. Complications have included non-Q-wave infarctions in 4.0%, Q-wave infarctions in 1%, urgent coronary surgery in 2%, and death in 0.8%. Long-term follow-up suggests a restenosis rate of 39%.

Laser Ablation. Laser technology has evolved from the "hot-tip" devices of the early 1980s, which produced thermal injury to intimal lesions, to the excimer lasers that deliver energy in short pulses. The lasers in current use emit ultraviolet or infrared light without the buildup of heat seen with continuous-wave lasers. Potential indications for coronary angioplasty with the excimer laser are long, diffuse, calcified, and vein-graft lesions, as well as total vascular occlusions that can be crossed with a guidewire. When combined with PTCA, the success rate of laser ablation is 90%. This figure is remarkable, given the difficult lesions against which the technique is used. Complications include coronary dissection in 16% of cases, acute occlusion in 7%, the need for coronary artery bypass grafting in 3.4%, embolism in 1.2%, and perforation in 0.4%.

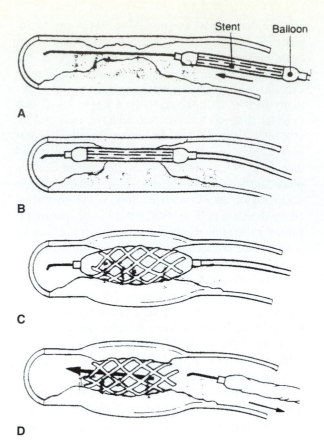

Figure 6–3. A coronary stent is a stainless steel mesh placed inside the coronary artery. **A.** To place a coronary stent within a vessel narrowing, physicians use a special catheter with a deflated balloon and the stent at the tip. **B.** The catheter is positioned so that the stent is within the narrowed region of the coronary artery. **C.** The balloon is inflated, causing the stent to expand and stretch the coronary artery. **D.** The balloon catheter is then withdrawn, leaving the stent behind to keep the vessel open.

Stents. Endovascular stents were designed to reduce the restenosis rates seen with conventional PTCA. Stents are metallic wire tubes that are implanted at the site of narrowing in a coronary artery to keep the vessel open (Figure 6–3.) When an acute occlusion occurs with PTCA, a stent can maintain vessel patency. In the case of arterial dissection, a stent can be used to compress the dissected intimal flap against the vessel wall (similar to placing a brace against a trap door) to oppose the elastic recoil and vasoconstriction that usually occur with dissection. Promising uses of stenting include the reduction of emergency CABG surgery after PTCA. In one large series, stent placement was successful in 98% of cases in which PTCA was done, and reduced the rate of restenosis to

25%. However, vascular injury or significant bleeding occurred in 16% of patients.

Nursing Care. Patients are prepared for one of the foregoing procedures in much the same way as they would be prepared for cardiac catheterization. Nursing responsibilities include patient assessment and teaching the patient and family about what can be expected during and after the procedure. Nursing care following the procedure is very similar to that following PTCA. Activities center on assessment of vital signs, cardiac and hemodynamic monitoring, and anticipation of potential complications. Distal pulses should be assessed frequently, since a thrombosis or hematoma may occur at the site of arterial puncture. Dressings should be checked frequently for any sign of bleeding. The contrast dye used in the new procedures is excreted through the kidneys, and patients should be encouraged to increase their fluid intake accordingly. Patients need to be at bed-rest for at least 6 hours after sheath or catheter removal.

SURGICAL TREATMENT

CABG surgery is performed when the coronary arteries have become critically stenosed. The procedure consists of suturing one end of a segment of a vessel (taken from the internal mammary artery or the saphenous vein of the patient's leg) to a small opening made in the aorta and the other end to a coronary artery. This graft bypasses the obstructed portion of a diseased artery and permits blood to pass from the aorta to the myocardium. For the operation to succeed in its purpose, the distal end of the graft must be attached to a portion of the coronary artery that is relatively free of advanced atherosclerotic disease (as determined preoperatively by coronary arteriography). If the disease process is diffuse and extends throughout the entire length of the artery, the bypass will not be effective. Fortunately, atherosclerotic narrowing is most likely to occur near the point of origin of an artery, thus permitting grafts to be applied in most patients with CAD.

Because more than one coronary artery is involved in the majority of cases of symptomatic CAD, usually two or three (or more) grafts are placed during the CABG procedure. The operation can be accomplished with a low surgical mortality; indeed, many large medical centers report an operative mortality of only 1%. Patency rates at 1 and 5 years are 98% and 96%, respectively, for CABG with internal mammary artery grafts.

Bypass surgery was conceived originally as a means of treating severe, disabling angina that could not be controlled medically; however, now it is also being used as a therapeutic as well as a prophylactic measure in many other situations, including stable angina pectoris, unstable angina, and AMI. In principle, the revascularization procedure produces an immediate increase in coronary blood flow (and myocardial oxygen supply), and in this way controls angina and may prevent serious complications of myocardial ischemia.

Extensive clinical experience during the past decade has clearly shown that CABG surgery is extremely effective in relieving angina pectoris. About 85% of patients describe symptomatic improvement after a bypass procedure and 65% show increased exercise tolerance. Much less certain is the value of the operation for other purposes. In fact there has been no evidence thus far to suggest that CABG surgery can inhibit the progression of ischemic heart disease. It can, however, reduce the most common complications of the disease (ie, heart failure and arrhythmias).

Research is currently being conducted to compare the outcomes of PTCA and CABG. Clearly the former is less expensive and less risky. Available data suggest that cardiac surgery is more likely to have fewer complications (eg, myocardial infarctions and arrhythmias) than PTCA. Surgically treated patients remain free of pain for longer periods, are more likely to have negative exercise stress tests, and achieve a better functional class than patients undergoing PTCA.

Researchers have also compared surgically treated patients to patients treated conventionally. They have identified certain subgroups (by virtue of their anatomy) that are more likely to benefit from surgical than from medical treatment. Patients with left main artery disease, two- or three-vessel disease, severe disease of the right coronary artery and left anterior descending artery, and isolated disease of the left anterior descending artery have better outcomes when treated surgically. Patients with large areas of jeopardized myocardium also form a distinct subgroup that benefits from surgical intervention.

Although CABG surgery has been effective in improving the quality of life of certain patients, it should be recognized that this (or any other) surgical method can have only limited application in terms of the overall problem of CAD throughout the world. This is not only because relatively few hospitals have facilities for open-heart surgery (13% in the United States), but also because the cost of such surgery is so high that economic considerations preclude its wide-use. The overall cost of CABG surgery in the United States, for example (about 100,000 operations per year), already exceeds $1 billion a year. Few societies can afford an expense of this magnitude for treating only a small percentage of their population.

Chapter 7

Heart Failure

Heart failure is a syndrome in which left ventricular function is impaired; the heart does not have enough "pumping power" to meet the metabolic needs of the body. Heart failure may result from any form of heart disease that can cause myocardial dysfunction. It is the principal manifestation of nearly every form of cardiac disease, including coronary atherosclerosis and myocardial infarction, cardiomyopathy (disease of the heart muscle), valvular heart disease, hypertension, congenital heart disease, and abnormalities of the pericardium. Although valvular heart disease and hypertension are not primary disorders of heart muscle, they impose a chronic load on the left ventricle, which ultimately may result in myocardial dysfunction leading to heart failure.

More than 400,000 new cases of heart failure develop in the United States each year, and the condition is the most common hospital discharge diagnosis for Medicare patients. The incidence of heart failure is almost 10% among persons more than 75 years old. This high incidence partly reflects the prevalence of CAD and hypertension in the older population, but it also reflects age-related changes in myocardial and peripheral vascular function that lead to heart failure. Moreover, as the population of the United States ages, heart failure will undoubtedly become an increasingly common reason for admission to the CCU.

Many patients are treated in the CCU for heart failure, either because it is a complication of AMI or because the symptoms of chronic heart failure (usually dyspnea and fatigue) become so severe that the patient requires hospitalization and intensive care. This chapter will review the mechanisms, clinical manifestations, and treatment of heart failure, with special emphasis on its relationship to AMI.

VENTRICULAR FUNCTION AND CARDIAC OUTPUT

The heart consists of two separate but closely related pumping systems: the *right* heart, which is the pump for the pulmonary circulation, and the *left* heart, which is the pump for the systemic circulation. The relationship of these two systems is shown in Figure 7–1.

Heart failure initially may involve the left or the right heart, depending on the underlying type of heart disease. However, the cardiovascular system is a closed circuit, and eventually both the left and right ventricles are affected. The reduction in ventricular pumping performance in heart failure is manifested by a decrease in ejection fraction, stroke volume, and cardiac output. The normal ejection fraction (which is a measure of the amount of blood pumped from the left ventricle compared to the total amount of blood in the ventricle before it contracts) is usually 60% to 70%. Patients with heart failure have an ejection fraction of less than 40%.

Stroke volume is the volume of blood ejected from the ventricle with each contraction. It is affected by preload, afterload, and contractility (Figure 7–2). Preload is the degree of ventricular muscle stretch present at the onset of myocardial contraction. It can be expressed as end-diastolic volume or pressure, and is measured by the pulmonary capillary wedge pressure. Afterload is the force against which the myocardium contracts in systole. It is a major determinant of ventricular wall stress and is measured by systemic vascular resistance. Contractility is the degree to which cardiac muscle fibers can shorten when

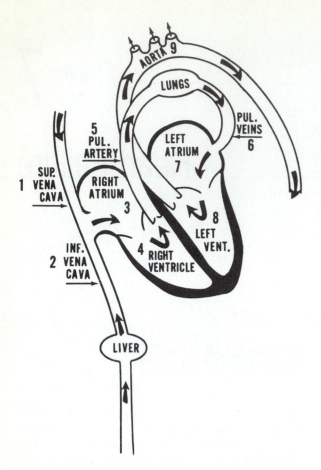

Figure 7–1. Circulation through the left and right heart. *Right heart (pulmonary circulation):* Blood collected from the entire venous system is returned by way of superior and inferior venae cavae (**1,2**) to the right atrium (**3**). From the right atrium, blood passes to the right ventricle (**4**) where it is pumped through the pulmonary artery (**5**) to the lungs. In the lungs, carbon dioxide is removed from the blood, and oxygenated blood returns by way of the pulmonary veins (**6**) to the left heart. *Left heart (systemic circulation):* Oxygenated blood from the pulmonary veins enters the left atrium (**7**) and passes to the left ventricle. Contraction of the left ventricle propels the blood through the aorta (**9**) into the systemic circulation.

activated by a stimulus, independent of either preload or afterload.

Cardiac output represents the total volume of blood pumped from the ventricle per minute. The relation between stroke volume and cardiac output is expressed as follows:

Cardiac output = stroke volume × heart rate

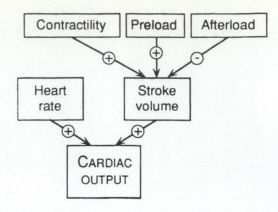

Figure 7–2. Four major mechanisms that regulate ventricular performance.

COMPENSATORY MECHANISMS

The cardiovascular system utilizes several neurohormonal compensatory mechanisms in an attempt to maintain an effective circulation and avert heart failure. These mechanisms are shown in Figure 7–3.

Sympathetic Nervous System

One of the main cardiovascular compensatory mechanisms for maintaining an effective circulation is an increase in sympathetic nervous system activity that occurs (through reflex means) as soon as cardiac output begins to fall. As a result of this sympathetic stimulation, the heart beats faster and the strength of myocardial contractions increases; both of these actions help to preserve an adequate cardiac output, at least temporarily. If, for example, the stroke volume falls after AMI to 40 mL, but the heart rate increases to 120/minute, cardiac output is maintained at a satisfactory level of 4,800 mL (40 × 120), or 4.8 L/minute despite the reduction in ventricular pumping ability. Thus, a rapid heart rate and several other characteristic signs of left ventricular failure (as described below) are actually compensatory mechanisms meant to limit the progression of heart failure. In addition to the indirect effects of the sympathetic nervous system are efforts by the heart itself to compensate for its diminished pumping performance. This is accomplished as follows: when the residual volume and pressure in the left ventricle increase during diastole, the ventricle dilates and its muscle fibers stretch (lengthen). This stretching has a beneficial effect because the strength of ventricular contraction depends on the length of the myocardial fibers just before they contract (in much the same way as the force of con-

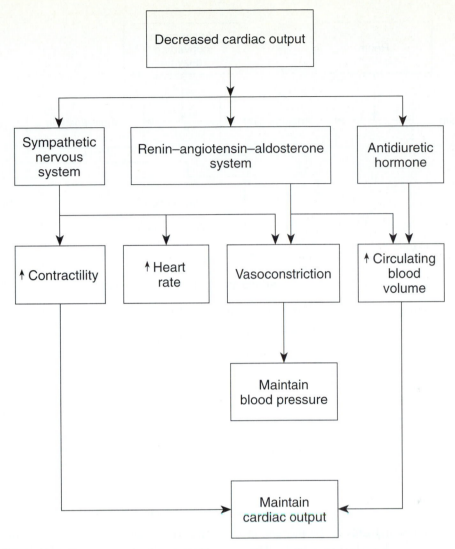

Figure 7–3. Neurohormonal compensatory mechanisms seen in response to the decreased cardiac output and blood pressure of heart failure.

traction of a rubber band depends on the extent to which it is stretched).

Renin–Angiotensin–Aldosterone System

A low cardiac output will trigger the renin–angiotensin–aldosterone system (depicted in Figure 7–4) to maintain a functional blood pressure. In response to decreased renal perfusion (secondary to a low cardiac output) and direct stimulation by the sympathetic nervous system, renin is secreted from the juxtaglomerular cells of the kidneys. Renin acts on circulating angiotensinogen to generate angiotensin I, which then (via angiotensin converting enzyme) forms angiotensin II, a potent vasoconstrictor. With increased levels of angiotensin II, blood

pressure is maintained. In addition to this, angiotensin II stimulates the patient's thirst mechanism (based in the hypothalamus) to increase fluid intake. Patients with advanced heart failure describe having a thirst that cannot be quenched.

The reduction in cardiac output that accompanies left heart failure results in a decrease in renal blood flow. This insufficiency in renal flow stimulates the adrenal cortex to secrete aldosterone, a hormone that acts to increase circulating blood volume by retaining sodium and water.

Antidiuretic Hormone

Secretion of antidiuretic hormone is the third compensatory mechanism in heart failure. This hormone

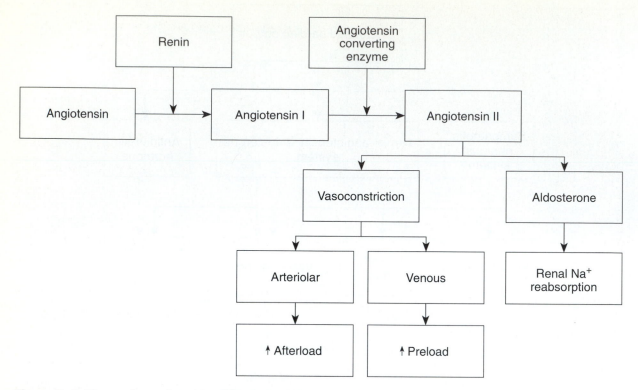

Figure 7–4. The renin-angiotensin-aldosterone system. Angiotensin is produced by the liver. It is cleaved by renin, which is released by the kidneys, to produce angiotensin I. Angiotensin I is cleaved in the circulation by angiotensin converting enzyme (ACE) to produce angiotensin II, a potent vasoconstrictor. Angiotensin II stimulates the release of aldosterone from the adrenal cortex, which in turn increases the reabsorption of sodium and water from the kidney.

increases water retention and adds to the increase in circulating blood volume described previously. This increase in blood volume initially causes cardiac output to improve (since an increase in ventricular end-diastolic pressure or volume leads to increased ventricular contractility via the Frank–Starling mechanism).

These (and other) compensatory mechanisms are effective up to a certain point, but finally become unable to counteract the effects of the failing heart, and in fact become self-defeating. At this stage, called *decompensation,* signs and symptoms of overt heart failure develop.

PATHOPHYSIOLOGY OF LEFT HEART FAILURE

In heart failure, the left ventricle is no longer able to eject the volume of blood it receives from the pulmonary circulation (right heart). This decrease in ejection fraction means that an excess of blood remains in the left ventricle after each contraction (sys-

tole). The residual volume of blood in the left ventricle gradually increases, since the uninjured right ventricle continues to pump its normal quota of blood into the pulmonary circulation, whereas the left ventricle is incompletely emptied by each systolic contraction. As a result, the pressure in the left ventricle gradually increases during diastole (the interval between contractions, during which the ventricles fill with blood). This increase in *ventricular diastolic pressure* impedes the subsequent flow of blood from the pulmonary circulation into the left heart, causing the pressure to increase in the left atrium and, in turn, in the pulmonary veins and pulmonary capillaries. In effect, a backward pressure develops throughout the pulmonary venous system. The engorged (congested) veins and capillaries impose on the available airspace within the lungs and also reduce the lungs' distensibility. More significantly, the increased pulmonary venous pressure forces fluid through the walls of the pulmonary capillaries into the lung tissues. This exudation of fluid into the lungs produces the clinical state known as *left ventricular failure.*

At first, the fluid forced into the lungs by an in-

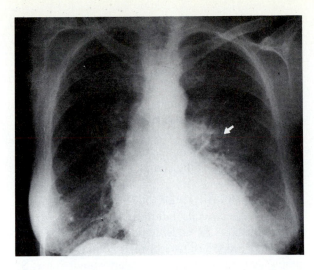

Figure 7–5. X-ray film of chest demonstrating interstitial edema. Interstitial edema is manifested as indistinctness of the pulmonary vessels (arrow) and redistribution of the vasculature so that the vessels supplying blood to the upper lobes of the lung are larger than those supplying the lower lobes.

creased ventricular diastolic pressure collects in the interstitial tissues that surround the air cells (alveoli) of the lungs, causing what is *called interstitial edema.* This early manifestation of left ventricular failure does not produce specific symptoms, nor can it be detected by physical examination of the chest. The presence of interstitial edema can, however, be identified by chest X-ray, as shown in Figure 7–5.

The threat of pulmonary congestion in heart failure is one reason why X-ray examination of the chest is a standard procedure in most coronary ICUs. As left ventricular failure progresses, fluid is forced into the alveoli themselves. This collection of fluid within the airspaces of the lungs is called *alveolar edema.* Unlike interstitial edema, alveolar edema produces distinct signs and symptoms and therefore is described as *overt left ventricular failure.* The chain of events leading to overt left ventricular failure is summarized in Figure 7–6.

CLINICAL MANIFESTATIONS OF LEFT VENTRICULAR FAILURE

Symptoms

Dyspnea. Shortness of breath (dyspnea) is the earliest and most common symptom of left ventricular failure. It results primarily from congestion of the

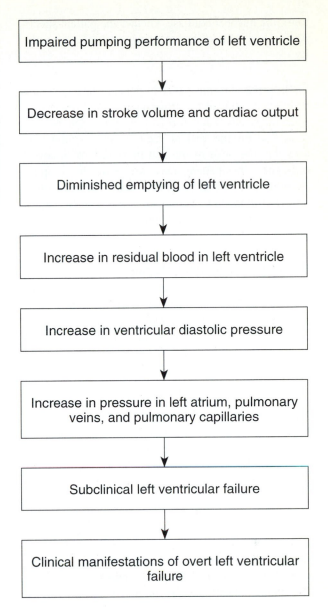

Figure 7–6. Chain of events leading to left ventricular failure.

pulmonary venous network, which reduces the elasticity (distensibility) of the lungs and diminishes the available pulmonary airspace. The problem is intensified when alveolar edema develops, because the edema fluid interferes with the exchange of oxygen for carbon dioxide in the alveoli, causing a reduction in the oxygen saturation of the blood. At first, dyspnea occurs only on exertion, and may not therefore be apparent except during physical activity (eg, when the patient gets out of bed or washes himself). As heart failure worsens, dyspnea occurs even at complete rest. Because mild dyspnea may be difficult for an observer to detect (since it is a subjective symptom), the nurse should ask whether the patient specifically feels short of breath, particularly during activity.

Orthopnea.

Dyspnea that is present during recumbency and relieved by sitting up is called *orthopnea*. This more advanced form of dyspnea can be suspected when the patient requests extra pillows or asks that the head of the bed be raised. With severe orthopnea the patient may prefer to be propped straight up in bed or to sit in a chair. These positions relieve orthopnea by diminishing pulmonary congestion and improving the ventilatory capacity of the lungs.

Paroxysmal Nocturnal Dyspnea.

For reasons that are not wholly clear, marked shortness of breath sometimes develops abruptly during sleep, and is therefore called *paroxysmal nocturnal dyspnea*. Episodes of such sudden dyspnea represent decompensation of the left ventricle following an acute increase in pulmonary venous congestion. The usual clinical setting in paroxysmal nocturnal dyspnea is sudden awakening with marked dyspnea and respiratory distress about an hour or two after falling asleep. The patient complains of suffocation, and usually exhibits great anxiety. Paroxysms of coughing associated with loud wheezing accompany the dyspnea. (Because of the wheezing, which resembles that in an asthmatic attack, the term cardiac asthma is sometimes used to describe such episodes.) Breathing is improved in the sitting position, and most patients assume this posture immediately or attempt to leave bed and reach a nearby window, believing that fresh air will help their breathing. The attack may subside after the patient sits for a few minutes, or may worsen progressively, with dyspnea, coughing, and wheezing becoming more intense. Although paroxysmal nocturnal dyspnea most often develops with dramatic suddenness, it is quite likely that subclinical left ventricular failure existed previously and progressed insidiously.

Physical Signs

Many patients with moderate to severe left heart failure have no physical findings, making identification of symptoms of the condition even more important. The most sensitive physical finding is a third heart sound (S_3), which is present in about two-thirds of patients. Rales are present in only about one-third of all patients with heart failure. Lateral displacement of the apical impulse may be seen in patients with long-standing heart failure who have developed enlarged hearts (cardiomegaly).

Rales.

The abnormal breath sounds known as *rales* are produced by fluid in the alveoli, and can be detected by auscultation of the chest. At first, rales are usually confined to the bases of the lungs (basilar rales), but as left ventricular failure progresses, the rales extend to increasingly high levels in the lung fields. Thus, the height of rales in the lungs provides a general index of the extent of heart failure. With acute pulmonary edema, coarse, bubbling rales may be heard throughout the entire chest.

Third and Fourth Heart Sound.

The first classic sign of left ventricular failure is S_3, which is identified by stethoscopic examination of the heart. Normally the heart has two distinct sounds, described simply as the first and second heart sounds (or as S_1 and S_2). They are related to the closure of the mitral and tricuspid valves (S_1) and aortic and pulmonic valves (S_2), respectively. When the left heart fails and the ventricle dilates (in order to accommodate the increased diastolic volume), a third heart sound usually can be heard. Because the cadence of the three sounds resembles the sound of a galloping horse, the heart rhythm in left ventricular failure is descriptively termed a *gallop rhythm*. The extra, S_3 heart sound occurs just after the second heart sound. It is best heard with the bell of the stethoscope placed over the apex of the heart. This type of gallop rhythm (known as a *ventricular gallop*) specifically indicates dilation of the left ventricle, and is a distinct sign of left ventricular failure even if rales cannot be heard.

A second type of gallop rhythm is known as an *atrial gallop*. It differs from a ventricular gallop in that the extra heart sound is heard just before the first heart sound rather than after the second sound. In this circumstance the extra sound is called a fourth heart sound (S_4), to distinguish it from the S_3 of a ventricular gallop. An atrial gallop (also described as an S_4 gallop) is a less serious finding than a ventricular gallop (an S_3 gallop), and may sometimes occur even in the absence of left ventricular failure. It is believed that an atrial gallop is caused by resistance to ventricular filling during diastole.

Apical Impulse.

The apical impulse is usually best palpated at the fifth intercostal space at the midclavicular line. In patients with heart failure, the heart becomes enlarged and the impulse shifts toward the patient's left side. When cardiomegaly is severe, sometimes it can even be palpated as far to the left as the midaxillary line.

Nonspecific Signs.

Although an S_3 and rales are the most sensitive diagnostic signs of left ventricular failure, other physical manifestations usually develop when the heart fails. For example, tachycardia, sweating, a reduction in blood pressure, and restlessness are often observed during acute left ventricular failure. Rather than being specific indications of left ventricular failure, these latter signs are usually part of the overall clinical picture. They may, however, be the earliest manifestations of left ventricular failure and are therefore important diagnostic clues to it.

Treatment of Left Ventricular Failure

Of the several methods now being used to control heart failure, four seem to hold the greatest promise: (1) detecting heart failure at its earliest stages so that treatment for it can be initiated promptly in an attempt to prevent its progression (particularly with the use of an angiotensin-converting-enzyme inhibitor); (2) improving the pumping efficiency of the heart by reducing its workload with drug therapy; (3) increasing left ventricular function (particularly in cardiogenic shock) by means of mechanical circulatory assistance (eg, intraaortic balloon pumping or external counterpulsation) and aggressive reperfusion; and (4) performing emergency bypass surgery if other methods are unsuccessful. Although the effectiveness of this multipronged approach must still be determined, it is fair to say that the possibility of reducing mortality from advanced left ventricular failure and cardiogenic shock is brighter than before, at least in selected patients.

The underlying objective of the treatment program for left ventricular failure is to increase cardiac output. This can be accomplished (up to a certain stage, at least) by correcting or adjusting the four principal mechanisms that normally govern left ventricular performance. To this end, the following four methods may be used singly or in combination.

Reduce Preload Volume. Since the injured left ventricle is unable to adequately empty itself (eject) of the volume of blood it receives, a logical step in treating left ventricular failure (in fact, usually one of the first steps) is to reduce venous return to the heart. This *preload volume reduction* decreases the filling volume of the left ventricle and in turn reduces pulmonary venous pressure. These desirable hemodynamic effects serve to increase stroke volume (and cardiac output) and relieve pulmonary venous congestion. In patients with a pulmonary artery catheter, preload is adjusted to maintain the PCWP below 15 mm Hg.

The simplest means for reducing preload is *diuretic therapy*. By promoting fluid loss, diuretics diminish the circulating blood volume and thus reduce venous return to the heart. (The use of diuretic therapy is discussed in the next section, on right heart failure.) In addition to diuretics, a second class of drugs, categorized as *vasodilating agents* or vasodilators, may also be used to reduce preload volume, particularly when left ventricular failure is severe or insufficiently responsive to diuretics alone. Vasodilating agents act by relaxing the tone and resistance of peripheral blood vessels, causing them to dilate. Some vasodilators are designed to dilate arterial vessels while others act predominately on the venous vessels; several of these agents exert an action on both types of vessel (Table 7–1).

Among these last-named vasodilators, which reduce both preload and afterload, the most important are the angiotensin-converting-enzyme (ACE) inhibitors. Drugs of this class work by blocking the conversion of angiotensin I to angiotensin II, thereby reducing the resistance against which the heart has to pump to eject blood, and increasing cardiac output. The ACE inhibitors also decrease aldosterone levels, thereby reducing intravascular volume and reducing congestion.

The ACE inhibitors (eg, enalpril or captropil) are the only drugs documented to reduce mortality

TABLE 7–1. VASODILATORS USED IN THE TREATMENT OF HEART FAILURE

Agent	Action Site	Administration Route	Usual Dose
Nitroglycerin	Venous	Sublingual, IV, ointment and transdermal	0.4 mg
Isosorbide dinitrate	Venous	Sublingual	2.5–10 mg
		Oral	20–40 mg
Phentolamine	Arterial	Intravenous	0.1–2.0 gm/minute
Hydralaine	Arterial	Oral	50–100 mg
Minoxidil	Arterial	Oral	10–40 mg
Sodium nitroprusside	Venous and arterial	Intravenous	25–200 gm/minute
Prazosin	Venous and arterial	Oral	5 mg
Captopril	Venous and arterial	Oral	50–150 mg

and increase functional status in patients with advanced heart failure. ACE inhibitors have also been shown to prevent heart failure after AMI. Because of this, they should be prescribed for all patients with ejection fractions of less than 40%, and should therefore constitute standard therapy for all patients with heart failure.

Preload reduction also can be achieved with vasodilators that act on the venous system. Nitroglycerin (administered intravenously, sublingually, or topically) and long-acting nitrates (isosorbide dinitrate) expand the venous bed and allow large quantities of blood to pool in the peripheral veins. As a result of this venous pooling, the amount of blood returning directly to the heart is decreased substantially, thus reducing preload.

Reduce Afterload.
In addition to reducing preload, another important aspect of the treatment of heart failure is to reduce ventricular afterload, or the resistance against which the heart must pump to eject blood. This resistance (impedance), although also dependent on other factors, reflects the systemic vascular resistance. In general, the greater the systemic vascular resistance the smaller the volume of blood ejected by the ventricle (stroke volume). Furthermore, in working harder to overcome impedance, the heart requires more energy and consumes more oxygen, further reducing cardiac output. It is therefore highly desirable to reduce systemic vascular resistance to within the normal range (ie, 800–1,200 dynes/sec/cm^{-5}) as a means of improving cardiac performance in patients with heart failure.

Afterload reduction is accomplished primarily with ACE inhibitors or arterial vasodilators. However, agents with a direct vasodilator effect on both the arterial and venous sides of the circulatory system (e.g., prazosin or nitroprusside) are often used for this purpose in critical care, since they permit concomitant reduction of both afterload and preload.

While this type of afterload reduction represents a major advance in therapy, its application may pose problems. To take but one example, excessive reduction of the blood pressure (to hypotensive levels) with vasodilators is not uncommon, and can compromise coronary artery blood flow, with a sudden deterioration in cardiac performance. The nurse is responsible for titrating all vasoactive drugs so that they effect an optimal cardiac output without producing complications. This responsibility requires a thorough understanding of the factors that influence cardiac output and the mechanisms of action of the various drugs used to support it.

Strengthen Myocardial Contractility.
In addition to unburdening the injured heart by means of reducing preload and afterload, the treatment program for heart failure includes the use of an inotropic drug (eg, digitalis or amrinone) to increase the strength of myocardial contraction. However, although inotropes have traditionally been cornerstones in the treatment of heart failure, some experts are now questioning the possible physiologic cost of their use, since the increase they may produce in contractility in the short run may come at the cost of increased morbidity and mortality in patients with chronic heart failure.

While waiting for the appropriate clinical trials of the effects of inotropic agents in heart failure, most clinicians believe that patients with advanced heart failure who continue to have symptoms despite treatment with an ACE inhibitor and diuretic should receive an inotrope such as digitalis. The object of strengthening myocardial contractility is to improve ventricular emptying, so that the volume of residual blood in the ventricle decreases while the stroke volume and cardiac output increase. Through these effects, inotropic therapy may substantially alleviate symptoms of dyspnea and fatigue in patients with heart failure.

Although the role of digitalis in chronic heart failure is still being defined, it is not used in the earliest stages of AMI. The increase in contractility brought about by digoxin is at the expense of myocardial oxygen consumption, and use of the drug in the early stages of an infarction may therefore increase the risk of arrhythmia and including ventricular fibrillation.

Control the Heart Rate.
Cardiac output, as noted earlier, is a function of heart rate (cardiac output = stroke volume × heart rate). As a general rule, in patients with AMI, heart rates that are either too fast or too slow reduce cardiac output and may lead to or worsen heart failure. With fast rates (eg, about 140/minute) the period of ventricular filling is shortened and stroke volume therefore falls. With slow rates (below 50/minute) cardiac output decreases because the stroke volume cannot increase sufficiently to counteract the rate. All of this indicates that in principle, part of the treatment program for heart failure should be directed at establishing an effective heart rate with drug therapy or cardiac pacing (as explained in subsequent chapters) in order to preserve cardiac output. Of the four determinants of left ventricular performance, heart rate control is in practice the most difficult to achieve and maintain. For this reason, attempts to correct preload, afterload, and myocardial contractility usually comprise the bulk of the treatment program.

ACUTE PULMONARY EDEMA

The most advanced stage of acute left heart failure is *pulmonary edema.* This condition develops because of a massive accumulation of fluid throughout the alveolar and interstitial tissues of the lungs. The fluid interferes with oxygenation of the blood and results in *hypoxia* (a decrease in the oxygen content of the blood). Unless this hypoxia is corrected, the vital organs become deprived of oxygen, irreversible arrhythmias develop, and death occurs.

The clinical picture in acute pulmonary edema is distinctive and seldom poses a problem in diagnosis. The condition is a horrifying experience for the patient and presents the nurse with an individual who is struggling to breathe. Its characteristic features are severe dyspnea, orthopnea, an incessant cough (producing frothy, blood-tinged sputum), and extreme anxiety. Cyanosis may be present, and gurgling sounds can often be heard, even without a stethoscope. In conjunction with these obvious signs of respiratory difficulty, the patient will have a rapid pulse rate and be cold and clammy, a response to the marked increase in sympathetic nervous activity that accompanies a decline in cardiac output. The total picture leaves no doubt that the patient is in acute distress and that emergency treatment is essential.

Treatment of Acute Pulmonary Edema

The methods and sequence of treatment of pulmonary edema depend primarily on the severity of the patient's left ventricular failure and urgency of the clinical situation. Patients with mild heart failure, for example may require only diuretic therapy, whereas in treating acute pulmonary edema, reflecting the most severe degree of left ventricular failure, several methods of treatment are combined.

Patient Position. The patient should be seated upright (in a Fowler's position) to permit pooling of blood within the systemic veins of the lower body. This position reduces venous return to the heart, decreasing preload.

Morphine. The administration of morphine should be one of the first steps in the treatment of acute pulmonary edema. Morphine has several beneficial effects in this circumstance: not only does it relieve the intense anxiety associated with pulmonary edema but, more significantly, it has a significant vasodilator effect. It decreases the volume of blood returning to the heart by reducing venous tone, which causes the pooling of blood in peripheral veins. At the same time, morphine depresses the respiratory center in the brain, thereby reducing the rate of respiration. This respiratory slowing in turn decreases the return of blood from the pulmonary circulation to the left ventricle. Morphine sulfate is usually given intravenously to patients with pulmonary edema, in doses of 4 to 10 mg (2 mg at a time until symptoms are relieved or patient becomes hypotensive).

Oxygen Therapy. During the period of acute respiratory distress in pulmonary edema, the concentration (saturation) of oxygen in arterial blood is usually markedly reduced. It is therefore it is essential to administer oxygen in order to preserve tissue function. The greatest oxygen concentration is provided by an intermittent positive pressure apparatus that delivers 100% oxygen through a well-fitted face mask (with a non-rebreathing bag). Nasal catheters or cannulas deliver only 30% to 40% oxygen and are therefore the least desirable means of supplying oxygen in this critical situation. Oxygen should always be humidified prior to its inhalation, in order to prevent drying of the airway. The humidification can be accomplished by bubbling oxygen through water.

Since the patient with acute pulmonary edema is already feeling a sense of suffocation, placing an oxygen mask over the nose and mouth may heighten this feeling. The nurse needs to instruct the patient about the need for oxygen and explain how the mask will feel before putting it in place.

Diuretics. Rapid-acting diuretics, such as furosemide (Lasix) or ethacrynic acid (Edecrin), administered intravenously, usually produce dramatic clinical improvement in acute pulmonary edema; dyspnea abates within minutes, after which there is a copious diuresis. Theoretically, the rapid-acting diuretics are effective because they promote the excretion of fluid, thereby reducing the volume of blood returning to the heart. However, the extraordinary rapidity with which these drugs act in controlling pulmonary edema (even before diuresis occurs) suggests that they also exert other pharmacologic effects. One of these is believed to be a direct effect on the venous system, causing the veins to dilate and hold a greater volume of blood. Furosemide is administered intravenously in doses of 40 to 80 mg. The usual intravenous dose of ethacrynic acid is 50 mg. (Diuretic therapy is described in greater detail in the discussion of right heart failure; see pp 106–107.)

Vasodilators. Severe dyspnea resulting from acute pulmonary edema can often be relieved promptly by the administration of 0.4 to 0.8 mg of nitroglycerin sublingually. Nitroglycerin, as already explained, acts as a venous dilator and substantially reduces preload. The left ventricular filling pressure begins to fall within 2 to 3 minutes after nitroglycerin is given, and this beneficial effect lasts for 15 to 30 minutes. Isosorbide dinitrate (eg, Isordil or Sorbitrate), given either sublingually or orally, produces the same effect, but has a somewhat slower onset of action (about 5 minutes) and much longer duration of action (2–4 hours). The proven effectiveness of both short- and long-term nitrate therapy has given these drugs a high ranking on the list of methods used to treat acute pulmonary edema. After its initial action in decreasing ventricular filling pressure, the administration of a nitrate is continued, at least during the period of hospitalization. The main limitations of nitrate therapy are its frequent causation of headaches (through its vasodilator effect) and excessive reduction of blood pressure (owing to postural hypotension). Consequently, titration of the dosage of a nitrate drug is essential to the successful management of heart failure. Vasodilators that act on both the arterial and venous networks, such as nitroprusside or prazosin, are usually reserved for patients with high arterial blood pressures or those who do not respond to preload reduction alone.

Inotropes. Inotropes play a minimal role in the management of acute pulmonary edema. As already noted, they are not used to treat pulmonary edema resulting from AMI. Research suggests that digitalis should not be given to patients with acute pulmonary edema associated with heart failure unless other treatment methods are ineffective or the heart failure is accompanied by a rapid-rate arrhythmia (eg, atrial fibrillation). Digitalis is generally administered in the form of digoxin at a starting dose of 0.25 to 0.5 mg.

Bronchodilators. Acute pulmonary edema is accompanied by spasm of the bronchial tree. This bronchospasm (which creates the loud wheezing sounds heard during the acute stage of the condition) interferes with ventilation. In an effort to relieve the bronchospasm, bronchodilator drugs are often used in conjunction with oxygen therapy. The most popular drug for this purpose is aminophylline, which is given intravenously at a dosage of 250 to 500 mg in 50 mL of sterile water injected *slowly* over a 15-minute period. The dose may be repeated every 3 to 4 hours if needed. In addition to dilating the bronchioles, aminophylline increases cardiac output and reduces venous pressure. The main disadvantage of the drug is that it may cause hypotension and arrhythmias, particularly if injected too rapidly.

Other Measures. The methods of treatment of acute pulmonary edema vary with the clinical response. On some occasions the precise benefit (and risk) of a particular means of treatment cannot be determined without continuous *hemodynamic monitoring,* as described in Chapter 3.

RIGHT HEART FAILURE

In most disease states, including AMI, the right heart usually fails as a consequence of left heart failure. Isolated right heart failure, as mentioned previously, is rare, save in the case of right ventricular infarction. Exceptions to this are provided by patients with chronic lung disease or disease of the tricuspid or pulmonic valves, all of which cause right heart failure.

The relationship between left and right ventricular failure is as follows: When the left heart fails, significant backward pressure develops in the pulmonary veins and capillaries, as already noted. Because of this, blood being pumped from the right ventricle through the pulmonary arteries meets resistance in the pulmonary capillaries, causing the blood pressure in the main pulmonary artery to increase. As the pulmonary artery pressure mounts, emptying of the right ventricle is impaired. The residual volume of blood within the right ventricle impedes the flow of blood into the ventricle from the right atrium. As a consequence, blood returning to the right atrium from the superior and inferior vena cavae meets resistance. This creates a backward pressure throughout the entire peripheral venous system, leading to congestion of the venous network.

The clinical picture that results from this overloading of the venous system is sometimes called *backward heart failure,* while the clinical picture that results from insufficient cardiac output from the left ventricle is called *forward heart failure.* Although the terms are logical and explain many of the clinical findings in right and left heart failure, the problem of the failing heart is infinitely more complicated. Thus, for example, the activation of the renin-angiotensin-aldosterone system described as part of the compensation that occurs with left heart failure results in the retention of sodium and water. The renal and hormonal changes that lead to this retention, which are stimulated by poor renal perfusion (ie, forward heart failure), also contribute to the total picture of right heart failure. Backward and forward heart failure coexist, and the various clinical findings in right heart failure result from both conditions.

Clinical Manifestations of Right Heart Failure

The signs and symptoms of right heart failure are related fundamentally to the retention of water and sodium within the body. The end result of this fluid entrapment is an overloading of the venous system that produces the clinical findings described in the following sections.

Distended Neck Veins (Jugular Venous Distention).

Increased venous pressure in the superior vena cava causes distention of the jugular veins in the neck. If the veins remain distended when the patient is placed in a semi-upright position (45-degree angle), right heart failure is very likely to be present. (Neck veins may distend in the absence of heart failure, but in this circumstance the veins empty immediately when the patient's head is raised, which is why observation of the neck veins should always be done with the patient in a semi-upright position.) Neck vein distention is one of the earliest signs of right heart failure.

Peripheral Edema.

Because of the increased venous pressure in right heart failure, fluid is forced from the capillaries into the subcutaneous tissues of the body. This fluid collection, called peripheral or subcutaneous edema, develops in dependent areas of the body as a result of gravity. In patients who are bedridden, the back (especially the sacral area) is dependent, and therefore edema is usually noted first in this area. In patients who are ambulatory the feet and ankles are the usual sites of edema. Rarely, peripheral edema is generalized and found throughout the entire body; this condition is called *anasarca*.

Edema can be identified by placing several fingertips firmly on the skin over a possibly affected area and seeing if indentations (or "pitting") are left when the fingertips are removed. The severity of peripheral edema is graded from 1+ to 4+. Mild edema (1+) is sometimes difficult to detect on physical examination; however, all forms of edema are accompanied by a gain in body weight, and daily weighing of the patient is therefore a useful method of estimating the extent of fluid accumulation in the body.

Pleural Effusion.

Edema fluid may also accumulate in the pleural cavity. Such an accumulation is described as a pleural effusion. It usually develops concurrently with peripheral edema, but can occur independently. Large pleural effusions compress the lungs and therefore may produce (or intensify) dyspnea. The presence of a pleural effusion can be suspected if diminished or absent breath sounds are noted while listening to the patient's lungs. The diagnosis is confirmed by X-ray examination of the chest (Figure 7–7).

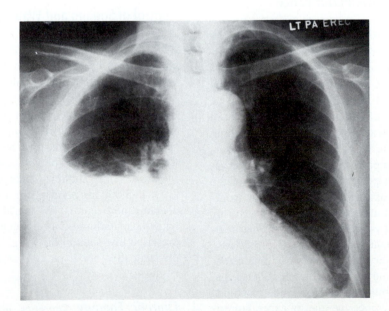

Figure 7–7. A very large pleural effusion in the right chest is noted in this X-ray film. In most instances pleural effusions are much less extensive than shown in this example.

Enlarged and Tender Liver. Backward pressure in the inferior vena cava and hepatic veins causes venous engorgement of the liver. As a result, the liver enlarges, becomes tender, and can be palpated on physical examination. Hepatic enlargement may produce discomfort in the right upper quadrant of the abdomen, and is often accompanied by loss of appetite and nausea. When the liver is engorged, pressure applied over the right upper quadrant of the abdomen causes the neck veins to distend. This phenomenon, known as the *hepatojugular reflux,* is a diagnostic sign of right heart failure. It occurs because abdominal compression increases the amount of blood returning to the heart, which, in the face of the inability of the right heart to handle the increased blood flow, raises venous pressure and intensifies neck vein distention.

Treatment of Right Heart Failure

Since right heart failure almost always coexists with left heart failure (especially in patients with AMI), the treatment programs for the two conditions overlap and share certain common features. Nevertheless, the management of right heart failure is based on specific objectives that differ in direction and emphasis from those in left ventricular failure. The two goals in treating right ventricular failure are: (1) to improve cardiac performance; and (2) to reduce sodium and water retention. The following measures are used in achieving these aims.

Improvement in Cardiac Performance

Reduction of Metabolic Needs of the Body. As stated previously, heart failure indicates that the cardiac output is insufficient to meet the metabolic demands of the body. Consequently, it is highly desirable to reduce the body's metabolic needs, if possible, as a means of assisting the failing heart in the acute stage of treatment for right heart failure. (Patients with chronic heart failure can safely exercise, and research supports the benefits of regular activity for this patient population.) Rest is one of the most effective ways of diminishing the cardiac workload. Consequently, limitation of physical activity by bed-rest or chair-rest is a basic element in the treatment program for right heart failure. Total bed-rest, however, is unnecessary, and patients can obtain adequate rest while sitting in a bedside chair. Also, patients should be permitted to use a bedside commode rather than a bedpan, since the energy expenditure is lower with a commode. Moreover, complete bed-rest is undesirable because it tends to increase the risk of thromboembolism, as explained later in this chapter.

For right heart failure, rest by itself is often remarkably effective in promoting diuresis, slowing the heart rate, and relieving dyspnea.

Vasodilator Therapy. Reducing afterload is very useful in the treatment of acute right heart failure. Just as with left heart failure, ACE inhibitors are the first line of therapy in treating right heart failure. Intravenous arterial dilators (eg, hydralazine), venous dilators (eg, nitrates), or vasodilators with a combined arterial and venous action (eg, nitroprusside) may be utilized in the critical-care setting; the choice depends on the overall hemodynamic picture. Patients with severe right heart failure will have to have their therapy optimized through the measurement of hemodynamic parameters (particularly systemic vascular resistance, PCWP and cardiac index).

Inotropes. The beta-adrenergic agonists, especially dobutamine and dopamine, are given intravenously to patients with acute right heart failure for temporary hemodynamic support. Their long-term use is limited by the lack of an oral form of either drug. Digitalis therapy remains a fundamental method of treatment for right heart failure. It increases the contractility of the heart and therefore enhances cardiac output. As previously described, digitalis does not have a role in the immediate treatment of AMI because of the cost it entails in myocardial oxygen consumption, but it is usually prescribed once the patient has moved out of the acute phase of the condition.

Control of Sodium and Water Retention

Restriction of Sodium Intake. Right heart failure is characterized by the retention of sodium and water, which in turn produces a volume overload. Consequently, it is highly important in treating right heart failure to rid the body of this excess of sodium and water, thus permitting a reduction in the circulating volume of blood. To this end, restriction of sodium in the diet is essential. When clinical signs of right heart failure develop, sodium intake is usually limited to 2,000 to 3,000 mg per day (the average American diet contains more than 10,000 mg of sodium daily). Even when heart failure is not evident, many practitioners prescribe low-sodium diets (eg, 3,000 mg daily) prophylactically for all patients with ejection fractions below 40%.

Diuretic Therapy. Diuretics are highly effective in promoting the renal excretion of sodium and water and, through this mechanism, in reducing the circulating fluid volume. In fact, edema and other manifestations of heart failure are in most instances so readily controlled with diuretics that these drugs have become the initial means of treatment for heart failure. Despite their ability to alleviate heart failure, however, diuretics alone are not sufficient for this purpose; they should be used in conjunction with ACE inhibitors, sodium restriction and, if necessary, digitalis. Diuretic agents fall into several classes with varying degrees of potency:

Thiazide diuretics. These drugs, which are moderately potent, act by blocking the reabsorption of sodium in the tubules of the kidneys. Fluid filtered through the glomeruli of the kidneys normally contains a large quantity of sodium; however, most of this sodium is reabsorbed by the renal tubules and returned to the bloodstream (in order to maintain an adequate sodium level in the body). Only the amount of sodium not reabsorbed by the tubules is excreted in the urine.

By inhibiting the customary return of sodium to the body, thiazide diuretics (eg, hydrochlorothiazide) allow large amounts of sodium and water to be excreted in the urine. These agents are administered orally and usually promote diuresis within 2 hours. The effectiveness of their action can be assessed by carefully measuring the patient's output of urine and fluid input, along with recording the patient's body weight daily. The main problem with the use of thiazide diuretics is potassium depletion, which happens because thiazides also block the tubular re absorption of potassium, causing excessive amounts of it to be excreted in the urine. The loss of potassium resulting from this drug-induced mechanism is of particular concern in patients with AMI because low potassium levels (hypokalemia) can increase myocardial excitability and cause serious ventricular arrhythmias. Hypokalemia is also dangerous in patients receiving digitalis, because potassium depletion sensitizes the myocardium to this drug and therefore predisposes to digitalis toxicity. Indeed, in the presence of hypokalemia, even small doses of digitalis may be toxic. In addition to these adverse effects on the heart, hypokalemia also has systemic effects. Marked potassium depletion often causes lethargy, anorexia, mental confusion, and a decrease in urine output. Hypokalemia can be identified by measuring serum potassium levels and, less dependably, by electrocardiography. If hypokalemia develops, replacement of potassium (either by intravenous infusion or orally, depending on the clinical circumstances) is essential.

Furosemide (Lasix) and Ethacrynic Acid (Edecrin). Furosemide and ethacrynic acid are the most potent of the available diuretics. They exert their effect in the same way as the thiazides, by blocking the renal tubular reabsorption of sodium. They can be administered intravenously or orally, and produce a rapid and profound loss of sodium and water, that far exceeds that achieved with the thiazide diuretics. Because of their extreme potency, which may produce marked hypokalemia and excessive fluid loss, both furosemide and ethacrynic acid should be reserved for urgent clinical situations (eg, acute pulmonary edema) or heart failure that is refractory to the thiazide diuretics. Potassium replacement is nearly always required in patients treated with furosemide or ethacrynic acid.

Aldosterone Antagonists. As mentioned earlier, congestive heart failure is accompanied by an excessive production of aldosterone, a hormone that causes the body to retain salt. Spironolactone (Aldactone) is an aldosterone antagonist and therefore promotes the excretion of sodium. This drug is far less potent than the thiazide diuretics, and has a very slow onset of action (usually 2-5 days). It is therefore used as a diuretic in non-urgent situations, particularly if other forms of therapy have failed. The main advantage of aldosterone antagonists is that they do not cause significant potassium loss, thus minimizing the risk of hypokalemia.

Fluid Restriction. It is usually not necessary to restrict the fluid intake of patients with mild or moderate heart failure. However, with more advanced failure it is beneficial to limit water intake to 1,000 mL daily. The reason for this is that excessive water intake tends to dilute the sodium content of body fluids and may produce a *low-salt syndrome* (hyponatremia). The latter condition, characterized by lethargy and weakness, most often results from the combination of a restricted sodium diet, increased sodium loss during diuresis, and excessive water intake. The diagnosis of hyponatremia is established by measuring serum sodium levels.

NURSING CARE OF THE PATIENT WITH HEART FAILURE

The multifaceted role of nursing in the management of patients with heart failure comprises four main functions: (1) detecting early heart failure; (2) evaluating the response to therapy, (3) initiating emergency treatment for acute pulmonary edema, (4) educating and counseling the patient and patient's family. These categories are discussed below.

Detecting of Early Heart Failure

There is good reason to believe that the sooner acute heart failure is treated the better will be the result. Consequently, recognition of the first signs and symptoms of heart failure is an important aspect in the total care of patients with AMI. Because the nurse is in constant attendance and has the opportunity to observe the patient's clinical course uninterruptedly, the detection of early heart failure has become an integral part of coronary-care nursing. The nurse is expected to assess the patient's clinical status frequently and advise the physician of significant findings. This nursing evaluation should be based on planned observation, careful physical examination, and thoughtful analysis of the patient's clinical data. The signs and symptoms discussed in the following sections may indicate early heart failure.

Respiration. The onset of overt heart failure is often accompanied by a gradual increase in the rate of respiration; therefore, ongoing measurement of the number of respirations per minute and comparison with preceding values may provide a valuable diagnostic clue to the condition. Dyspnea and orthopnea, the classic symptoms of left ventricular failure, cannot always be recognized by observation alone, especially with mild or early heart failure. Consequently, it is important to ask the patient (while vital signs are being obtained) whether he or she feels short of breath or is more comfortable propped up in bed than lying down. Coughing, another manifestation of heart failure, should also be noted, along with whether its frequency has increased and whether it is productive of sputum.

Heart Rate and Rhythm. A heart rate persistently greater than 100 per minute is cause for suspicion of left ventricular failure. (This possibility becomes even more likely when other causes of tachycardia, such as temperature elevation, pain, or anxiety are absent.) In addition to observing the heart rate, monitoring the cardiac rhythm is also essential, because arrhythmias develop very frequently during heart failure, and premature ventricular contractions puts the patient at high risk for sudden cardiac death.

Sweating. Perspiration is another manifestation of early heart failure. It results from the increased sympathetic nervous activity that accompanies a declining cardiac output. In this circumstance sweating is usually mild or moderate rather than drenching (as it is with acute pulmonary edema).

Restlessness and Insomnia. Although restlessness, anxiety, and disturbed sleep patterns are often the result of emotional turmoil among patients in the CCU, these symptoms may also represent subtle warnings of early left ventricular failure. The indiscriminate use of tranquilizers or sedatives without consideration of the underlying cause of restlessness or a sleep disturbance is unwise and may mask a useful clue to the early diagnosis of heart failure.

Physical Examination. The nurse should conduct careful, frequent physical examinations to detect evidence of heart failure. The following physical findings should be noted specifically:

1. Rales in the lungs. Indicate whether the rales are heard only at the bases of the lungs (mild failure) or extend higher in the lung fields (moderate failure).
2. Gallop rhythm. Is the extra sound an S_3 gallop (a definite sign of heart failure) or an S_4 gallop (a less specific sign)?
3. Distention of the neck veins (with the patient in a semi-upright position of 45 degrees).
4. Hepatojugular reflux (neck vein distention while pressure is applied to the area over the liver).
5. Peripheral edema, especially of the sacral area and back of the patient at bed-rest in the ICU
6. Abdominal tenderness in the right upper quadrant, resulting from venous engorgement of the liver.
7. Diaphoresis or pallor resulting from activation of the sympathetic nervous system and hypoxemia.

Evaluating the Response to Therapy

After beginning the treatment program for heart failure, it is essential to evaluate the patient's clinical status at regular intervals in order to determine further appropriate measures. Should vasodilators be administered? Is digitalis therapy indicated? Is oxygen still necessary? Should the dosage of the patient's diuretic agent be increased or decreased? These are just a few of the questions that the health-care team must answer on the basis of the patient's response to treatment.

As with the detection of early heart failure, repeated clinical assessment by the nurse is a major component of the overall treatment program for heart failure. Moreover, the nurse is responsible for titrating all intravenous drugs, and must therefore be highly knowledgeable about the actions and side effects of such drugs and the treatment goals to be obtained through their use.

The nursing assessment includes the following procedures:

1. Recording vital signs (every 1 to 4 hours, depending on the clinical status of the patient), with particular emphasis on changes in heart rate, respiration, and blood pressure. If a pulmonary artery catheter is in place, the patient's right atrial pressure, PCWP, and cardiac output also need to be measured frequently. If the catheter permits measurement of $S\bar{v}O_2$, oxygenation should also be assessed.

2. Examining the patient frequently to determine improvement or worsening of the clinical signs of heart failure.

3. Questioning the patient about dyspnea and other symptoms that may be difficult to assess objectively.

4. Recording accurate intake and output measurements to assess fluid balance, and weighing the patient daily in order to detect fluid retention that otherwise might not be apparent. The patient should be weighed at the same time each day.

5. Recognizing the side-effects of the various drugs used in the treatment program. Many drugs affect the heart rate and blood pressure, causing changes in vital signs. For example, vasodilators (eg, nitrates) may reduce blood pressure to hypotensive levels if cardiac output (flow) is not sufficiently increased.

6. Monitoring the heart to identify arrhythmias that may result from heart failure itself or from drug therapy for it (eg, arrhythmias caused by hypokalemia from diuretic therapy).

7. Obtaining laboratory data (eg, electrolyte and arterial blood gas results) in a timely fashion so that changes in these results can be readily noted.

Initiating Emergency Treatment for Acute Pulmonary Edema

In beginning emergency treatment for acute pulmonary edema, the following steps should be taken:

1. Recognize the complication, examine the patient, and notify the physician promptly. The clinical picture of acute pulmonary edema is so distinctive that its diagnosis is seldom a problem. Every critical-care unit should have a standard protocol for the treatment of pulmonary edema, and should immediately initiate treatment when it occurs.

2. Administer humidified oxygen by face mask. Make sure that there are no leaks around the side of the face mask. The flow rate should be adjusted to 8 to 10 L/minute. Face masks are usually frightening to patients in respiratory distress, and the nurse should reassure the patient that the mask will not interfere with breathing. Intermittent positive-pressure ventilation (IPPB) may be required.

3. Raise the head of the bed so that the patient is in a sitting (Fowler's) position. This position facilitates breathing by lowering the diaphragm and allowing the lung capacity to expand.

4. Prepare and administer drug therapy as ordered by the physician (or in accordance with the standard protocol of the CCU). The customary treatment program for acute pulmonary edema involves the immediate administration of morphine and a rapid-acting diuretic.

5. If the patient has a pulmonary artery catheter in place, monitor the patient's pulmonary artery pressure and PCWP. Obtain a reading of the parient's cardiac output. Titrate vasodilators to maintain the PCWP at 12 to 15 mm Hg and the systemic vascular resistance at 800 to 1,200 dynes/sec/cm^{-5}.

6. Observe the cardiac monitor for the development of arrhythmias. Reduced tissue oxygenation and electrolyte disturbances resulting from heart failure commonly precipitate serious arrhythmias during acute pulmonary edema.

7. Collect arterial blood samples for blood gas determinations, as appropriate.

8. Help the patient and family understand what has happened and describe the treatment program for it. Acute pulmonary edema is an extremely frightening experience, and most patients who experience it feel that death is near. The nurse should reassure the patient that prompt improvement can be anticipated after treatment is started. A calm, confident attitude is often the best form of reassurance. Each step in the treatment program should be explained briefly to the patient and family members, particu-

larly when it involves the use of equipment (eg, positive-pressure breathing devices).

CARDIOGENIC SHOCK

Cardiogenic shock is a condition involving a severely decreased cardiac output (less than 2.0 L/minute) and hypotension (systolic blood pressure less than 90 mm Hg), which leads to inadequate perfusion of peripheral tissues. It is the most severe manifestation of impaired left ventricular pumping function, and occurs in 10% to 15% of patients hospitalized with AMI. Until recently, more than 80% of patients who developed the clinical syndrome of cardiogenic shock could be expected to die during the period of hospitalization. Now there is hope that this awesome rate of mortality can be reduced by the application of new treatment methods for this condition.

Although the precise cause of cardiogenic shock remains uncertain, it is known that this complication of AMI is associated with extensive destruction of the left ventricle. Autopsy studies have shown that in most patients who die of cardiogenic shock, more than 40% of the myocardium is destroyed. This does not necessarily mean that the initial infarction produces all of this damage; it may be that the infarcted area continues to enlarge during the course of cardiogenic shock. In any case, a downward spiral in cardiac function often occurs because hypotension leads to decreased coronary artery perfusion, which exacerbates ischemic damage to the myocardium. The decreased stroke volume in cardiogenic shock increases left ventricular size (preload) and therefore myocardial oxygen demand.

Thrombolytic and other drug therapy is designed to limit the damage that occurs within the first few hours after a myocardial infarction. As new treatment techniques make it increasingly possible to limit the ultimate size of an evolving myocardial infarct, the incidence of cardiogenic shock (and left ventricular failure) may decline.

The effects of the severe myocardial damage resulting from cardiogenic shock are shown in Figure 7–8. As a result of extensive injury to the myocardium, the stroke volume and cardiac output are reduced greatly. (This is accompanied by an increased pressure in the left atrium, pulmonary capillaries, and pulmonary arteries, as noted in the discussion of left ventricular failure.) The marked decrease in cardiac output causes the systemic arterial blood pressure to fall (hypotension). In an effort to preserve effective circulation, the small arterioles throughout the body constrict, in effect confining the volume of circulating blood to the vital organs at the expense of peripheral tissues. This *generalized vasoconstriction,* mediated through the sympathetic nervous system, is beneficial at first; ultimately, however, it cannot compensate for the very low cardiac output in cardiogenic shock, and sustained hypotension develops. When the systolic arterial blood pressure falls below a critical level, the vital organs fail to receive an adequate supply of blood and oxygen to sustain normal cellular metabolism; this is called *inadequate perfusion.* This generalized perfusion deficit affects all of the organs of the body and produces the clinical findings of cardiogenic shock. Of particular importance is the effect of inadequate perfusion on the heart itself. During shock, blood flow through the coronary arteries decreases and the myocardium is further deprived of oxygen. This decrease in the myocardial oxygen supply impairs the contractility of the uninjured segment of the ventricle and at the same time promotes additional tissue destruction (thus increasing the size of the infarction). Consequently, the cardiac output falls even more, and a vicious cycle of inadequate perfusion and progressive failure is created. In summary, cardiogenic shock develops because the damaged left ventricle cannot maintain the cardiac output at a level necessary for adequate tissue perfusion.

Unless adequate perfusion can be restored promptly, the body cells deteriorate and die. It is believed that this results from irreparable damage to certain enzyme systems involved in the tissues' utilization of oxygen. Once the vital organs are destroyed in this way, treatment is to no avail and death must be anticipated. This latter state is known as *irreversible shock.* The exact point at which shock becomes irreversible is unknown, but it appears that reversibility is related primarily to the duration of a major perfusion deficit. The end stage of cardiogenic shock is associated with profound vasodilation (circulatory collapse), and finally with the development of ventricular fibrillation or ventricular standstill that are unresponsive to treatment.

Clinical Manifestations of Cardiogenic Shock

Inadequate tissue perfusion produces a combination of clinical findings that collectively define cardiogenic shock. Because this underperfusion affects all of the major organs of the body, the clinical picture of cardiogenic shock is characterized by involvement of multiple organ systems. The most important manifestations of cardiogenic shock are as follows.

Hypotension. A marked decrease in arterial blood pressure is an outstanding feature of acute circulatory insufficiency. In nearly all instances of cardiogenic

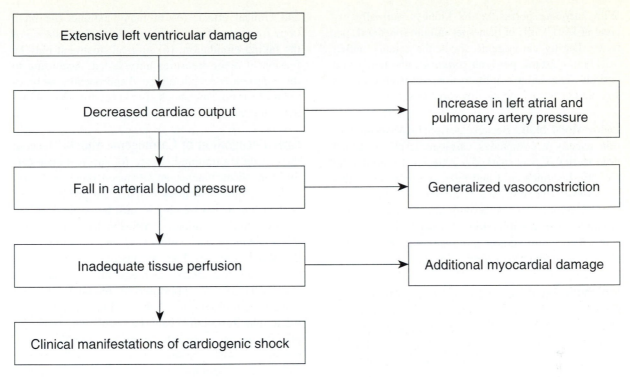

Figure 7–8. Mechanism of cardiogenic shock.

shock the systolic blood pressure falls below 90 mm Hg. However, it must be clearly understood that hypotension by itself is not synonymous with cardiogenic shock. Unless hypotension is accompanied by other clinical findings of inadequate perfusion (eg, diminished urinary output or mental confusion, as described below), the diagnosis of cardiogenic shock is not justified. If, for example, a patient has a blood pressure of 84/50 mm Hg but lacks a rapid pulse rate, has a normal urinary output, and shows no evidence of mental confusion, cardiogenic shock is not present. A more reasonable diagnosis in the face of such findings is hypotension, a common occurrence in the early stages of AMI and of much less importance than cardiogenic shock. Patients receiving vasodilator therapy also have low blood pressure without being in cardiogenic shock.

When cardiogenic shock develops, the systolic pressure declines before the diastolic pressure; it is not unusual to record a blood pressure of 70/60 mm Hg, for example. The numerical difference between the systolic and diastolic pressures is called the *pulse pressure* (eg, a blood pressure of 120/80 mm Hg yields a pulse pressure of 40 mm Hg). Since a decline in the pulse pressure is often an early sign of cardiogenic shock, it is essential to measure the systolic and diastolic pressures accurately in order to detect insidious changes in the patient's condition. When cardio-

genic shock worsens, the diastolic pressure falls along with the systolic pressure, and the blood pressure often becomes unobtainable.

In taking blood pressure readings, it is necessary to realize that the customary cuff-stethoscope method of measurement may produce spuriously low readings, particularly in the presence of cardiogenic shock. Therefore, when blood pressure readings are very low or cannot be obtained, *direct* blood pressure measurement may be required. This is accomplished by inserting an indwelling catheter into the patient's arterial system and recording the intraarterial pressures directly.

Mental Changes. One of the earliest features of cardiogenic shock is mental apathy and lassitude: the patient seems uninterested in his or her surroundings and often stares off into space. Other common concurrent or later findings are disorientation, confusion, agitation, and restlessness. All of these mental changes reflect ineffective perfusion of the brain. As the shock state progresses, seizures may occur, leading ultimately to coma.

Oliguria. As a result of diminished renal blood flow, the kidneys fail to function effectively in cardiogenic shock, and the urinary volume decreases markedly.

With adequate perfusion the kidneys normally excrete at least 1 mL of urine per minute (or 60 mL per hour). During cardiogenic shock the urinary output falls below 20 mL per hour *(oliguria)* and may cease entirely. This latter condition *(anuria)* is an ominous sign and generally signals irreversible shock.

Cold, Moist Skin.

Because peripheral vasoconstriction usually accompanies cardiogenic shock, blood flow to the skin is markedly reduced. Consequently the skin becomes cold and pale. Accompanying this vasoconstrictive response is an increase in sympathetic nervous system activity that causes profuse sweating. The combination of vasoconstriction and sympathetic stimulation produces the cold, pale, clammy skin that characterizes cardiogenic shock.

Metabolic Acidosis.

Adequate oxygenation is essential for normal cellular metabolism and function. In cardiogenic shock the supply of oxygen available to the tissues is drastically reduced. In an attempt to preserve cellular function and life, the body employs a temporary, alternate metabolic pathway that does not demand oxygen; this is called *anaerobic* metabolism, in contrast to the normal *aerobic* pathway of metabolism, which uses oxygen. The end product of aerobic metabolism is carbonic acid, which is excreted as carbon dioxide by the lungs; the end product of anaerobic metabolism is *lactic acid.* Unlike carbon dioxide, which is readily removed from the body, lactic acid cannot be excreted by the lungs or kidneys, and therefore accumulates in the blood. This retention of lactic acid results in *lactic acidosis.* It can produce lethal arrhythmias that are refractory to treatment.

Treatment of Cardiogenic Shock

Over the years a variety of methods have been used to treat cardiogenic shock. That the present mortality rate in this complication of AMI remains above 80% clearly indicates that no mode of therapy has been consistently successful in combating it. However, ongoing research has provided several important leads regarding an improved plan of treatment for cardiogenic shock.

The plan is based on the following concepts: (1) the earlier cardiogenic shock is recognized and treated, the greater is the chance for survival; (2) therapeutic decisions must be based on repeated assessment of the patient's hemodynamic status; (3) a standardized treatment program for all patients is self-defeating because the clinical course of the condition has many variations; (4) drug therapy should be selected and altered according to its hemodynamic

and clinical effect; (5) in many patients the main hope for survival rests with mechanical assistance of the failing circulation; (6) surgical treatment may be feasible if other measures have failed. According to these current concepts, a logical approach to the treatment of cardiogenic shock should involve the following components.

Early Recognition of Cardiogenic Shock.

Because there is only a minimal chance for survival once cardiogenic shock reaches an advanced stage (eg, complete cessation of urinary output), the primary focus of the program for treating it must be on its early detection and treatment. Occasionally cardiogenic shock develops soon after AMI, but far more often the shock state evolves gradually, usually several hours after the attack. Consequently, in most instances there is an opportunity to recognize the first clinical manifestations of shock. Early detection of these manifestations can be achieved only by planned, repeated observation of the patient's clinical condition. Any evidence suggesting impending shock, such as diminished mental alertness, a modest reduction in blood pressure, a decrease in the pulse pressure, a gradual decrease in urinary output, or coolness and paleness of the skin is cause for prompt investigation of the patient's physiologic status and the initiation of supportive treatment.

Hemodynamic and Physiologic Measurements.

In order to assess the extent of cardiogenic shock and plan a logical treatment program for it, hemodynamic and physiologic measurements are necessary. All of these can now be made quickly and safely at the bedside.

Arterial Blood Pressure.

It is advantageous to insert an intraarterial catheter (usually by way of the radial or brachial arteries) to permit direct measurement of the blood pressure. In this way the blood pressure can be monitored continuously and samples for blood-gas analysis can be taken frequently from the arterial catheter.

PCWP and Cardiac Output.

Left ventricular pumping performance can be determined indirectly by measuring PCWP with a pulmonary artery catheter. An increase in left ventricular end-diastolic pressure (LVEDP) is one of the earliest and most important expressions of diminished left ventricular function. Cardiac output can be measured with a pulmonary thermodilution artery catheter. It is highly desirable to measure both of these pressures as a means of evaluating the severity of cardiogenic shock, as well as the effects of treatment for it.

Urinary Output. Accurate measurement of urinary output is of such great importance in assessing the physiologic status of the patient in cardiogenic shock that an indwelling (Foley) catheter should be inserted into the bladder in the early stages of shock. The urinary volume is measured at 30-minute intervals.

Arterial Blood Gases. As noted earlier, cardiogenic shock is accompanied by inadequate oxygenation and metabolic acidosis. The extent of these two disturbances is determined by arterial blood-gas studies (Pao_2 and pH).

Supportive Therapy. With the first signs of cardiogenic shock, several general measures are undertaken to preserve vital-organ function until specific treatment can be instituted to improve cardiac performance (based on the results of hemodynamic studies). These initial steps, categorized as supportive therapy, include the following procedures.

Administration of Oxygen. Oxygen is administered initially by means of a tight-fitting face mask. Arterial blood gas studies should be performed while the patient is receiving oxygen. If the results indicate inadequate arterial oxygenation (Pao_2 levels below 75 mm Hg), the patient should be intubated and placed on a positive-pressure ventilator.

Relief of Pain. Patients with cardiogenic shock often develop ischemic chest pain because of reduced coronary blood flow and inadequate myocardial perfusion. Small doses of morphine (5–1.0 mg) should be given intravenously to relieve this pain. (Intramuscular or subcutaneous injections are not advisable in cardiogenic shock, since drug absorption may be very slow in the presence of diminished circulation.)

Correction of Acidosis. As explained previously, inadequate tissue perfusion leads to lactic acidosis, a condition that even when only moderately severe adversely affects cardiac performance and contributes to the development of lethal arrhythmias. Consequently, it is essential to promptly detect and correct lactic acidosis. This is done by measurement of the arterial blood pH. (The normal arterial blood pH is 7.35–7.45; levels below 7.35 indicate acidosis.) Lactic acidosis is treated with intravenous sodium bicarbonate (an alkali).

Specific Treatment (Drug Therapy)

Infusion of Fluids. Hypotension, oliguria, and other signs of cardiogenic shock sometimes develop in AMI as the result of a reduction in the circulating blood (plasma) volume. This volume depletion, called *hypovolemia,* is usually caused by a combination of factors, including inadequate fluid intake, anorexia, vomiting, profuse sweating, and excessive fluid loss from vigorous diuretic therapy. Hypovolemic shock is characterized by a *normal or low PCWP* (in contrast to the high pressures that are expected with typical cardiogenic shock). The condition can be corrected by the administration of intravenous fluids to expand the plasma volume. Consequently, if the patient in cardiogenic shock does not exhibit an elevated PCWP, plasma-volume expansion should be undertaken as the first step in treatment. Usually, 200 mL of 5% dextrose in water (D_5W) is administered intravenously over a 10-minute period (20 mL/minute). If hypovolemia is a contributing factor to shock, this trial of fluid loading usually causes the blood pressure and urinary volume to increase promptly. Additional fluids are then infused according to the patient's clinical and hemodynamic responses. With marked volume depletion, albumin, whole blood, or low-molecular-weight dextran may be required to expand the intravascular volume sufficiently. As a general rule, patients who respond to volume expansion have a good chance for recovery.

Inotropic Drugs. Unless cardiogenic shock responds to plasma-volume expansion (which happens in approximately 10% of cases), drug therapy is initiated in an attempt to increase the strength of myocardial contraction (and to raise the blood pressure). A variety of drugs are available for this purpose, but none is ideal. The main problem with inotropic drugs in treating cardiogenic shock is that in achieving their effect they increase myocardial oxygen consumption. An increase in myocardial oxygen consumption is especially dangerous in the presence of cardiogenic shock, since the additional oxygen deprivation it incurs may further reduce the pumping function of the heart. Despite this (and other) adverse physiologic effects, inotropic drugs must be used, at least temporarily, when the blood pressure is very low and perfusion of vital organs cannot be maintained. One or more of the following drugs may be administered in this circumstance: norepinephrine (Levophed), dopamine (Inotropin), and dobutamine (Dobutrex). Although it is beyond the scope of this discussion to describe the precise pharmacologic effects and methods of administration of each of these agents, several general statements about inotropic therapy are pertinent. First, its results vary from one patient to another, and trials with different drugs (or different dosages) may therefore be necessary. Second, no attempt should be made to restore blood pressure to its normal, preshock levels. As a general rule the systolic pressure should be maintained in the range of 90 to 100 mm Hg; higher levels create an excessive myocardial oxygen demand. Third, inotropic drugs often induce serious arrhythmias, and careful ECG monitoring is therefore mandatory during the period of treatment. Fourth, inotropic drugs usually act promptly, and if definite improvement does not occur within an hour after their administration, mechanical assistance of the circulation may be required.

Vasodilator Drugs. As noted previously, cardiogenic shock is accompanied by constriction of the peripheral arterioles (as a compensatory mechanism) to preserve adequate circulation to the vital organs. Although this vasoconstriction is highly desirable at first, it may ultimately reduce in cardiac output because the left ventricle must pump against strong resistance in the arterial system (peripheral vascular resistance), thus impeding ventricular emptying. On this basis it has been proposed that vasodilator drugs be used to improve cardiac output if there is evidence of increased systemic vascular resistance (ie, greater than 1,200 dynes-sec-cm^{-5} as calculated from hemodynamic measurements). Unfortunately, this concept has limited application in the treatment of cardiogenic shock because vasodilator drugs tend to substantially reduce the blood pressure. Occasionally, however, patients with cardiogenic shock exhibit systolic blood pressures above 90 mm Hg, in which case vasodilating agents may be cautiously administered. The two agents that appear most effective at increasing cardiac output in the presence of marked vasoconstriction are sodium nitroprusside and phentolamine. It must be emphasized that these vasodilating agents should *not* be used if the systolic blood pressure is below 90 mm Hg.

Regulation of Heart Rate. An important process in the treatment of cardiogenic shock is to maintain the heart rate at more than 60/minute but less than 120/minute if possible. Heart rates beyond this range are ineffective and reduce the cardiac output. Therefore, every effort must be made to control abnormally slow or fast heart rates as a means of improving cardiac output. This is achieved through the use of drugs or by electrical means (cardiac pacing or cardioversion), as described in subsequent chapters.

Mechanical Assistance of the Circulation

As is apparent from the foregoing discussion, drug therapy in cardiogenic shock is designed primarily to increase cardiac output. In order for such therapy to succeed, however, the heart must receive an amount

of oxygen adequate to preserve myocardial function, or the size of the infarcted area will increase and treatment will be to no avail. Consequently, the outcome of cardiogenic shock ultimately depends on the amount of oxygen available to the myocardium.

Attempting to increase myocardial perfusion with inotropic drugs is often a lost cause because these agents also increase myocardial oxygen consumption. For this reason patients in cardiogenic shock who do not respond promptly to drug therapy should receive mechanical circulatory assistance to increase their coronary blood flow and decrease the workload of the heart. This can at least temporarily maintain myocardial function.

Intraaortic Balloon Pump. The best known and probably the most effective method of mechanical cardiac assistance involves the use of the intraaortic balloon pump. The principle of intraaortic balloon pumping (IABP) is as follows: When blood is ejected from the left ventricle into the aorta during systole, only a small amount of the aortic blood flows through the coronary arteries. By far the greatest flow through the coronary circulation occurs during diastole (when the myocardium is in a resting state). The underlying purpose of IABP is to increase momentarily the diastolic pressure in the aorta after each contraction, so that a larger volume of blood will flow through the coronary arteries. This is achieved by inserting a

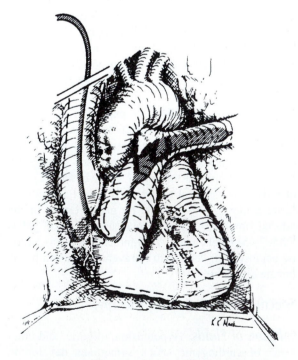

Figure 7–9. Intraaortic balloon pump.

TABLE 7–2. CRITERIA FOR ISOLATED RIGHT OR LEFT VENTRICULAR FAILURE

Isolated Right Ventricular Failure
Right atrial pressure >20 mm Hg
Pulmonary artery wedge pressure <10 mm Hg
Cardiac index <1.8 L/minute/meter^2

Isolated Left Ventricular Failure
Pulmonary artery wedge pressure >20 mm Hg
Arterial systolic pressure <90 mm Hg
Cardiac index <1.8 L/minute/m^2

long, narrow balloon through a femoral artery and into the thoracic aorta (Figure 7–9) and inflating it rapidly (with helium) at the onset of diastole. At the end of diastole (just before systole) the balloon is instantly deflated by a vacuum pump. The sudden decrease in aortic pressure reduces the resistance to left ventricular pumping, thereby reducing the workload of the ventricle. The inflation-deflation system is automatically synchronized with the heart beat, and IABP can be continued for many hours if necessary. Drug therapy is used concomitantly with IABP, and if the patient's condition stabilizes, IABP is gradually decreased (ie, the patient is weaned) and finally withdrawn.

Ventricular Assist Device. The ventricular assist device allows blood to bypass the right ventricle, left ventricle, or both, thereby reducing myocardial oxygen demand by allowing the heart to rest. It is used when IABP has proven ineffective or when the patient's shock state is related to isolated right or left ventricular failure (see Table 7–2). A cannula is placed surgically in the right or left atrium (or in both, for biventricular failure) and the blood is routed through this and through an assist pump (or two pumps in the case of biventricular assistance). Total systemic blood flow (which includes both native ventricular output and assisted ventricular flow) is maintained at 2.2 L/minute/m^2. The left atrial pressure or pulmonary artery wedge pressure is maintained at 5 to 15 mm Hg by adjusting the flow volume. Most critical-care units have policies requiring that a thoracic surgeon (or surgical resident), two critical-care nurses, and a perfusionist constantly attend patients receiving ventricular assistance.

Effect on Prognosis. Unfortunately, clinical experience has shown that many patients with cardiogenic shock have difficulty being weaned from an intraaortic balloon pump or ventricular assist device. In these cases signs of shock reappear as soon as either technique is diminished or stopped.

Thus, the IABP and ventricular assist device

have not had a significant impact on mortality from cardiogenic shock. Nevertheless, they are sometimes the only hope of survival for patients who have not responded to aggressive pharmacologic treatment. The IABP and ventricular assist device also provide time to search for potentially reversible causes of pump failure and to attempt emergency cardiac surgery or cardiac transplantation in selected patients.

Acute Cardiac Surgery. Patients in cardiogenic shock who do not respond to drugs or who cannot be weaned from IABP may be candidates for emergency cardiac surgery. The principal hope in such cases is that a coronary bypass operation, usually in conjunction with resection of a noncontractile portion of the myocardium (or other lesion), can restore adequate pumping performance. Toward this end, emergency cardiac catheterization and ventriculography are performed first, while cardiac function is being sustained with IABP. Surgery is then done to provide a blood supply to the infarcted area. Researchers have shown that mortality at 1 year after this procedure is significantly improved if the infarct-related blood vessel is patent (open).

Cardiac Transplantation. Cardiac transplantation provides an important chance for survival to heart-disease patients who would otherwise have no hope. Patients in cardiogenic shock may be candidates for transplantation if they meet the age requirement (most centers require patients to be less than 65 years of age), have no irreversible organ damage or life-threatening illness (eg, cancer), are mentally competent, and have adequate social support. The annual rate of survival following transplantation is 90% and the 5-year rate is 50%. However, the role of cardiac transplantation in the treatment of cardiogenic shock is severely limited by the lack of donor hearts.

PATIENT AND FAMILY EDUCATION AND COUNSELING

Heart failure is a chronic condition. It is vital that patients and their families understand the condition and that patients be involved from the beginning in the plan for their care. This philosophy begins in the CCU. Nurses have many opportunities to provide critical information about heart failure and to answer questions about the treatment plans for it. Patient and family education about any intervention (eg, surgery, pharmacologic therapy, the intraaortic balloon pump) should be designed to help patients arrive at realistic expectations about the outcome of their condition while still supporting hope. Patient- and family-

TABLE 7–3. SUGGESTED TOPICS FOR PATIENT AND FAMILY EDUCATION AND COUNSELING ABOUT HEART FAILURE

General Counseling	**Activity Recommendations**
Explanation of heart failure and reason for symptoms	Recreation, leisure, and return to work
Probable cause of heart failure	Exercise
Symptoms to watch for as signs of worsening heart failure	Sexual activity, sexual difficulties, and coping strategies
What to do if symptoms worsen	**Dietary Recommendations**
Explanation of treatment plan	Low-sodium diet (2–3 g)
Clarification of patient's responsibilities	Alcohol restriction
Role of family members in treatment plan	Fluid restriction (if required)
Importance of cessation of tobacco use	**Medications**
Availability and value of qualified local support group and other resources (dietician, social worker, cardiac rehabilitation nurse)	Review of all medication actions
	Potential side effects and what to do if they occur
Prognosis	Dosing
Life expectancy	Coping mechanisms for complicated medical regimens
Advance directives	Availability of lower cost medications or financial assistance
Advice for family members in the event of a cardiac emergency	**Importance of Compliance with Cardiac Risk Factor Reduction and Treatment Plan**

education material can be very useful in clarifying information and enhancing the understanding of heart failure and its management. A list of suggested topics for discussion is presented in Table 7–3.

It is impossible for patients to absorb all the information they need to have while in the CCU. Much of the information provided by nurses and physicians in the CCU will have to be repeated in an outpatient setting. Visiting or home-health nurses can be especially useful in clarifying misconceptions and encouraging compliance with the complicated regimen entailed in treating heart failure.

Chapter 8

Electrocardiographic Interpretation of Arrhythmias

Arrhythmias may occur without noticeable symptoms or cause the severe symptoms that accompany an extremely low cardiac output or myocardial ischemia. Because they can be identified specifically only by means of an ECG, it is absolutely essential for the CCU nurse to acquire a basic, usable knowledge of electrocardiography as it pertains to the recognition of arrhythmias. The object of this and the following chapters is to describe the electrocardiographic basis for detecting and interpreting arrhythmias.

FUNDAMENTALS OF ELECTROCARDIOGRAPHY

Disorders of heart rhythm result from an alteration in cardiac impulse formation, impulse conduction, or both.

Impulse Formation

Each normal heartbeat is the result of an electrical impulse that originates in a specialized area in the wall of the right atrium called the sinoatrial (SA) node. This island of tissue serves as a "battery" for the heart and normally discharges an electrical force at a rate of 60 to 100 times per minute in rhythmic fashion. Because the SA node controls the heart rate, it is designated the *pacemaker*. Most other areas of the heart also have the potential ability to initiate impulses (an inherent property of cardiac muscle), but they assume this role only under abnormal circumstances. Whenever the SA node is displaced as the

pacemaker, the new site of impulse formation is called an *ectopic pacemaker.*

Impulse Conduction

Each original impulse from the SA node is transmitted from the atria to the ventricles along a network of specialized cells called the *conduction system.* When the impulse reaches and stimulates the ventricular muscles, myocardial contraction occurs.

The pathways of electrical conduction from the SA node to the contractile tissues of the ventricle are shown in Figure 8–1. The His-bundle system delivers the wave of depolarization to the endocardial surfaces of both ventricles, where it spreads to the ventricular myocardium by the Purkinje fibers. The Purkinje fibers are small fibers that penetrate the ventricular myocardium, conducting the electrical impulses rapidly.

The Cardiac Cycle

When an impulse from the SA node (or an ectopic pacemaker) stimulates the cells of the myocardium, it causes them to discharge electrical forces that have been stored across their cell membranes. This electrical process is called *depolarization,* and results in myocardial contraction. Following depolarization, the myocardial cells recover and have their electrical charges restored. This recovery process is called *repolarization.* Under normal circumstances the next impulse from the SA node arrives when repolarization has been completed, after which activation of the

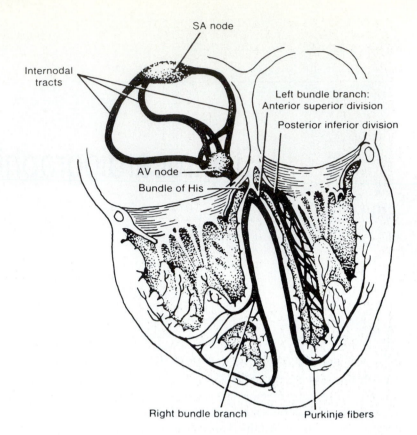

Figure 8–1. The conduction system of the heart. (Reproduced with permission from Greene HL, Humphries JC. Cardiac arrhythmias. In: Harvey AM, Johns RJ, MsKusick VA, et al, eds. *Principles and Practice of Medicine.* New York: Appleton-Century-Crofts, 1980.)

myocardial and Purkinje-fiber cells can occur again. The combined periods of stimulation (depolarization) and recovery (repolarization) constitute the electrical events of the cardiac cycle. The discharge and storage of electrical forces within the myocardial cells during depolarization and repolarization are associated with a chemical process involving the exchange of sodium and potassium ions across the cell membrane.

THE ELECTROCARDIOGRAM

The electrical activity associated with the depolarization and repolarization of cardiac muscle can be recorded and analyzed by means of electrocardiography. The basis of this technique is that electrical currents emanating from the heart are transmitted through surrounding tissues to the body surface, where they can be detected by electrodes placed on the extremities (or the chest wall). These electrical forces are then directed through a sensitive galvanometer (the basic component of an electrocardiograph machine), which produces a series of upward and downward deflections according to changes in the heart's electrical activity. The resulting waves

are then amplified (for greater visibility) before being inscribed on a moving strip of graph paper in the recording known as an electrocardiogram (ECG). Analysis of the wave forms in the ECG permits the identification of cardiac arrhythmias and the diagnosis of AMI (among many other conditions).

Electrocardiography Leads

Because the electrical forces generated in the heart create currents that travel in multiple directions simultaneously, it is necessary to record the flow of current in several different planes if a comprehensive view of the heart's electrical activity is to be obtained. The three major planes for detecting the electrical activity of the heart are called lead I, lead II, and lead III. The currents in these planes are recorded by placing electrodes on the right arm, left arm, and left leg. (In practice, a fourth electrode is placed on the right leg; it serves as a ground electrode and is not a part of an electrical lead.) Each of the three ECG leads records the difference in electrical forces between two electrode sites. As shown in Figure 8–2, lead I is derived from electrodes on the right arm and left arm; lead II from electrodes on the right arm and left leg; and lead

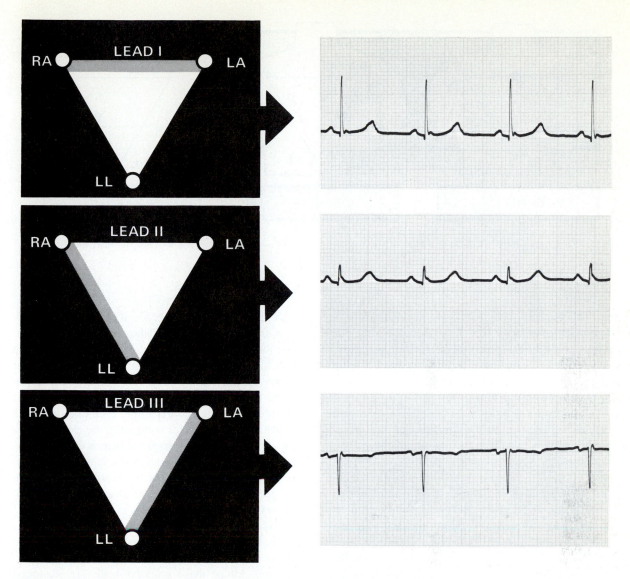

Figure 8–2. Electrocardiographic patterns as recorded from leads I, II, and III. RA, right arm; LA, left arm; LL, left leg.

III from electrodes on the left arm and left leg. From an electrical standpoint, these three leads form a hypothetical triangle (called the Einthoven triangle) with the heart in its center. In other words, each lead is electrically equidistant from the heart.

Since these leads record electrical forces in three different planes, it is understandable that an ECG obtained from each of the leads will have a different appearance. An example of the variation of electrocardiographic patterns in leads I, II, and III (recorded simultaneously) is shown in Figure 8–2.

To understand why the electrocardiographic deflections (waves) differ in the three ECG leads, it is necessary to consider briefly a fundamental principle of electricity: electrical current flows between two poles (or electrodes), one of which is positive (+) and the other negative (−). The respective positions of the positive (+) and negative (−) poles or electrodes in ECG leads I, II, and III are shown in Figure 8–3. Consequently, the deflections (waves) observed in an ECG depend on which lead is recorded. When the current flows toward a positive pole, the electrocardiograph will record an upward (positive) deflection in the ECG tracing (Figure 8–4). Conversely, when the current flows away from a positive electrode, the electrocardiograph will record a downward (negative) deflection (Figure 8–5).

The 12-Lead Electrocardiogram

A complete (12-lead) ECG consists of three standard (limb) leads, three augmented leads, and six chest (precordial) leads. When the ECG was first invented, the recording was made by dunking the patient's arms and legs into large buckets of electrolyte solu-

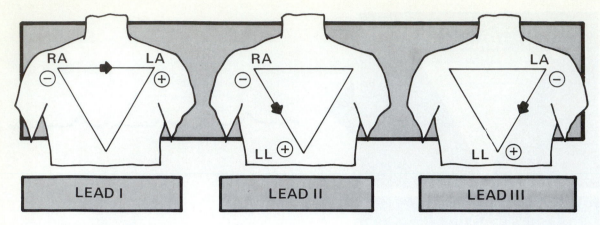

Figure 8–3. Positions of positive (+) and negative (−) electrodes for leads I, II, and III.

tion. The buckets were wired to the electrocardiograph machine and provided an assessment of the difference in electrical potential between the various limbs. Luckily for patients, technology has come up with a less cumbersome technique, using electrodes placed directly on the skin.

ECG leads I, II, and III, known as standard leads, are *bipolar* leads. This means that they measure the *difference* in electrical potential between two recording sites. Lead I measures the difference in potential between the right-arm and left-arm electrodes. Lead II measures the difference in potential between the right-arm and left-leg electrodes, while lead III measures the difference between the left-arm and left-leg electrodes.

The development of *unipolar* ECG leads (in the early 1930s) permitted the routine measurement of actual electrical potentials at various electrode sites, and in doing so expanded the scope and accuracy of the electrocardiographic diagnosis of ischemia and arrhythmias.

The concept of unipolar leads is as follows: the heart is considered to lie in the center of the equilateral triangle (described earlier) formed by the three limb leads of the ECG. Although the direction and magnitude of the electrical forces generated by the

heart differ in these three leads, these differences balance each other, so that if they are added together, their sum at any moment is zero. Thus, if the three limb leads are connected to a neutral electrode (or central terminal, as it is also called) the electrical potential of neutral electrode will be zero. Since this electrode has no electrical force, it can be used as a standard of reference for comparing the electrical potentials at other sites, which are detected with an exploring electrode (see Figure 8–6). It is this arrangement, in which there is a zero-potential electrode at one end and an exploring electrode at the other, that is described as a unipolar lead.

The exploring electrode of the unipolar-lead system is attached to the limbs and to the chest wall to record actual electrical potentials from these particular sites. All of these unipolar leads are identified (prefaced) by the letter V, and are called *V leads*. Unipolar leads recorded from the extremities are of low voltage and are therefore electrically augmented for ECG recording. Hence, unipolar limb leads are called *augmented unipolar leads* and are designated by the symbol aV ("a" standing for "augmented" and "V" for "unipolar"). There are three augmented unipolar limb leads: aVR (right arm), aVL (left arm),

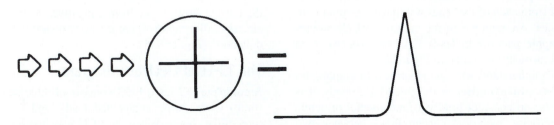

Figure 8–4. The relationship of current flow and inscription on an ECG. When the current flow is toward the positive pole, the ECG will record a positive (upward) deflection.

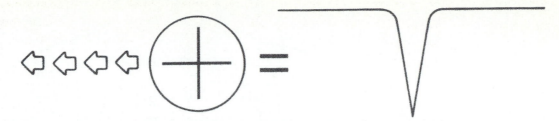

Figure 8–5. The relationship of current flow and inscription on an ECG when the current flow is toward the negative pole. The electrocardiogram records a negative (downward) deflection.

and aVF (left leg). The six unipolar leads recorded from the chest (precordium) are designated V1 to V6, depending on the particular location of the electrode on the chest wall (Figure 8–7).

Thus, the complete 12-lead ECG consists of the three standard limb or bipolar leads (I, II, and III), three modified (augmented) unipolar leads (aVR, aVL, and aVF), and six unipolar leads positioned across the chest wall (V1–V6). A full 12-lead ECG is reproduced in Figure 8–8. Note that each lead produces a different electrocardiographic pattern because of the differences in the electrode positions.

Each of the 12 leads of the ECG has a positive electrode. As described earlier, the position of this electrode affects the direction in which the wave forms are deflected on the ECG. The average of the electrical forces generated during atrial or ventricular depolarization is called the *electrical axis* of depolarization. If this axis is in the direction of the positive electrode of a particular lead, a positive deflection will be inscribed in the ECG. If the electrical axis is directed away from the positive electrode, a negative deflection will be recorded. If the electrical axis runs perpendicularly to the axis of a lead, no deflection will be recorded.

Monitoring Leads

Cardiac monitors depict one or more electrocardiographic leads. Lead II is often chosen as a monitoring lead because the normal axis of cardiac depolarization is in the same direction as the axis of this lead (ie, the positive electrode in lead II is on the left leg and the mean axis of depolarization in the heart [runs from the base (top) to the apex (bottom) of the heart toward the left leg]). Both atrial and ventricular depolarization are easily seen in lead II.

A modified chest electrode position is used as a second monitoring lead or (in the case of a single-lead monitoring system) as an alternate lead. The positive electrode is this lead is usually placed at the fourth intercostal space at the right sternal border, so that it is equivalent to lead V1. This lead is called modified chest lead 1 (MCL$_1$). It is particularly useful for monitoring ischemic changes in the myocardium.

While lead II and MCL$_1$ are the two most useful ECG leads for detecting the majority of arrhythmias, they can by no means reveal all disturbances in cardiac rhythm. It is important to recognize this limitation of cardiac monitoring, and to understand that

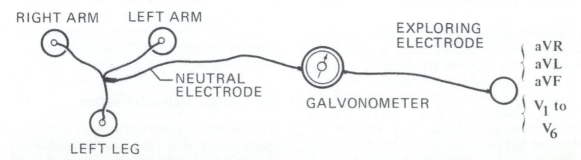

Figure 8–6. Arrangement for a unipolar lead. The exploring electrode is attached to the limbs (lead aVR, aVL, and aVF) and the chest wall (leads V1–V6).

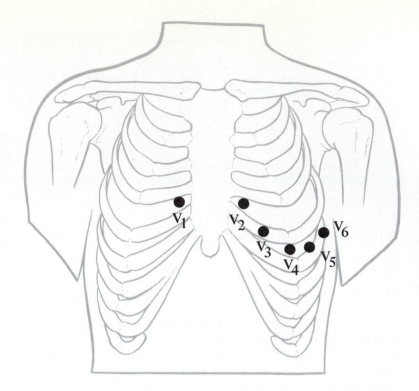

Figure 8–7. Location of unipolar chest leads (V1–V6).

when the interpretation of an arrhythmia is in doubt, the chest leads may have to be repositioned (to obtain a more distinctive lead) or a 12-lead ECG recorded.

It must also be understood that the ECG seen on the monitor will depend on which particular lead is being used; therefore, attempting simply to memorize certain patterns as a means of identifying arrhythmias is of no avail. For example, the ECGs shown in Figure 8–9 were recorded simultaneously from lead II and MCL_1. The difference in the appearance of the wave forms in the two leads makes it readily apparent that memorizing patterns is not a useful way to learn the interpretation of arrhythmias.

ELECTROCARDIOGRAPHIC WAVE FORMS

The electrical activity during the cardiac cycle is characterized by five separate waves or deflections, designated as P, Q, R, S, and T (these letters were arbitrarily selected and have no additional meaning). Before considering the meaning of each of these deflections, it is necessary to discuss two key features of electrocardiographic waves: their amplitude (or voltage) and their duration.

The *amplitude* (voltage) of a wave is measured by a series of horizontal lines on the ECG. Each horizontal line is 1 millimeter apart and represents one-

tenth of a millivolt (the basic unit of intensity of the heart's electrical activity). In Figure 8–10, for example, we see that the deflection extends seven lines (7 millimeters) above the baseline; this indicates that the voltage of the wave is 0.7 millivolt. The amplitude of the wave reflects only its voltage, or electrical magnitude, and has no relation to the muscular strength of ventricular contraction.

The *duration* of a wave is measured by a series of vertical lines, also 1 millimeter apart. The time interval between each vertical line is 0.04 second because the paper used in ECG recording travels at 25 mm/second. Accordingly, the width of the first deflection (the QRS complex) shown in Figure 8.10 extends for 2 millimeters and represents 0.08 second (0.04×2).

To simplify the measurement of the wave forms in the ECG, every fifth line, both horizontally and vertically, is inscribed boldly, producing a series of large squares. These large squares thus represent 0.5 millivolt vertically and 0.20 second horizontally, as shown in Figure 8–11.

The Normal Electrocardiogram

A normal ECG consists of a series of five successive waves. The P wave represents electrical activation (depolarization) of the atria; the QRS complex represents depolorization of the ventricles; and the T wave reflects recovery (repolarization) of the ventricles.

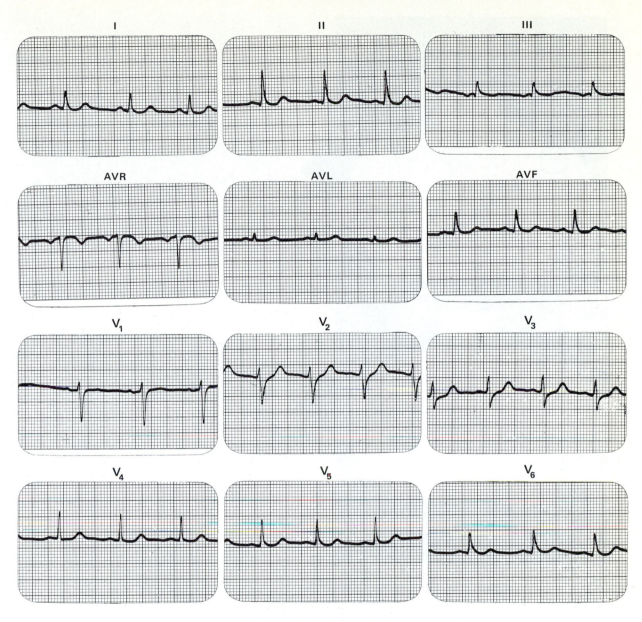

Figure 8–8. A 12-lead ECG.

The atria also have a recovery period, but the wave for atrial repolarization is hidden in the QRS complex. The distances between the waves in the ECG are called intervals or segments (eg, the *PR interval,* the *ST segment,* and the *QT interval*). The configuration of one complete ECG complex demonstrating both the waves and intervals normally seen in the ECG is shown in Figure 8–12.

P Wave. The P wave represents the electrical activity associated with the original impulse emanating from the SA node and its passage through the atria. If P waves are present in the ECG and are of normal size and shape, it can be assumed that the

stimulus for cardiac contraction began in the SA node. Absence or abnormal positioning of these waves implies that the impulse for contraction originated outside the SA node. Therefore, the identification of P waves is of critical importance in differentiating normal sinus rhythm from *ectopic rhythms.*

P–R Interval. The period from the beginning of the P wave to the beginning of the QRS complex is designated the P–R interval. It represents the time taken for an original impulse to pass from the SA node through the atria and AV node and to the ventricles.

With normal conduction the duration of this in-

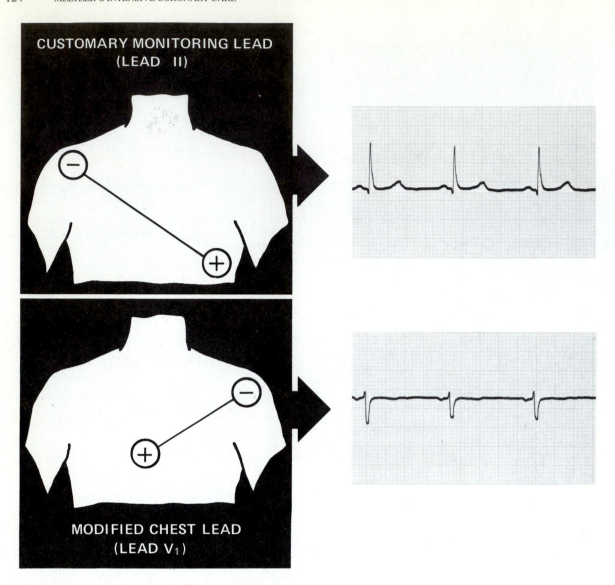

Figure 8–9. ECGs recorded simultaneously from Lead II and MCL₁.

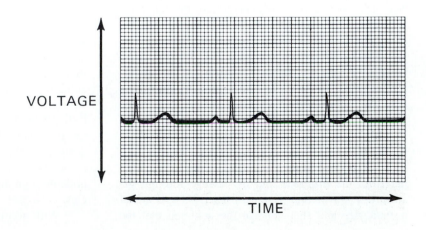

Figure 8–10. Relationship between voltage and time in ECG.

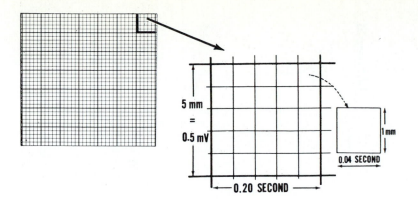

Figure 8–11. Electrocardiographic measurements.

terval is from 0.12 to 0.20 second. If the duration of the P–R interval exceeds 0.20 second it can be reasoned that a conduction delay (block) exists in the area of the AV node (or less likely, below the AV node). In some instances the P–R interval is unusually short (less than 0.10 second).

A shortened P-R interval may indicate that an impulse has reached the ventricle through a shorter-than-normal *(accessory)* pathway. Abnormally short P–R intervals are observed in the Wolff-Parkinson-White syndrome and the Lown-Ganong-Levine syndrome (as described in Chapter 13, on conduction disorders). An accessory pathway provides a connection between the atria and ventricles that bypasses the AV node and therefore stimulates the ventricles prematurely. Syndromes characterized by accessory conduction pathways are also known as *pre-excitation syndromes.*

A junctional rhythm is generated in the area of the AV node instead of the SA node. In the case of a junctional rhythm, the atria are depolarized in a retrograde direction. The P wave may be inverted or buried in the QRS. Depending on where in the AV node it generated a junctional rhythm, it can cause a shortened P–R interval.

QRS Complex. The waves of the QRS complex represent depolarization of the ventricular muscle. The depolarization process starts at the endocardium of the ventricle and progresses outward to the epicardial surface. This results in a complex consisting of an initial downward deflection (Q wave), a tall upward deflection (R wave), and a second downward deflection (S wave). These three deflections comprising the QRS complex vary in size according to the lead being

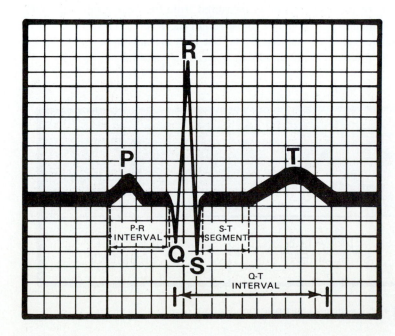

Figure 8–12. Normal cardiac cycle on the ECG.

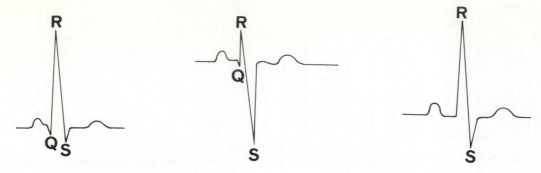

Figure 8–13. Various configurations of the QRS complex.

recorded. There may, for example, be a tall R wave and a small S wave (Figure 8–13A) or a small R wave and a deep S wave (Figure 8–13B). In many instances, again depending on lead placement, one or more of the three components of the QRS complex may not be seen. The complex shown in Figure 8–13C, for example, does not include a Q wave.

The QRS interval is measured from the beginning of the Q wave to the end of the S wave. (If a Q wave, R wave, or S wave is absent, the QRS complex is measured from the beginning to the end of the remaining waves.) The normal duration of the QRS complex is always less than 0.12 second. A duration of the complex of 0.12 second or more indicates that the ventricles have been stimulated in a delayed or abnormal manner (eg, a bundle branch block).

ST Segment. The ST segment of the ECG reflects the period between the completion of depolarization and the beginning of repolarization (recovery) of the ventricular cells. Normally this segment is *isoelectric,* meaning that it is neither elevated nor depressed, because the positive and negative electrical forces

within the ventricular myocardium are equal to one another during this period. Elevation or depression of the ST segment indicates an abnormality in the onset of recovery of the ventricular muscle, usually because of injury (eg, acute myocardial infarction or ischemia). Examples of isoelectric, depressed, and elevated ST segments are shown in Figure 8–14.

T Wave. The T wave represents the major portion of the recovery phase after ventricular depolarization. Any condition that interferes with normal ventricular repolarization (eg, myocardial ischemia) may cause T-wave inversion. Examples of inverted T waves are shown in Figure 8–15.

Q-T Interval. The Q-T interval defines the total duration of the combined phases of depolarization and repolarization of the ventricular muscle. In other words, it represents the total period of ventricular stimulation and recovery (see Figure 8–12). The Q-T interval is measured from the beginning of the QRS complex to the end of the T wave. The interval varies with heart rate, but with normal sinus rhythm its duration seldom exceeds 0.40 second.

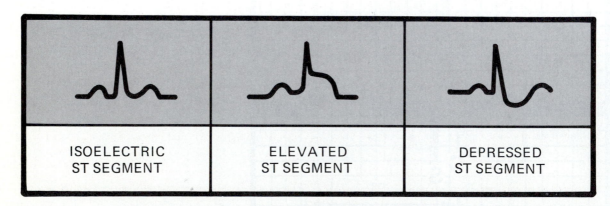

Figure 8–14. ST segment morphology (form).

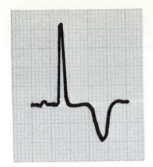
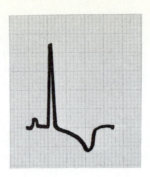
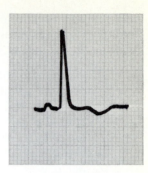

Figure 8–15. Illustrations of inverted T waves.

SIGNIFICANCE OF THE ELECTROCARDIOGRAM

Analyzing the wave forms and intervals just described permits certain deductions to be made that offer indirect information about the heart. It is important to realize that the ECG does not depict the actual physical condition of the heart or its function; it simply reveals the electrical activity of the heart. Thus, an ECG may be normal in the presence of heart disease unless the disease process disturbs the electrical forces within the heart. In the case of a patient with coronary atherosclerosis that has not produced myocardial ischemia or injury, for example, no abnormality will be seen in the ECG.

The ECG, however, can be correlated with the systolic and diastolic phases of ventricular action, as shown in Figure 8–16. Note that ventricular contrac-

tion (systole) begins at the peak of the QRS complex, after electrical stimulation has occurred, and ends near the completion of the T wave. Diastole commences at this time and continues until the next R wave.

Although electrocardiography has many valuable uses in clinical practice, its major importance is in the identification of abnormal cardiac rhythms (Chapters 9 through 13), the diagnosis of AMI (Chapter 14), and the evaluation of thrombolytic therapy.

The Normal Electrocardiogram

A normal cardiac mechanism is characterized by normal sinus rhythm and normal conduction of impulses. *Normal sinus rhythm* means that the SA node controls the heart beat, discharging impulses regularly at a rate of 60 to 100 per minute. *Normal conduction* indicates that there is no obstruction to or delay in the

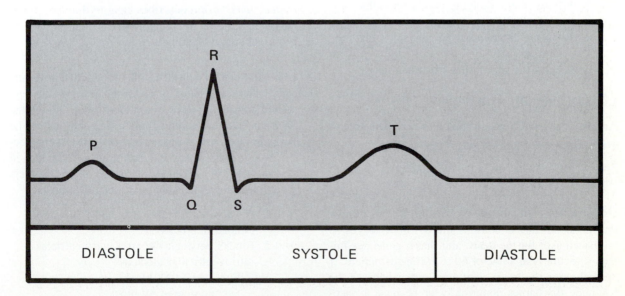

Figure 8–16. Relationship of the ECG to diastole and systole.

passage of impulses from the SA node through the AV node and ventricles. Therefore, among the main features of a normal ECG are:

1. A heart rate within the normal range of 60 to 100 per minute
2. Regularity of the cardiac rhythm
3. Normal P waves, each of which is followed by a ventricular (QRS) complex
4. A P-R interval of 0.12 to 0.20 second in duration
5. A QRS complex ranging from 0.04 to 0.12 second in duration, indicating that impulses from the SA node are reaching both ventricles on schedule.

ARRHYTHMIAS

When the heart rate, rhythm, or conduction fails to conform to normal standards, the resulting disorder is called an *arrhythmia*. In a strict sense, the term "arrhythmia" indicates an absence of rhythm, and, therefore, might be restricted to only the disorders that are characterized by irregular rhythms. In practice, however, the term has been used collectively for many years to describe all clinical disorders affecting the heart beat, including disturbances in rate, rhythm, and conduction. The term *dysrhythmia* is more appropriate and should be used instead, but the more common usage has been adopted here.

When confronted with an arrhythmia, the nurse should ask the following questions:

1. What is the rhythm?
2. What is the mechanism that caused it?
3. What is the underlying condition(s) that provoked it?
4. What are the symptoms and signs that accompany it?
5. What is the appropriate treatment for it?

Classification of Arrhythmias

Arrhythmias can be categorized into two main groups according to their underlying mechanism:

1. Disturbances in impulse formation
2. Disturbances in impulse conduction

Disturbances in Impulse Formation. We know that under normal conditions the SA node serves as the pacemaker for the heart, and that it generates impulses regularly at a rate of 60 to 100 beats/minute. If normal sinus rhythm is disrupted, either because the SA node discharges abnormally or because a pacemaker at another site (an ectopic pacemaker) gains

control of the heartbeat, the resulting disorder is called a *disturbance in impulse formation.*

Arrhythmias in this category are classified according to the site of impulse formation, as follows:

1. Disturbances arising in the SA node (sinus rhythms)
2. Disturbances arising in the atria (atrial arrhythmias)
3. Disturbances arising in the AV junction (AV junctional arrhythmias)
4. Disturbances arising in the ventricle (ventricular arrhythmias)

These disorders of impulse formation may be further subdivided according to the mechanism of the arrhythmia. There are six major arrhythmic mechanisms, as follows:

1. Tachycardia (heart rate greater than 100/minute)
2. Bradycardia (heart rate less than 60/minute)
3. Premature (ectopic) beats
4. Escape beats
5. Flutter
6. Fibrillation

On the basis of this combined classification (involving the site of impulse formation and mechanism of arrhythmia), the term *sinus tachycardia* indicates that its causative impulse originates in the SA node but produces a heart rate exceeding 100/minute (tachycardia). By contrast, the term *ventricular tachycardia* signifies impulses that originate in the ventricles (rather than the SA node), again at a rate exceeding 100/minute. Similarly, the term *supraventricular tachycardia* describes an arrhythmia originating in the atria or AV junction and which produces a heart rate above 100/minute.

Disturbances of Conduction. A conduction disturbance refers to a block or abnormal delay in the passage of cardiac impulses from the SA node through the AV node and left and right bundle branches and to the Purkinje-fiber system in the ventricles. Blocks may occur at any point along the course of the conduction system, but it is customary to classify these disorders according to three main anatomic sites, as follows:

1. Blocks within the SA node or atria (sinoatrial blocks)
2. Blocks between the atria and ventricles (atrioventricular blocks)
    First-degree AV block
    Second-degree AV block
    Third-degree (complete) AV block

3. Blocks within the ventricles (intraventricular blocks)
    Left bundle branch blocks
    Right bundle branch blocks
    Bilateral bundle branch blocks
    Ventricular asystole

CLASSIFICATION OF ARRHYTHMIAS BY PROGNOSIS

In addition to the method just described, arrhythmias can also be classified in a general way (but not categorically) according to their seriousness or prognosis. This division of arrhythmias is useful to nurses caring for patients with heart disease, since it considers the relative importance of various arrhythmias from a clinical standpoint. It is essential to realize, however, that this classification is only a broad index and is not truly dependable in assessing the actual prognosis in an individual case of arrhythmia. Using this classification, three prognostic categories of arrhythmias can be established:

1. *Minor arrhythmias.* These disorders are not of **immediate** concern because they usually do not affect the circulation, nor do they warn of the development of more serious arrhythmias.
2. *Major arrhythmias.* These disturbances either reduce the pumping efficiency of the heart or herald the onset of lethal arrhythmias. They require prompt treatment.
3. *Lethal arrhythmias.* These arrhythmias require immediate resuscitation in order to prevent death.

The classification of arrhythmias according to their seriousness or prognosis is shown in Table 8–1.

Interpretation of Arrhythmias from the Electrocardiogram

Electrocardiographic interpretation of specific arrhythmias involves a deliberate analysis of cardiac rate, rhythm, and conduction. Most arrhythmias can be correctly identified by following the five basic steps described below. Attempting to interpret arrhythmias without adhering to this type of orderly process can only lead to confusion and error.

Step 1. Calculate the Heart Rate.
Three methods may be used to determine the heart rate from the ECG:

1. Count the number of R waves in a 6-second strip of the ECG tracing. Multiply this number by 10 to get the heart

TABLE 8–1. CLASSIFICATION OF ARRHYTHMIAS ACCORDING TO PROGNOSIS

Minor Arrhythmias
    Sinus tachycardia
    Sinus bradycardia
    Sinus arrhythmia
    Wandering pacemaker
    Premature atrial contractions
    Premature junctional contractions
    Premature ventricular contractions (infrequent)

Major Arrhythmias
    Sinus tachycardia (when persistent)
    Sinus bradycardia (rate < 50/minute)
    Sick sinus syndrome
    Sinoatrial arrest (and SA block)
    Paroxysmal supraventricular tachycardia
    Atrial flutter
    Atrial fibrillation
    Premature junctional contractions
    Junctional rhythm
    Paroxysmal junctional tachycardia
    Nonparoxysmal junctional tachycardia (accelerated junctional rhythm)
    Premature ventricular contractions (when frequent)
    Accelerated idioventricular rhythm
    First-degree AV heart block
    Second-degree AV heart block
    Third-degree AV heart block
    Intraventricular blocks (bundle branch blocks)

Lethal Arrhythmias
    Ventricular tachycardia
    Ventricular fibrillation
    Ventricular asystole

rate per minute. Since all electrocardiography paper is marked at 3-second intervals (along the top margin), the approximate heart rate can be estimated very quickly with this simple method, as shown in Figure 8–17. The 6-second ECG strip contains nine R waves. Therefore the heart rate is approximately 90/minute (9 × 10).

2. Place a commercially available rate calculator, which measures the distance between R waves, on the ECG and read the heart rate directly from the rate scale.

3. Count the number of large squares between two R waves and divide this sum into 300 to obtain the rate per minute. For example, the ECG shown in Figure 8–18 has four large squares between two consecutive R waves. Dividing 300 by 4 indicates that the heart rate is 75/minute. Three large squares would

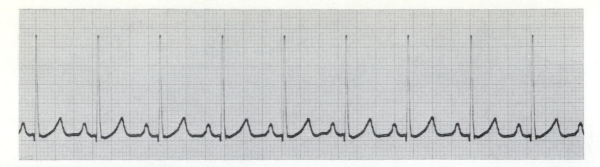

Figure 8–17. Calculation of heart rate from the ECG.

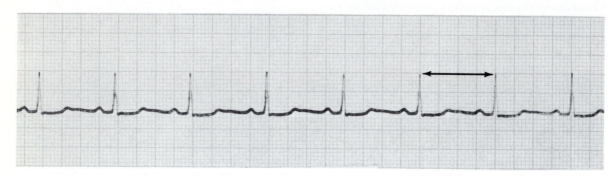

Figure 8–18. Normal ECG of lead II. The arrow demonstrates four large squares (each square = 0.20 second) between R waves.

indicate a heart rate of 100/minute. Two large squares would indicate a heart rate of 150/minute.

On the basis of heart rate determination alone, arrhythmias can be classified as: (1) slow rate or *bradyarrhythmias,* in which there are less than 60 beats/minute; (2) normal-rate arrhythmias, in which the rate is between 60 and 100 beats/minute; and (3) fast-rate or *tachyarrhythmias,* in which there are more than 100 beats/ minute. Since many arrhythmias are characterized only by changes in rate, rate calculation is essential in interpreting any ECG.

Step 2. Determine the Regularity (Rhythm) of the R Waves. The regularity of the heart beat can often be determined by simply looking at the ECG: If the R–R intervals are equal, without any obvious variation in their length, it can be concluded that the ventricular rhythm is regular. In many instances, however, scanning is unreliable and it is necessary to measure the R–R intervals precisely with ECG calipers to ascertain whether the R waves are in fact regular. When the difference between R–R intervals is more than 0.12 second, the ventricular rhythm is

described as abnormal or irregular. Many arrhythmias are characterized by either regular or irregular rhythms, and this single finding is therefore an important step in the process of interpretating arrhythmias. An example of a regular ventricular rhythm is shown in Figure 8–19. Note that there are 19 small squares between each R wave.

An example of an irregular ventricular rhythm is depicted in Figure 8–20. The R–R intervals vary from 1.02 second to 1.40 second.

Step 3. Identify and Examine the P Waves. Although usually less conspicuous than the other waves of the cardiac cycle, P waves often provide more information than any of the other ECG wave forms about the type and mechanism of a cardiac arrhythmia. For this reason it is mandatory to search for P waves and to examine their size, shape, and position. A normal P wave (as seen in lead II) is upright, smoothly rounded, and precedes each QRS complex. These findings indicate that the heart beat originates in the SA node and sinus rhythm is present. In contrast, the absence of P waves or an abnormality in their configuration or position indicates that impulses are arising outside the SA node and that

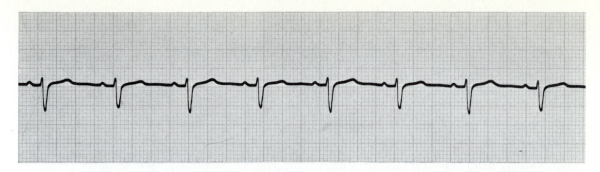

Figure 8–19. An example of a regular ventricular rhythm.

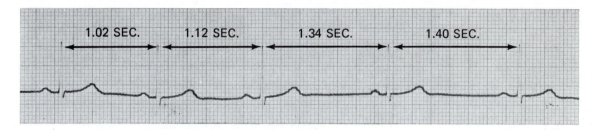

Figure 8–20. An example of an irregular ventricular rhythm.

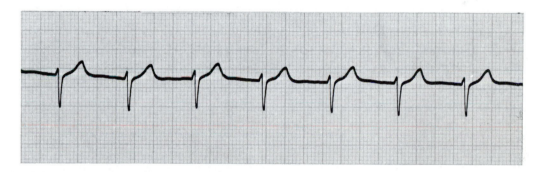

Figure 8–21. Rhythm strip demonstrating absence of P waves.

an ectopic pacemaker is in control of the heart rhythm. In Figure 8–21 the P waves cannot be identified, reflecting an ectopic pacemaker below the SA node.

Step 4. Measure the P–R Interval. Normally the duration of this interval should be between 0.12 and 0.20 second. Prolongation of the P–R interval beyond 0.20 second indicates a delay in the passage of impulses from the SA node to the ventricle. Conversely, a P–R interval of less than 0.12 second indicates that impulses from the SA node are reaching the ventricles sooner than expected, through an abnormal pathway (ie, an accessory pathway). The P–R interval of the ECG shown in Figure 8–22 is within normal limits (0.16 second).

Step 5. Measure the Duration of the QRS Complexes. The width of the QRS complex represents the time required for a stimulus to activate both ventricles. The normal duration of the QRS complex is no more than 0.12 second. If there is an obstruction in one of the bundle branches, activation of the ventricles will be delayed, as manifested electrocardiographically by widening of the QRS complex beyond 0.10 second. Two examples of abnormally widened (beyond 0.12 second) QRS complexes are depicted in Figures 8–23 and 8–24.

Interpretation of Specific Arrhythmias

The application of the five-step process just described for identifying and interpreting specific arrhyth-

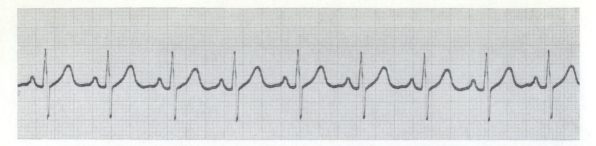

Figure 8–22. The P-R interval in this ECG is within normal limits, at 0.16 second.

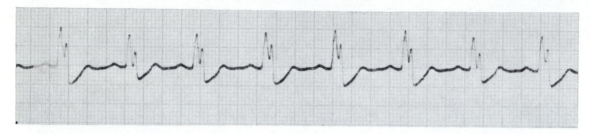

Figure 8–23. The QRS complex is abnormally wide, at more than 0.12 second.

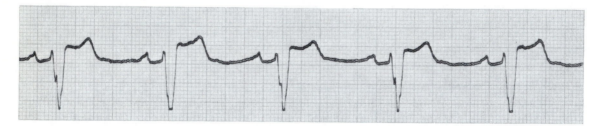

Figure 8–24. An abnormally wide QRS complex, of more than 0.12 second.

mias is considered in the following paragraphs, using the ECG shown in Figure 8–25 as the first example.

Analysis of ECG

1. *Heart rate.* There are four R waves in the 6-second ECG strip. This means that the heart rate is approximately 40/minute. (Since the R–R intervals consist of 37 small squares, the heart rate, according to the rate conversion table, is actually 41/minute.)
2. *Rhythm.* The R–R intervals are essentially equal (varying by only one small square, a normal finding). We know therefore that this arrhythmia is marked by a regular rhythm.
3. *P waves.* A P wave occurs before each QRS complex and is normal in configu-

ration. This indicates that the impulses originated in the SA node.

4. *P-R interval.* This interval measures 0.16 second (four small squares), which is within normal limits (0.12–0.20 second). Consequently, we can infer that conduction from the SA node to the ventricles is not disturbed.
5. *QRS complexes.* These complexes of ventricular activation measure 0.06 second, indicating that there is no conduction disorder in the bundle branches or the Purkinje network.

Interpretation. Analyzing the foregoing facts, we can conclude that the only abnormality detected in the ECG is a rate of about 40/minute, which is distinctly below the lower limits of normal (60/minute). Since there are no disturbances in conduction (both

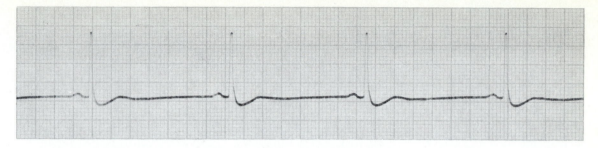

Figure 8–25. Rhythm strip for analysis.

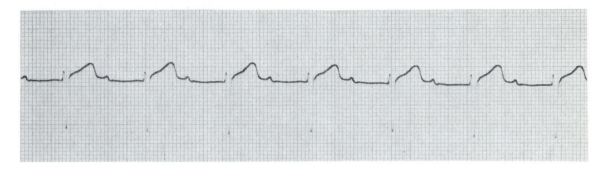

Figure 8–26. Rhythm strip for analysis.

the P–R interval and the QRS complexes are normal), we know that the slow heart rate is due to a disturbance in impulse formation. The presence of a normal P wave before each QRS complex tells us that the site of impulse formation is in the SA node itself. However, the SA node is discharging too slowly, which accounts for the heart rate of 40/minute. Thus the interpretation of this arrhythmia is *sinus bradycardia.*

Another demonstration of the five basic steps used in arrhythmia interpretation is presented in Figure 8–26.

Analysis of ECG

1. *Heart rate.* That there are seven R waves in 6 seconds indicates that the heart rate is approximately 70/minute. (Since the R–R intervals comprise 21 small squares, the precise heart rate is 72/ minute.)
2. *Rhythm.* The R waves occur at very regular intervals and therefore the rhythm can be categorized as regular.
3. *P waves.* A normal P wave precedes each QRS complex, indicating a sinus rhythm.

4. *P–R interval.* The time from the beginning of a P wave to the onset of a QRS complex is 0.44 second (11 small squares). This interval is markedly prolonged, far exceeding the maximum normal P–R interval (0.20 second).
5. *QRS complexes.* These complexes are 0.06 second in duration and show no abnormalities.

Interpretation. On the basis of the information obtained from the ECG, it can be concluded that impulse formation is normal: the impulses originate in the SA node at a rate of 70/minute, with a regular rhythm that is the criterion of normal sinus rhythm. However, conduction is not normal: the P–R interval is distinctly prolonged (0.44 second), indicating a delay in the passage of impulses somewhere between the SA node and the ventricles. Since the QRS complexes are of normal duration (0.06 second), we know that once the delayed impulses reach the bundle branches, they proceed normally and stimulate the ventricles. The delay is at the level of the AV node. This particular disturbance in conduction is called a first-degree atrioventricular (AV) block, the details of which are described in later chapters.

Chapter 9

Arrhythmias Originating in the Sinoatrial Node

SINUS TACHYCARDIA
SINUS BRADYCARDIA
SICK SINUS SYNDROME
WANDERING PACEMAKER
SINOATRIAL ARREST (AND SA BLOCK)

The group of arrhythmias named above results from disturbances of impulse formation in the SA node.

In these arrhythmias, the SA node retains its normal role as the cardiac pacemaker, but instead of discharging impulses from 60 to 100 times/minute at regular intervals, it discharges them at a rate that either exceeds 100/minute (sinus tachycardia) or is below 60/minute (sinus bradycardia), or does not discharge rhythmically (sick sinus syndrome). In some instances the pacemaker site wanders from the SA node to nearby areas (wandering pacemaker). The arrhythmia that results from failure of the SA node to discharge an impulse at the expected time is called sinus arrest, and leads to an escape rhythm by more distal latent pacemakers (in the AV node or ventricles).

Impulse formation in the SA mode is under the control of the sympathetic and parasympathetic nervous systems. Overactivity of one of these normally balanced forces leads to disturbances in heart rate, rhythm, or the site of impulse formation. When the sympathetic nervous system predominates, the heart rate accelerates, whereas control by the parasympathetic system (vagal influence) slows the heart rate.

Respiration causes a normal variant of sinus rhythm (termed sinus arrhythmia). The sinus rate increases during inspiration and decreases with expiration because of alterations in vagal tone.

The SA node itself is seldom the source of arrhythmic disturbances. However, coronary atherosclerosis or myocardial infarction can cause ischemic damage to the node. Sick sinus syndrome occurs when the function of the SA node is disturbed and the output from the node becomes highly variable, causing bradycardia alternating with tachycardia.

As a general rule, disorders of the SA node are not dangerous and their effects can be considered as minor arrhythmias. However, if the heart rate is very slow (less than 50/minute) or very fast (greater than 130/minute), the risk of more ominous arrhythmias is significantly increased.

SINUS TACHYCARDIA

Mechanism

As the cardiac pacemaker, the SA node may discharge impulses regularly at a rate exceeding 100/minute. This acceleration in heart rate often reflects overactivity of the sympathetic nervous system resulting from fever, anxiety, hyperthyroidism, or physical activity. Of greater importance is that sinus tachycardia may be a manifestation of heart failure. In this situation the heart rate increases through reflex mechanisms to compensate for reduced stroke volume.

Significance

1. Tachycardia tends to increase the work of the heart and its oxygen consumption. This may lead to heart failure, myocardial ischemia (angina), or an increase in the size of an infarction, particularly if the rapid rate is persistent.
2. *Risk:* The danger in sinus tachycardia depends primarily on the etiology of the rapid heart rate. The risk of complications from sinus tachycardia due to anxiety, fever, hyperthyroidism or physical activity, is usually not great. The danger is distinctly greater if sinus tachycardia develops as a consequence of heart failure or hypoxemia, in which case the prognosis varies with the cardiac reserve and the duration of the tachycardia.

Clinical Features

1. In most instances sinus tachycardia does not produce any symptoms. However, tachycardia that is very rapid or sustained may lead to angina or dyspnea.
2. The only pertinent physical finding in sinus tachycardia is a rapid, regular heart rate, usually of 100 to 150/minute. An ECG is required to distinguish sinus tachycardia from other tachyarrhythmias.
3. Sinus tachycardia terminates gradually, in contrast to other tachycardias (eg, paroxysmal supraventricular tachycardia), which cease abruptly.

ECG FEATURES IDENTIFYING SINUS TACHYCARDIA

1. Rate:	Usually 100 to 150 beats/minute.
2. Rhythm:	Regular.
3. P waves:	Normal, and precede each QRS complex.
4. P–R interval:	Normal, indicating that conduction from the SA node through the ventricles is not disturbed.
5. QRS:	Normal.

Sinus Tachycardia (Figure 9–1)

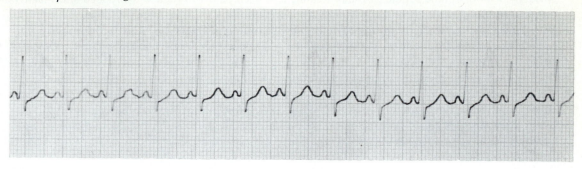

Rate:	About 130/minute (actual rate: 125/minute).
Rhythm:	Regular.
P waves:	Normal, and precede each QRS complex.
P–R interval:	Normal (0.12 second).
QRS:	Normal (duration 0.08 second).
Comment:	Other than the rapid heart rate, no abnormalities are present.

Sinus Tachycardia (Figure 9–2)

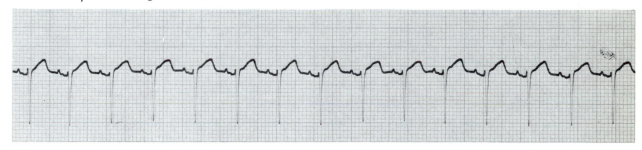

Rate:	About 140/minute (136/minute).
Rhythm:	Regular.
P waves:	Normal.
P–R interval:	Normal (0.12 second).
QRS:	Normal (0.04 second).
Comment:	Note the difference in the configuration of the QRS complexes in the two examples shown. The tracing shown in Figure 9–1 was recorded with a conventional monitoring lead (lead II), while the tracing in Figure 9–2 was recorded with a modified chest lead (MCL$_1$).

Treatment

1. The first step in treating sinus tachycardia is to identify its underlying cause rather than attempt to slow the heart rate. Always to be considered is the possibility that sinus tachycardia represents a sign of early left ventricular failure.
2. Once the cause of sinus tachycardia is recognized, treatment is directed at correcting the underlying problem. When the rapid rate is due to temperature elevation, aspirin may be effective, whereas thyroid surgery will reduce the heart rates in tachycardia secondary to hyperthyroidism. Patients bothered by tachycardia as a result of anxiety can be taught relaxation techniques.

3. It is vital to immediately treat chest pain from unstable angina or an evolving myocardial infarction (usually with morphine sulfate). Prompt treatment of such pain will reduce the related sinus tachycardia and avoid increasing myocardial oxygen consumption.

4. If a patient with ischemic heart disease and sinus tachycardia is highly anxious in relation to being admitted to the CCU, it may be wise to have family members stay. If this cannot be done, a tranquilizer or sedative may be indicated.

5. If sinus tachycardia produces ischemic pain, opiates should be given.

6. When sinus tachycardia is due to left ventricular failure, administration of digitalis is usually effective in controlling the heart rate (as well as increasing the force of myocardial contraction).

7. Drug therapy aimed solely at reducing the heart rate, without consideration of the underlying cause of sinus tachycardia, is ill advised.

Nursing Responsibility

1. Identify the rapid-rate arrhythmia as sinus tachycardia and document it with an ECG rhythm strip.

2. Examine the patient at regular intervals, always seeking possible causes for the arrhythmia (eg, pain, elevated temperature, apprehension).

3. When the source of sinus tachycardia cannot be readily identified, suspect the possibility of left ventricular failure and attempt to elicit other evidence of early heart failure (eg, orthopnea, cough, restlessness).

4. If the patient develops symptoms secondary to the arrhythmia, or if the clinical signs change, notify the physician.

5. Based on the identified cause, discuss the use of sedatives, tranquilizers, aspirin, or digitalis with the physician.

6. If anxiety seems to be the cause of sinus tachycardia, attempt to alleviate the emotional stress through nursing intervention.

CASE HISTORY

A 42-year-old male has been in the CCU for 2 days with a stable pulse rate ranging from 75 to 90/minute. An ECG showed an acute anterior infarction with normal sinus rhythm. The patient experienced chest pain (with an intensity of 6 on a scale in which 10 represented the most severe pain). The monitor showed sinus tachycardia at a rate of 130/minute. The nurse assessed the clinical condition of the patient and could find no significant change. A 12-lead ECG showed no changes from ECGs on the previous 2 days. The nurse immediately gave morphine sulfate as ordered for pain, and called the physician. The nurse also calmed the patient by talking with him, and continued to assess the patient's heart rate. One hour later the patient's pulse rate was 90/minute.

SINUS BRADYCARDIA

Mechanism

Sinus bradycardia exists when the SA node discharges regularly at a rate below 60/minute. The underlying cause of the slow rate is parasympathetic (vagal) dominance of the SA node. This can occur in well-trained athletes or elderly individuals. Patients with hypothermia (eg, immediately after coronary revascularization surgery) or hypothyroidism will also have sinus bradycardia. Certain drugs (eg, the beta blockers and verapamil) can also cause sinus bradycardia. Sinus bradycardia occurs more frequently with acute inferior myocardial infarction than acute anterior infarction (because of ischemia of the SA node).

Significance

1. The main threat of sinus bradycardia is that it may allow a more rapidly discharging ectopic focus to take over the role of cardiac pacemaker from the SA node. Ventricular rates below 50/minute predispose to serious ventricular and atrial arrhythmias.
2. The slow heart rate in sinus bradycardia may also reduce cardiac output, particularly in elderly patients, thus reducing coronary and cerebral blood flow. In this circumstance, angina, syncope or heart failure may develop.
3. *Risk:* Sinus bradycardia with heart rates of less than 50/minute can lead to several arrhythmic and hemodynamic complications (particularly in the first hours after infarction), and for this reason must be regarded as a warning arrhythmia in a patient admitted for AMI. When the heart rate exceeds 50/minute, sinus bradycardia is usually well tolerated and classified as a minor arrhythmia.

Clinical Features

1. Sinus bradycardia seldom produces symptoms unless the heart rate is sufficiently slow to reduce cardiac output. In this case patients may complain of fatigue or experience syncope.
2. The only physical sign of sinus bradycardia is a slow, regular heart rate, usually of 40 to 60/minute.

ECG FEATURES IDENTIFYING SINUS BRADYCARDIA

1. **Rate:** Usually 40 to 60/minute, but may be slower.
2. **Rhythm:** Regular.
3. **P waves:** Normal, and precede each QRS complex.
4. **P–R interval:** Normal.
5. **QRS:** Normal.

Sinus Bradycardia (Figure 9–3)

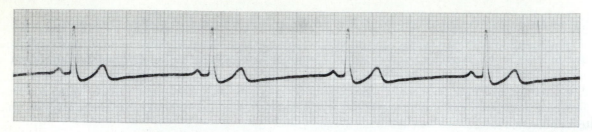

Rate:	About 40/minute (43/minute).
Rhythm:	Regular.
P waves:	Normal.
P–R interval:	Normal (0.16 second).
QRS:	Normal (0.08 second).
Comment:	Sinus bradycardia differs from normal sinus rhythm only in that the heart rate is less than 60/minute.

Sinus Bradycardia (Figure 9–4)

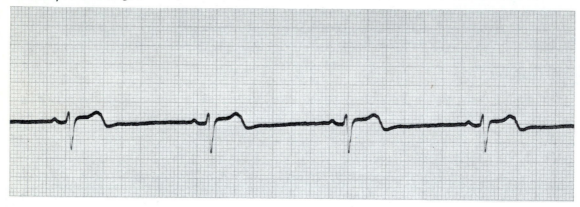

Rate:	About 40/minute.
Rhythm:	Regular.
P waves:	Normal; each P wave is followed by a QRS complex.
P–R interval:	Normal (0.12 second).
QRS:	Normal (0.08 second).
Comment:	The usual cause of sinus bradycardia is increased vagal tone, which slows discharges from the SA node.

Treatment

1. Sinus bradycardia should be treated only under the following circumstances:
   a. If there are any signs or symptoms of a reduction in cardiac output (syncope, hypotension, angina, or heart failure)
   b. If premature ventricular contractions develop during the period of bradycardia
   c. If the heart rate is persistently less than 50/minute, particularly in elderly patients or those with previous myocardial damage.

2. Atropine, which blocks the vagal effect on the SA node, is usually effective in accelerating the heart rate and should be the initial therapy for sinus bradycardia. The drug is given intravenously at a dosage of 0.5 to 1.0 mg.
3. If drug therapy fails or if its effect is short-lived, temporary transvenous pacing may be required to maintain a normal heart rate, particularly if heart failure is present.
4. Drugs with known bradycardic effects such as digitalis, reserpine, morphine, and beta-blocking agents, should be avoided or discontinued in the presence of sinus bradycardia.

Nursing Responsibility

1. Carefully review the ECG to ascertain that the slow heart rate is due to sinus bradycardia rather than another cause, such as heart block or junctional rhythm. Document the arrhythmia.
2. Record the heart rate at frequent intervals for comparative purposes; this is particularly important when drug therapy is used in an attempt to increase the rate.
3. Assess the patient's clinical course regularly to determine if there are signs or symptoms of decreased left ventricular performance.
4. Observe the ECG pattern repeatedly for evidence of premature ventricular contractions. If these occur, notify the physician.
5. If the heart rate falls below 50/minute, give atropine intravenously according to the standing orders, and advise the physician.

CASE HISTORY

A 78-year-old man was brought to the CCU 1 hour after an episode of severe chest pain. At the time of the patient's admission his blood pressure was 90/60 mm Hg and his pulse rate was 48/minute. Frequent premature ventricular beats were noted on the cardiac monitor, but the patient denied any fatigue or dizziness. The nurse notified the physician of these findings. Atropine (0.5 mg) was administered intravenously, and within 5 minutes the patient's blood pressure rose to 114/76 mm Hg; the heart rate increased to 76/minute, and the premature ventricular contractions became less frequent.

SICK SINUS SYNDROME

Mechanism

In sick sinus syndrome, impulses arise from the SA node, but without a completely regular rhythm. The irregularity of discharge is due to ischemia of the SA node, resulting in alternating periods of slow and rapid heart rates. The most common form of sick sinus syndrome occurs in elderly patients and is a bradycardia-tachycardia syndrome in which an atrial tachyarrhythmia (atrial fibrillation or flutter) is followed by sinus bradycardia.

Significance

1. If the periods of bradycardia are significant, sick sinus syndrome can cause an intermittent reduction of cardiac output, with a reduction in cerebral and coronary blood flow.
2. *Risk:* In an individual with low cardiac output as a result of advanced heart failure or an evolving myocardial infarction, sick sinus syndrome can result in serious atrial and ventricular rhythms.

Clinical Features

1. The pulse in sick sinus syndrome is irregular, alternating between tachycardia (often irregular) and bradycardia.
2. The diagnosis of sick sinus syndrome can be verified with an ECG, but the condition may be suspected clinically from a change in heart rate that occurs independently of the rate of respiration.

Treatment

1. Treatment of the sick sinus syndrome usually requires a combination of antiarrhythmic drug therapy directed at the tachyarrhythmia and a permanent pacemaker for the bradyarrhythmia.
2. In the case of the sick sinus syndrome accompanying an evolving inferior myocardial infarction, the pathology affecting the SA node may not be permanent, and treatment of the syndrome may initially involve the use of a temporary pacemaker.

Nursing Responsibility

1. Ascertain that the irregular rhythm is due to sick sinus syndrome and document the rhythm with an ECG strip, capturing both the tachy- and bradyarrhythmias.
2. Make certain that the irregularity in rhythm is not a manifestation of sinus arrhythmia.
3. Notify the physician immediately.
4. Treatment parameters are the same as for sinus bradycardia, with the administration of intravenous atropine being the initial treatment.
5. A temporary pacemaker is required if there are signs of decreased cardiac output or increased ventricular irritability.

CASE HISTORY

A 70-year-old woman was admitted to the CCU with a typical history of AMI. The patient's heart rate was 108/minute and an ECG showed the heart rhythm to be alternating between sinus rhythm with frequent premature atrial contractions and atrial fibrillation. Fifteen minutes after the patient's admission the nurse noted that the patient's heart rate had suddenly decreased, and was now a sinus and regular rhythm, but with a heart rate of only 44/minute. The blood pressure had dropped from 130/86 to 94/60 mm Hg. The patient complained of dizziness. Atropine (0.6 mg) was administered intravenously. Within 5 minutes the blood pressure rose to 135/80 mm Hg with a heart rate of 65/minute. The arrhythmia persisted and the patient received a permanent pacemaker and drug treatment for her atrial fibrillation.

WANDERING PACEMAKER

Mechanism

With a wandering pacemaker, impulses arise in a normal manner in the SA node, but the pacemaker occasionally wanders from the SA node to the atria or AV nodal area. This shifting of the pacemaker from the SA node to adjacent tissues is manifested electrocardiographically by transient changes in the size, shape, and direction of the P waves. A wandering pacemaker is usually caused by varying vagal tone (just as in the case of sinus arrhythmia). With increased vagal tone the rate of impulse discharge from the SA node slows, allowing a pacemaker in the atria or AV nodal area, which may emit impulses at a slightly greater rate than the SA node under these conditions, to briefly take over control of the heart rate. As soon as vagal tone decreases, the SA node accelerates its rate of impulse discharge and regains control of the heartbeat.

Significance

1. There is no particular danger from a wandering pacemaker. The arrhythmia usually reflects fluctuating depression of the SA node as a result of vagal input.
2. *Risk:* None.

ECG FEATURES IDENTIFYING A WANDERING PACEMAKER

1. Rate:	Usually normal, but may be slow (because of vagal dominance).
2. Rhythm:	Essentially regular, but the R–R intervals may vary as the pacemaker site shifts.
3. P waves:	As the pacemaker wanders to the atria or AV nodal area, the shape, position, or direction of the P waves changes, reflecting the different sites of origin of the cardiac impulse. However, a P wave precedes every QRS complex.
4. P–R interval:	The conduction time to the ventricle depends on the site of impulse formation. On this basis the P–R interval may vary slightly with changes in the pacemaker location.
5. QRS:	Normal. Because conduction from the AV node to the ventricle is unaffected, the QRS complex is normal regardless of the size, shape, or position of the P waves.

Wandering Pacemaker (Figure 9–5)

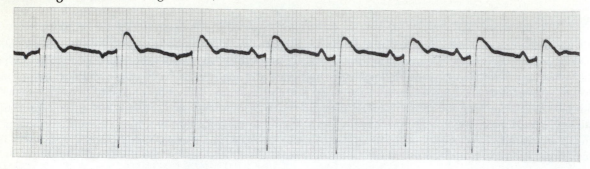

Rate:	About 80/minute.
Rhythm:	Nearly regular.
P waves:	In the first three complexes the P waves are inverted (indicating an atrial pacemaker). When the pacemaker shifts back to the SA node (the last five complexes) the P waves return to normal.
P–R interval:	Normal (0.16 second).
QRS:	Normal (0.08 second).
Comment:	The pacemaker shifts from the SA node to the atria.

Wandering Pacemaker (Figure 9–6)

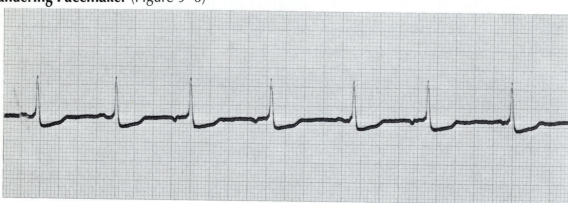

Rate:	About 70/minute.
Rhythm:	Regular.
P waves:	The size, shape, and direction of the P waves vary as the pacemaker changes position.
P–R interval:	Normal (0.20 second).
QRS:	Normal (0.06 second).
Comment:	The pacemaker moves back and forth between the SA node and the atria.

Treatment

1. No treatment is needed in most instances of a wandering pacemaker.
2. If depression of the SA node permits the AV nodal area to dominate as pacemaker, atropine can be used to block the vagal influence on the SA node.
3. If a wandering pacemaker develops during digitalis therapy, the drug may be temporarily withheld to see whether the arrhythmia is drug-related and will disappear with the cessation of digitalis.

Nursing Responsibility

1. When a wandering pacemaker is noted on the monitor, the arrhythmia should be documented with a rhythm strip.
2. The ECG should be subsequently observed to verify that the SA node has not relinquished complete control to the atria or AV nodal area.

CASE HISTORY

On the second day after admission to the CCU a 56-year-old man with an acute infarction of the inferior wall developed ECG evidence of a wandering pacemaker. The nurse noted that the configuration of the P waves varied at different times, and realized that the pacemaker site was changing during these periods. Because these episodes were infrequent and the SA node remained the dominant pacemaker, the nurse concluded that the problem was not serious and no treatment was given.

SINOATRIAL ARREST AND BLOCK

Mechanism

Under certain circumstances the SA node fails to initiate an impulse at the expected time in the cardiac cycle. In the absence of an impulse from the SA node, neither the atria or the ventricles are stimulated, and an entire PQRST complex therefore drops out of the ECG for one heartbeat (or more). This is called *sinoatrial (SA) arrest.* In other instances the impulse is initiated normally but is blocked within the SA node and never reaches the atria or ventricles. Again, the PQRST sequence is absent from the ECG. This condition is designated *SA block* or, more specifically, *SA exit block.* Although SA arrest is a disturbance of impulse formation and SA exit block a disturbance of conduction, it is often impossible to determine from an ECG alone which of the two mechanisms is responsible for a dropped beat. For this reason the terms SA arrest and SA block are used interchangeably, or are grouped together and called *sinus pauses.* Sinoatrial arrest (or block) may result from excessive vagal dominance of the SA node or from digitalis or quinidine toxicity; however, neither of these factors is probably as important in causing the condition as ischemic injury to the SA node secondary to coronary atherosclerosis or AMI.

Significance

1. When infrequent, SA arrest (or block) is not of great importance and usually reflects excessive vagal activity.
2. Repeated episodes of SA arrest or very prolonged pauses between beats suggest ischemic damage to the SA node, a condition that is potentially dangerous.
3. When related to overdosages of digitalis (or quinidine), SA arrest assumes special significance, since either drug may further depress SA nodal activity and produce atrial standstill.
4. *Risk:* SA arrest is usually not serious, but is potentially dangerous when the episodes are repetitive or prolonged as the result of ischemic damage or drug overdosage.

Clinical Features

1. The patient with SA arrest (or block) may notice pauses in the heartbeat and describe this sensation; however, most patients are unaware of the arrhythmia.
2. The only physical finding in SA arrest is a pause in the pulse or heartbeat.
3. If the missed beats in SA arrest occur frequently or consecutively, cerebral insufficiency may develop, as manifested by syncope or vertigo.

ECG FEATURES IDENTIFYING SINOATRIAL ARREST (AND SA BLOCK)

1. Rate:	Usually slow (40–70/minute), but may be normal.
2. Rhythm:	The basic heart rhythm is normal except for the missing beats.
3. P waves:	The P wave is absent with the missed beat since the SA node either does not discharge or the impulse fails to reach the atrium.
4. P–R interval:	The entire PQRST complex is missing for one or more beats, with a resulting absence of the P–R interval during SA arrest or block.
5. QRS:	No QRS complex is produced when the SA-nodal impulse is absent or blocked.

SA Arrest (or Block) (Figure 9–7)

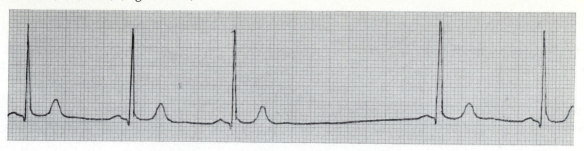

Rate:	About 50/minute.
Rhythm:	Regular except for a sinus pause between every third and fourth QRS complex.
P waves:	The P wave anticipated after the third complex is absent.
P–R interval:	No P–R interval during SA arrest; other P–R intervals are normal.
QRS:	No QRS complex for one beat; other QRS complexes normal.
Comment:	The duration of the pause in sinus rhythm in this case is exactly twice the R–R interval of the two previous beats, suggesting that the SA node continued to discharge normally but that one impulse was blocked within the node (SA block).

SA Arrest (or Block) (Figure 9–8)

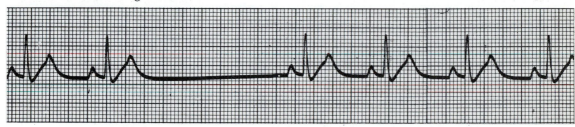

Rate:	About 60/minute.
Rhythm:	Regular except for one period of sinus arrest.
P waves:	Absent with missed beat; otherwise normal.
P–R interval:	Absent with missed beat; otherwise normal (0.16 second).
QRS:	Absent when SA node failed to discharge; otherwise normal (0.08 second).
Comment:	The duration of the pause in this case is not an exact multiple of the other R–R intervals. This implies that the SA node failed to discharge during this period (SA arrest) and then suddenly started to discharge once again.

Treatment

1. SA arrest (or block) that occurs only occasionally is usually self-limiting and requires no treatment.
2. If periods of SA arrest are frequent or prolonged, atropine (0.5–1.0 mg intravenously) will frequently restore normal SA impulse formation or conduction by inhibiting the causative vagal effect on the SA node. Isoproterenol can also be used for this purpose.
3. If SA arrest does not subside spontaneously or fails to respond to drug therapy, a transvenous pacemaker may be required.
4. If SA arrest occurs in patients receiving digitalis or quinidine, these drugs should be discontinued promptly.

Nursing Responsibility

1. When SA arrest (or block) is noted, the arrhythmia should be documented with a rhythm strip.
2. If SA arrest occurs frequently or if more than two consecutive beats are missed during an episode of the condition, notify the physician promptly.
3. If SA arrest develops in patients receiving digitalis or quinidine, further dosages of these drugs should be withheld until reordered by the physician.

CASE HISTORY

A 61-year-old man was admitted to the CCU with an acute inferior infarction. On examining the patient the nurse noted that his pulse was 50/minute and occasionally irregular. The ECG revealed sinus bradycardia with episodes of SA arrest. In some instances there were as many as three missed beats in a row. Atropine 1 mg was given intravenously, and promptly accelerated the heart rate and restored normal sinus function. No other treatment was initiated, and the rest of the patient's hospitalization was uneventful.

OTHER ARRHYTHMIAS ORIGINATING IN THE SINOATRIAL NODE

The ECG strips shown in Figures 9–9 through 9–18 are meant to:

1. Provide additional examples of the arrhythmias discussed in the preceding pages.
2. Demonstrate certain variations of the ECG patterns of these arrhythmias.
3. Illustrate that more than one arrhythmic disorder may be present at the same time.
4. Introduce other details in the interpretation of arrhythmias.

Normal Sinus Rhythm with Inverted T Waves (Figure 9–9)

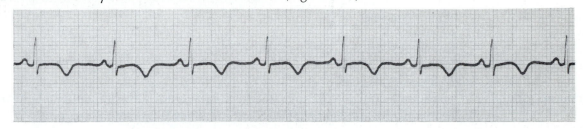

Rate:	About 80/minute (actual rate: 75/minute)
Rhythm:	Regular.
P waves:	Normal.
P–R interval:	Normal (0.12 second).
QRS:	Normal (0.04 second).
Comment:	The T waves are inverted, a common manifestation of myocardial ischemia. However, abnormalities of T waves or ST segments do not affect the interpretation of an arrhythmia, and this ECG shows normal sinus rhythm (NSR).

Sinus Tachycardia (Figure 9–10)

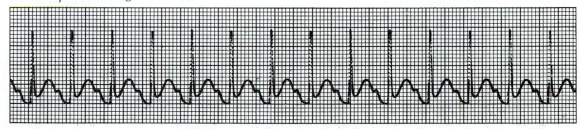

Rate:	About 140/minute.
Rhythm:	Regular.
P waves:	Because of the rapid rate, the P waves encroach on the preceding T waves.
P–R interval:	Normal (less than 0.20 second, but not clearly measurable).
QRS:	Normal (0.06 second).
Comment:	A careful search for P waves, often hiding in the preceding T waves, is an essential step in interpreting arrhythmias.

Sinus Bradycardia with Prominent U Waves (Figure 9–11)

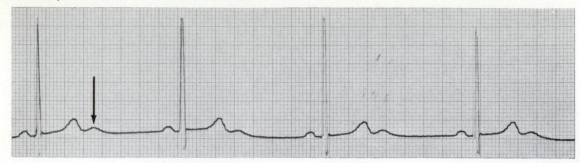

Rate:	About 40/minute.
Rhythm:	Regular.
P waves:	Normal. A P wave precedes each QRS complex.
P–R interval:	Normal (0.16 second).
QRS:	Normal (0.06 second).
Comment:	Immediately after each T wave is another wave called a U wave (arrow). U waves, particularly when prominent, often reflect low serum potassium levels.

Sinus Bradycardia with Conduction Disorder (Figure 9–12)

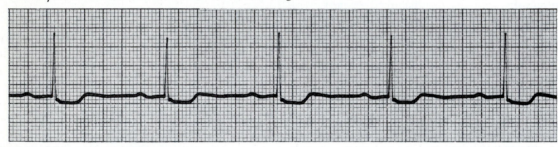

Rate:	About 50/minute.
Rhythm:	Regular.
P waves:	Normal.
P–R interval:	Prolonged (0.32 second), indicating a first-degree AV heart block.
QRS:	Normal (0.04 second).
Comment:	This ECG shows both a disturbance in impulse formation (sinus bradycardia) and a disturbance in conduction (first-degree AV block).

Sinus Arrhythmia (Figure 9–13)

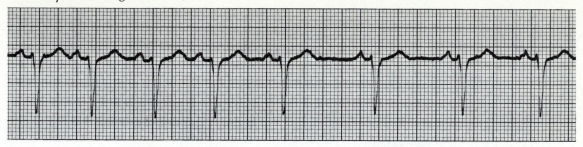

Rate:	About 80/minute.
Rhythm:	Irregular. There is a variation of at least 0.12 second between the longest and shortest R–R intervals.
P waves:	Normal. Each P wave is followed by a QRS complex.
P–R interval:	Normal (0.16 second).
QRS:	Normal (0.08 second).
Comment:	The rate increases during inspiration and slows during expiration, owing to variation of vagal influence on the SA node.

Sinus Arrhythmia (Figure 9–14)

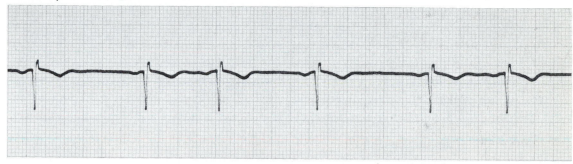

Rate:	About 60/minute.
Rhythm:	Irregular. The R–R intervals vary by more than 0.12 second.
P waves:	Normal but inverted (because of the particular monitoring lead being used).
P–R interval:	Normal (0.20 second).
QRS:	Normal (0.08 second).
Comment:	The key feature of sinus arrhythmia is the irregularity of the rhythm with otherwise normal wave forms. The heart rate varies between fast and slow, but usually is synchronized with respirations.

Sinus Arrhythmia and Sinus Bradycardia (Figure 9–15)

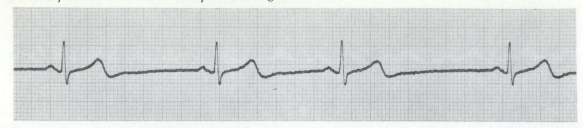

Rate:	About 40/minute.
Rhythm:	Irregular.
P waves:	Normal.
P–R interval:	Normal (0.16 second).
QRS:	Normal (0.08 second).
Comment:	Sinus bradycardia and sinus arrhythmia often occur together, with both resulting from increased vagal tone. This condition does not lead to a more serious arrhythmia.

Wandering Pacemaker (Figure 9–16)

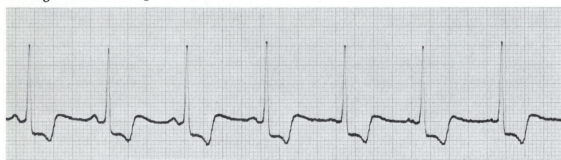

Rate:	About 70/minute.
Rhythm:	Regular.
P waves:	The P waves are normal with the first four beats, but their size and shape then change as the pacemaker wanders to the atria.
P–R interval:	Normal (0.20 second) during normal sinus rhythm.
QRS:	Normal duration (0.08 second).
Comment:	Marked (4-mm) ST-segment depression and T-wave inversion, as seen in this tracing, reflect myocardial disease.

Sinoatrial (SA) Arrest (Figure 9–17)

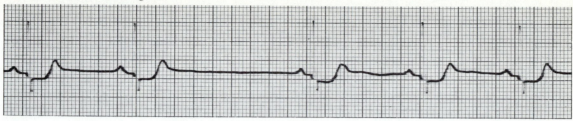

Rate:	About 50/minute.
Rhythm:	Regular except for one missed beat.
P waves:	Normal.
P–R interval:	Normal (0.16 second).
QRS:	Normal (0.06 second).
Comment:	This sinus pause, manifested by the absence of one PQRST complex, is not a multiple of the other R–R intervals, and therefore represents SA arrest rather than SA block.

Sinoatrial Pause with Sinus Arrhythmia (Figure 9–18)

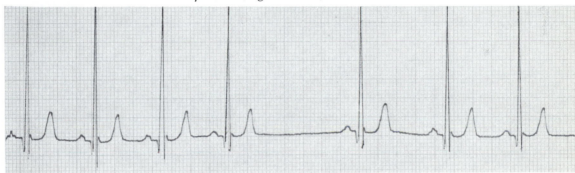

Rate:	About 70/minute.
Rhythm:	Irregular as the result of the sinoatrial pause and sinus arrhythmia.
P waves:	Normal.
P–R interval:	Normal (0.16 second).
QRS:	Normal (0.10 second).
Comment:	After four normal beats the SA node fails to discharge (or the impulse is blocked in the node), creating a pause before the sinus node discharges again. Sinus arrhythmia is evident after the pause in SA nodal discharge, suggesting that both the pause and arrhythmia were the result of increased vagal tone.

Chapter 10

Arrhythmias Originating in the Atria

PREMATURE ATRIAL CONTRACTIONS
PAROXYSMAL SUPRAVENTRICULAR TACHYCARDIA
ATRIAL FLUTTER
ATRIAL FIBRILLATION
ATRIAL STANDSTILL

As noted previously, the atria, the AV nodal area, and the ventricles all have the potential capacity to serve as pacemakers, but under normal circumstances the SA node retains control of the heart rate because it discharges impulses at an inherently faster rate than these other sites. If for some reason a focus in the atrial wall initiates impulses more rapidly than those arising from the SA node, the ectopic atrial site will replace the SA node as the cardiac pacemaker. This may occur as briefly as a single beat (premature atrial contraction) or continuously (atrial tachycardia, atrial flutter, or atrial fibrillation), depending on the degree and persistence of irritability of the abnormal focus.

When impulses originate in the atria outside the SA node at rates of less than 200/minute, P waves are usually visible but are distorted in shape, indicating that the SA node is not in command of the heart rate. In this situation each impulse nevertheless reaches the AV node and passes through it to the ventricles without difficulty. Consequently, a normal QRS complex follows each P wave (atrial tachycardia).

When the atria are stimulated at rates of 200 to 400 times per minute, the AV node is unable to accept each impulse and blocks every second, third, or fourth atrial beat. The impulses that do pass the AV node are conducted normally thereafter to the ventricles. In atrial flutter, for example, the rate of atrial contraction is two, three, or four times greater than the ventricular response, and there are two, three, or four P waves between each normal QRS complex.

If the atria are stimulated at extremely rapid rates (400 to 1,000 times per minute), the atrial muscle becomes unable to respond to the repetitive impulses and the individual fibers comprising the muscle merely twitch, or fibrillate, rather than contracting in an orderly and coordinated manner. Because the atria do not contract under these circumstances, P waves are not seen. As a result of the chaotic atrial activity, impulses reach the AV node at a rapid, irregular rate. The node blocks most of these rapid impulses, and those that do pass to the ventricles do so at irregular intervals. Consequently, the ventricular rhythm is irregular (atrial fibrillation).

Atrial arrhythmias result primarily from irritability of the atrial muscle, usually caused by ischemic damage to the muscle or overdistention (stretching) of the atrial wall. Atrial arrhythmias associated with a rapid ventricular rate are categorized as major arrhythmias because they increase myocardial oxygen demand and reduce the pumping efficiency of the heart. Because the atria contribute approximately 20% to cardiac output, atrial fibrillation severely decreases cardiac output. This situation is described clinically as "losing the atrial kick." Ordinarily, patients may be able to tolerate atrial flutter or fibrillation without experiencing symptoms of low cardiac output, but in the face of an AMI or advanced heart failure such arrhythmias can be extremely deleterious.

155

PREMATURE ATRIAL CONTRACTIONS

Mechanism

When an ectopic focus in the atrium discharges before the SA node, a premature atrial contraction (PAC) results. Because the impulse arises outside the SA node, the P wave of the ectopic beat is abnormally shaped or inverted. Conduction from the AV node to the ventricles is not affected, and therefore the QRS complex is normal. Following the premature beat there is a slight pause before the next normal sinus impulse arises. This pause, called an *incomplete compensatory pause,* occurs because the ectopic impulse discharges the nearby SA node and the node must recover before it can discharge again. (The compensatory pause is discussed in more detail in the discussion of premature ventricular contractions.)

If the ectopic focus fires shortly after the previous normal beat, the AV node may still be in a refractory state. In this case the impulse will not be conducted to the ventricles, and only a premature P wave with abnormal morphology will appear on the ECG. If the ectopic focus fires slightly later, the resulting impulse may be conducted through the AV node in a normal manner but may then encounter portions of the His-Purkinje system that are in their refractory period. The impulse would then be conducted through these portions and to the ventricles more slowly than normal, resulting in a QRS complex that is "aberrantly" wide (ie, greater than 0.12 second).

PACs usually reflect irritability of the atrial musculature, and may be provoked by hypoxemia, myocardial ischemia, atrial distention, or various drugs.

Significance

1. By themselves, PACs have no particular significance; they are common in healthy as well as diseased hearts. However, in patients with evolving myocardial infarctions or advanced heart failure, they indicate atrial irritability and may warn of impending serious atrial arrhythmias (eg, paroxysmal supraventricular tachycardia or atrial fibrillation). When PACs increase to a frequency exceeding 6/minute, the risk of serious arrhythmia increases.
2. *Risk:* PACs pose no immediate danger, but may herald the onset of atrial fibrillation or other sustained atrial arrhythmias, particularly when they occur frequently.

Clinical Features

1. Normally the patient is unaware of PACs, but occasionally a sensation of palpitation accompanies them.
2. PACs occur sooner than normal atrial contractions, and therefore increase the loudness of the first heart sound (S_1) because the atrioventricular valve leaflets are further apart when they close than they would normally be.
3. PACs can be positively identified only by ECG.

ECG FEATURES IDENTIFYING PREMATURE ATRIAL CONTRACTIONS

1. **Rate:** Usually normal.

2. **Rhythm:** After a PAC there is a slight delay (incomplete compensatory pause) before the next normal beat. This pause creates a mild irregularity in the cardiac rhythm.

3. **P waves:** Either abnormally shaped or inverted, and different from normal P waves originating in the SA node.

4. **P–R interval:** Usually normal, but may be short or prolonged.

5. **QRS:** Usually normal, indicating that there is no disturbance in conduction from the AV node to the ventricles.

Premature Atrial Contractions (Figure 10–1)

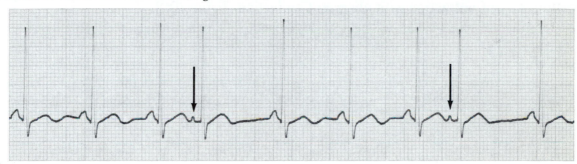

Rate:	About 90/minute.
Rhythm:	The two PACs (arrows) and the pauses that follow them create an irregular rhythm.
P waves:	The size and shape of the P waves of the PACs (arrow) are different from those of the P waves of normal beats. However, a P wave precedes each QRS.
P–R interval:	Normal (0.16 second).
QRS:	Normal (0.08 second).
Comment:	The most distinguishing feature of an ectopic beat arising in the atria (a PAC) is that the configuration of the P wave differs from that of other P waves.

Premature Atrial Contraction (Figure 10–2)

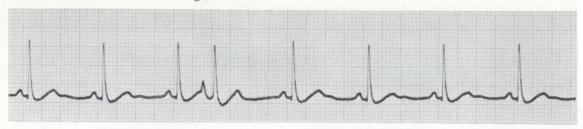

Rate:	About 70/minute.
Rhythm:	Irregular.
P waves:	The P wave of the PAC is hidden in the T wave of the preceding complex, producing a sharp pointed wave that differs from the other P or T waves.
P–R interval:	Normal (0.12 second).
QRS:	Normal (0.08 second).
Comment:	P waves are often obscured by the preceding T waves, particularly if the PAC occurs soon after the previous beat.

Premature Atrial Contraction with Aberrant Conduction (Figure 10–3)

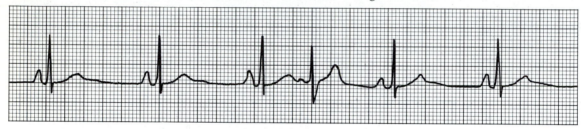

Rate:	About 60/minute.
Rhythm:	The otherwise regular rhythm is interrupted by the PAC.
P waves:	The P wave of the atrial premature beat differs in size and shape from the normal P waves of the other beats.
P–R interval:	Normal (0.12 second).
QRS:	The QRS complex of the PAC is wider and of a somewhat different configuration than the other ventricular complexes. This variation is due to abnormal conduction of the premature atrial impulse through the ventricles (aberrant conduction).
Comment:	In this example the degree of aberration is only moderate. However, in other instances aberrant conduction may be far more pronounced, resulting in a wide, distorted QRS complex that can resemble a premature ventricular contraction (PVC).

Treatment

1. If PACs occur rarely and do not increase in frequency, they do not usually indicate a need for treatment.
2. If the number of PACs increases during a period of observation, it is advisable to use antiarrhythmic drugs to control these ectopic beats. Digitalis alone or in combination with quinidine is usually effective in this circumstance.

Nursing Responsibility

1. Distinguish PACs from other causes of irregular heart rhythm and document their presence on an ECG.
2. Observe the frequency of these premature beats and note any change in their frequency over time.
3. Be aware that atrial fibrillation or other serious atrial arrhythmias may develop abruptly in the presence of frequent PACs, with a consequent decrease in cardiac output.
4. Distinguish aberrantly conducted PACs from premature ventricular contractions (PVCs).

CASE HISTORY

A 69-year-old man exhibited occasional PACs during the first day after his admission to the hospital. These ectopic beats occurred at a rate of 2 to 4/minute, and were recorded on hourly rhythm strips. On the second hospital day the frequency of the patient's PACs increased to 10 to 20/minute, and some of them occurred consecutively for two to three beats. The nurse advised the physician of these changes and treatment with digoxin was begun to suppress this increasing atrial ectopic activity. Within 8 hours after this the number of PACs had diminished greatly, and by 24 hours the arrhythmia was almost completely suppressed.

PAROXYSMAL SUPRAVENTRICULAR TACHYCARDIA

Mechanism

Paroxysmal supraventricular tachycardia (PSVT) originates from an impulse generated above the ventricles. It is caused by one of two mechanisms: *increased automaticity* in the discharge of an ectopic site in the atria, or *reentry*. Increased automaticity is responsible for only 10% of all PSVTs. In this case, the rapid discharge of the ectopic focus, occurring at a regular rate of 150 to 250/minute, replaces the SA node as pacemaker. Originally this mechanism was thought to be responsible for all supraventricular tachycardias, and the term paroxysmal atrial tachycardia (PAT) was coined to describe it. However, knowledge gained from electrophysiologic studies has shown the important role of reentry as another source of supraventricular tachycardias.

In reentry, the "loop" of tissue that carries the reentrant impulse is localized to the SA node, atria, or AV node, or consists of an accessory bypass tract (a tract that bypasses the AV node and connects the atrium and the ventricle). For a reentry loop to occur, two functionally different tracts or pathways must exist in the myocardium. One pathway must conduct slowly and have a short refractory period. The second pathway must conduct more rapidly but have a long refractory period. Impulses from above conduct down both pathways, but at different rates. An impulse can be conducted down the rapidly conducting tract, rendering that path refractory. If a second impulse then follows prematurely, it may find the second pathway repolarized and be conducted in a retrograde direction along this pathway. A reentrant loop is initiated (Figure 10–4).

In both types of mechanism the ventricles respond to each atrial impulse, and therefore the atrial and ventricular rates are identical.

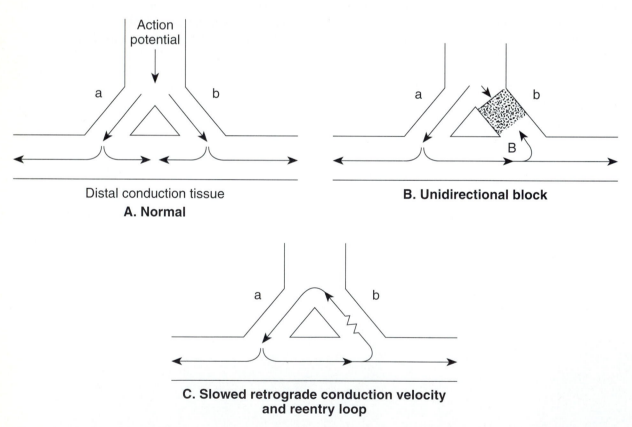

Figure 10–4. Reentry mechanisms in supraventricular tachycardia. **A.** Normal conduction. The action potential travels down both pathways a and b to excite distal myocardial cells. **B.** Effects of unidirectional block (perhaps caused by ischemia). When the action potential reaches the area of block, the impulse is conducted down the a pathway but not down the b pathway. **C.** The impulse is conducted backward (retrograde) through the pathway and finds the a pathway ready to depolarize again. A reentry loop is established.

Significance

1. The rapid heart rate tends to reduce cardiac output because the volume of blood ejected with each contraction (stroke volume) is decreased as a result of the very short ventricular filling time between beats. The decrease in cardiac output may lead to left ventricular failure, particularly if the tachycardia is sustained. Cerebral circulation can also be affected, resulting in syncope.
2. The fast ventricular rate increases the demand for and consumption of oxygen by the myocardium. Consequently, additional myocardial ischemia or angina may result. The longer that PSVT persists, the greater the threat of further myocardial injury.
3. *Risk:* PAT is a dangerous arrhythmia with acute myocardial infarction or heart failure but not a direct cause of death. The risk is directly proportional to the duration of the arrhythmia.

Clinical Features

1. Characteristically, paroxysmal supraventricular tachycardia occurs suddenly, sometimes without warning, but is usually preceded by a premature atrial contraction.
2. Most patients are immediately aware of the rapid heart action and frequently describe a fluttering sensation in the chest, lightheadedness, angina, or dyspnea.
3. The arrhythmia may be transient and end abruptly, even without treatment. In patients with underlying heart disease or in the elderly, PSVT may not be tolerated and may rapidly lead to pulmonary edema, syncope, or myocardial infarction.

ECG FEATURES IDENTIFYING PAROXYSMAL SUPRAVENTRICULAR TACHYCARDIA

1. **Rate:**   150 to 250/minute.

2. **Rhythm:**   Regular.

3. **P waves:**   An abnormal P wave precedes each QRS complex. However, the P waves can seldom be identified because they are buried in the preceding T waves.

4. **P–R interval:**   In most instances the P-R interval cannot be measured because the P waves are obscured.

5. **QRS:**   Usually normal.

Paroxysmal Supraventricular Tachycardia (Figure 10–5)

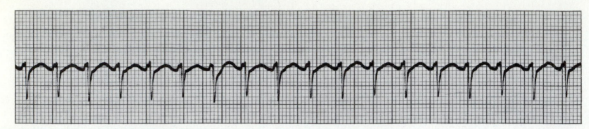

Rate:	About 180/minute.
Rhythm:	Regular.
P waves:	Not identifiable; probably buried in preceding T waves.
P–R interval:	Not measurable, since P waves cannot be identified specifically.
QRS:	Normal, indicating that all atrial impulses are conducted to the ventricles in a normal manner.
Comment:	Atrial tachycardia substantially increases the work of the heart, but fortunately often terminates spontaneously after a few minutes.

Paroxysmal Supraventricular Tachycardia (Figure 10–6)

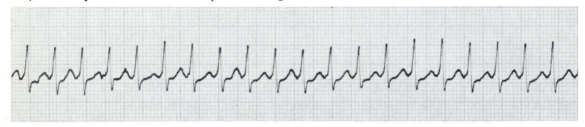

Rate:	About 200/minute.
Rhythm:	Regular.
P waves:	Cannot be identified specifically; probably superimposed on preceding T waves.
P–R interval:	Not measurable, since P waves cannot be delineated.
QRS:	Normal (0.08 second), indicating that all atrial impulses are conducted normally through the ventricles.
Comment:	In this typical example of PSVT, the ventricles respond regularly to each atrial impulse (ie, a QRS complex follows every P wave on a 1:1 basis). However, under certain conditions (especially digitalis toxicity), some atrial impulses are blocked in the AV node and not conducted to the ventricles. As a result, every P wave is not followed by a QRS complex, and the 1:1 relationship no longer exists. This latter arrhythmia is called *PAT with block*.

Treatment

1. Initially an attempt should be made to terminate the PSVT by reflex vagal stimulation (eg, carotid sinus massage). Vagal maneuvers increase parasympathetic stimulation of the AV node, decreasing AV nodal conduction and breaking the reentry circuit responsible for PSVT. This technique is ineffective for PSVT caused by increased automaticity.

2. If PSVT cannot be terminated by vagal stimulation, and the patient describes angina or symptoms of left ventricular failure, elective precordial shock (cardioversion) should be used promptly; this method seldom fails to restore sinus rhythm.

3. If the rapid rate in PSVT does not produce obvious symptoms, drug therapy can be attempted. Although several different drugs can be used for terminating PSVT, intravenous adenosine appears to be the most effective (see Chapter 16). Among other drugs that may be used in this situation are calcium-channel-blocking agents, particularly verapamil, and beta-blocking agents such as propranolol. These drugs slow conduction and block reentrant circuits in the AV node. Rapid-acting digitalis preparations can also be used, but are less effective in an acute episode of PSVT because of the relatively slow onset of action of the drug.

4. Digitalis toxicity should be suspected in the case of PSVT caused by an ectopic focus in the atria (rather than reentry). Digitalis should be discontinued and the patient should be assessed for hypokalemia which, if present, should be treated with potassium supplements.

5. Prophylactic antiarrhythmic therapy is advisable for PSVT that occurs repeatedly.

Nursing Responsibility

1. Examine the patient and verify the rapid pulse rate.
2. Document the arrhythmia with a rhythm strip.
3. Notify the physician immediately.
4. Assess the patient's clinical signs, with particular reference to the presence of angina or signs of left ventricular failure. Document the patient's blood pressure.
5. Working within the treatment protocol, perform carotid massage or other vagal maneuvers.
6. Patients who have signs or symptoms related to the rapid heart rate in PSVT, should be prepared for precordial shock (elective cardioversion).
7. Assist in giving appropriate intravenous drug.

CASE HISTORY

A 55-year-old woman with an AMI had been in normal sinus rhythm for 48 hours after admission. At 4 PM on the day of admission her pulse rate was 82/minute and regular, and the cardiac monitor showed a normal sinus rhythm. At 4:10 PM the tachycardia alarm sounded and the monitor showed a heart rate of 160/minute. At the patient's bedside the nurse confirmed the rapid rate. The patient complained of chest pain and was obviously frightened. She had no syncope or dyspnea. The nurse diagnosed the patient's arrhythmia as PSVT and called the physician immediately. Prior to the physician's arrival, however, the aberrant rhythm abruptly converted to sinus rhythm. A rhythm strip demonstrated that the PSVT had lasted for less than 3 minutes.

ATRIAL FLUTTER

Mechanism

Atrial flutter manifests the existence of a rapidly discharging ectopic atrial pacemaker or a reentry circuit involving intraatrial loops. The atrial rate is 250 to 400/minute. The AV node cannot conduct all of these impulses, but usually allows every second, third, or fourth impulse to reach the ventricles and cause contraction. The ventricular rate is therefore determined by the extent of the block in the AV node. If, for example, the atrial rate is 300/minute and the AV node blocks every second impulse (2:1 block), the ventricular rate will be 150/minute. If the AV node passes every third impulse, the ventricular response rate will be 100/minute. Atrial flutter usually occurs with preexisting heart disease (eg, heart failure or mitral stenosis).

Significance

Atrial flutter may last for weeks without significant consequences, or can lead precipitously to atrial fibrillation. It becomes more dangerous when the heart rate slows enough to allow 1:1 conduction through the AV node. Consider, for example, a patient with a heart rate of 300, who may have a 2:1 AV block and a ventricular response of 150 that is well tolerated. If the heart rate then decreases to 220/minute because of drug treatment, the AV node may be able to transmit every impulse that reaches it, which could lead to rapid degeneration of cardiac output and oxygenation.

1. When atrial flutter is associated with a rapid ventricular rate, cardiac output usually decreases and myocardial oxygen consumption increases (as with other rapid-rate arrhythmias; eg, PSVT). This impairment predisposes to left ventricular failure and myocardial ischemia.
2. If the ventricular rate is not increased, left ventricular performance may not be affected significantly.
3. *Risk:* Atrial flutter is a serious arrhythmia because of its potential hemodynamic consequences. It is usually more persistent than PSVT and therefore a greater threat.

Clinical Features

1. The occurrence of symptoms in atrial flutter depends fundamentally on the ventricular rate. If the ventricular response is rapid (eg, 150/minute or greater), the patient may describe palpitations, angina, or dyspnea. If the ventricular rate is normal (e.g., with a 4:1 block), the arrhythmia may produce no signs or symptoms.
2. Atrial flutter can be identified only by means of an ECG. It is characterized by a coarse "sawtooth" pattern for atrial activity.

ECG FEATURES IDENTIFYING ATRIAL FLUTTER

1. Rate: The ventricular atrial flutter rate may range from 60 to 160/minute, depending on the number of atrial impulses passing through the AV node. The atrial rate is 250 to 400/minute.

2. Rhythm: The ventricular rhythm is most often regular. However, as a result of varying degrees of block in the AV node from time to time, the ventricular rhythm may become slightly irregular.

3. P waves: Rather than P waves, there are characteristic atrial oscillations described as "sawtooth waves" that are easily identifiable. These waves (called F waves or flutter waves) occur regularly at a rate of 250 to 400/minute.

4. P–R interval: The P–R interval (actually the F–R interval) has no meaning and is not measured.

5. QRS: The QRS complex is normal, indicating that conduction beyond the AV node is not disturbed. However, only one-half, one-third, or one-fourth of the atrial impulses are conducted through the AV node and reach the ventricle. The resulting disparity between atrial and ventricular rates is described as atrial flutter with 2:1, 3:1, or 4:1 block.

Atrial Flutter (Figure 10–7)

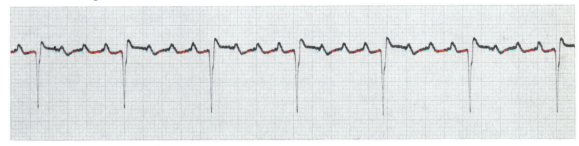

Rate: The ventricular rate is 65/minute and the atrial rate 260/minute.
Rhythm: Regular.
P waves: There are four F waves between each R wave. Note the typical sawtooth appearance of these atrial waves.
P–R interval: In the absence of P waves there is no P–R interval. The F–R interval has no significance.
QRS: Normal (0.06 second). Every fourth atrial impulse is conducted to the ventricle producing a QRS complex.
Comment: Note that there are four flutter waves for each QRS complex. This is called atrial flutter with 4:1 block.

Atrial Flutter (Figure 10–8)

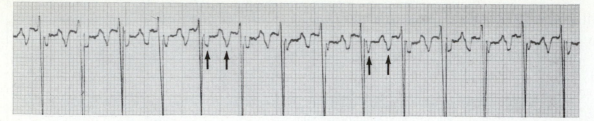

Rate:	The ventricular rate is about 140/minute. The atrial rate is about 280/minute.
Rhythm:	Regular.
P waves:	There are two F waves between ventricular complexes. These waves, which are inverted in the lead (arrows), have a sawtooth appearance, but not as distinctively as in atrial flutter with 4:1 block (as in Figure 10–7).
P–R interval:	Not determinable.
QRS:	Every second atrial impulse is conducted to the ventricle. This is called atrial flutter with 2:1 block. The QRS complexes are normal.
Comment:	Atrial flutter with 2:1 block should always be suspected when there is a regular ventricular rate of 140 to 160/minute. A careful search for F waves should be made in this circumstance.

Treatment

1. Atrial flutter can be instantly terminated by precordial shock (cardioversion) with very low discharge energies (less than 50 watt-seconds). Because of its predictable effectiveness, cardioversion should be the initial treatment for atrial flutter when the ventricular rate is rapid and the patient is symptomatic. It can also be used for atrial flutter that has not responded to other therapy.
2. Drug therapy may be successful in restoring normal sinus rhythm in patients with atrial flutter. A sodium-channel-blocking agent may convert the rhythm or reduce the flutter rate. To prevent an acceleration of the ventricular rate as the atrial rate slows, digitalis, beta-blockers, or calcium-channel-blocking agents (verapamil) are often used to control the ventricular rate (by increasing the degree of AV block).
3. A temporary artificial pacemaker can be used to break the reentry circuit responsible for atrial flutter and recapture a normal atrial rhythm.

Nursing Responsibility

1. When atrial flutter develops, the high-rate alarm on the cardiac monitor may or may not sound, depending on the ventricular rate.
2. Identify the arrhythmia on the monitor and document it with a rhythm strip.
3. Assess the patient's clinical status. Determine whether the patient has angina or dyspnea. Record the blood pressure.
4. If the patient complains of angina or if there is evidence of left ventricular failure, prepare for elective cardioversion (see Chapter 14).
5. Discuss treatment methods with the physician, implement them, and record the patient's response.

CASE HISTORY

Six hours after admission to the CCU, a 71-year old man developed atrial flutter. The rhythm was noted by the nurse when the high-rate alarm sounded on the patient's cardiac monitor. The ventricular rate was 150/minute. The nurse went to the bedside and noted that the patient was apprehensive, dyspneic, and ashen in color. She immediately notified the physician, recorded the patient's blood pressure and pulse rate, and documented the arrhythmia. Anticipating that precordial shock would be used because of the circulatory impairment induced by the arrhythmia, the nurse prepared for the procedure. Cardioversion restored normal sinus rhythm, and the patient's symptoms promptly disappeared.

ATRIAL FIBRILLATION

Mechanism

In atrial fibrillation, the atria (via multiple reentrant loops) discharge impulses at a rate of 400 to 600/minute. The atrial myocardium cannot respond uniformly to this very rapid, irregular stimulation. Instead, the individual muscle fibers respond on their own in a wholly disorganized way. The net effect is a mere twitching of the atrial walls rather than true atrial contraction. In a sense the atria are no more than quivering tubes connecting the great veins to the ventricles, and they provide no assistance in filling the ventricles.

The extremely rapid, irregular impulses coming from the atria in atrial fibrillation bombard the AV node, but the node can conduct only a small percentage of them to the ventricles; the rest are blocked. The impulses that pass through the AV node do so at irregular intervals, creating an irregular ventricular rhythm.

The ventricular rate during atrial fibrillation can vary from 40 to 160/minute, depending on the number of impulses conducted to the ventricles and the degree of AV block. When the ventricular response rate is more than 100/minute, atrial fibrillation is classified as rapid, and when the ventricular response is less than 60/minute the fibrillation is classified as slow.

Atrial fibrillation rarely occurs in healthy individuals. It is usually a result of atrial dilitation secondary to mitral regurgitation or stenosis, chronic ischemic heart disease, pulmonary disease, or thyrotoxicosis.

Significance

1. The major danger of atrial fibrillation is a reduction in the pumping efficiency of the heart (decreased cardiac output). This loss of efficiency results not only from the rapid, irregular ventricular response to atrial fibrillation but also from the loss of effective atrial contraction. (Normally the atrium serves as a booster pump for ventricular filling, and the loss of atrial contraction can cause a 20% reduction in cardiac output.) The resulting hemodynamic deficit may lead to left ventricular failure and worsen existing myocardial ischemia.
2. With atrial fibrillation there is a propensity for clots to form within the noncontracting atria. Mural thrombi, with subsequent embolization of the circulatory system, may develop and cause serious complications, including stroke.
3. *Risk:* Atrial fibrillation is a dangerous arrhythmia from a hemodynamic standpoint, especially when the ventricular rate is rapid.

Clinical Features

1. Most patients with atrial fibrillation are aware of the irregular heart action and describe palpitations or "skipping" of the heartbeat. This disturbing sensation is usually more pronounced when the ventricular rate is rapid.
2. If the patient has a left atrial or pulmonary artery catheter, the "a" wave (representing atrial contraction) will not be seen on the monitor.
3. The grossly irregular rhythm in atrial fibrillation is so characteristic as to be by itself almost diagnostic of this arrhythmia.
4. In most instances the peripheral pulse rate is slower than the heart (apical) rate. This pulse deficit results from variations in the volume of blood ejected with each ventricular contraction; at times the stroke volume is inadequate to produce a peripheral pulse.
5. If the ventricular rate is persistently rapid, evidence of left ventricular failure may be anticipated.

ECG FEATURES IDENTIFYING ATRIAL FIBRILLATION

1. Rate: The ventricular rate in atrial fibrillation may be normal (60–100/minute), rapid (greater than 100/minute), or slow (less than 60/minute), depending on the number of atrial impulses conducted to the ventricles.

2. Rhythm: The ventricular rhythm is totally irregular. This irregularity is the most typical finding in atrial fibrillation.

3. P waves: P waves are not present because of the chaotic atrial activity. They are replaced by small, irregular, rapid oscillations called f (fibrillatory) waves.

4. P–R interval: There is no P–R interval.

5. QRS: The QRS complex is normal but occurs at irregular intervals. Most of the atrial impulses that bombard the AV node are blocked, but those that do pass through are conducted normally through the ventricles. Thus, atrial fibrillation is manfested electrocardiographically by the absence of P waves and the presence of normal QRS complexes that occur at totally irregular intervals.

Atrial Fibrillation (Figure 10–9)

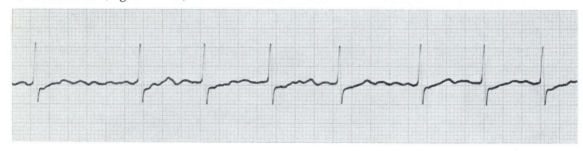

Rate:	The ventricular rate is about 80/minute.
Rhythm:	Irregular.
P waves:	Absent. Fibrillatory waves of different sizes and shapes are present instead.
P–R interval:	Not determinable.
QRS:	Of normal duration (0.08 second), but complexes occur irregularly.
Comment:	The most characteristic feature of atrial fibrillation is the irregular ventricular rhythm. This finding, in conjunction with the absence of P waves, confirms the diagnosis of atrial fibrillation.

Rapid Atrial Fibrillation (Figure 10–10)

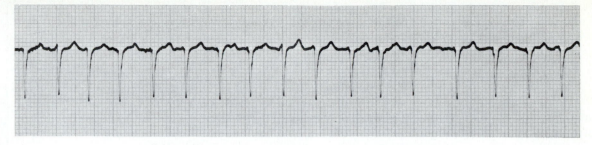

Rate:	The average ventricular response is about 170/minute.
Rhythm:	Irregular.
P waves:	Absent. (Note the variation in the shape and size of the T waves, resulting from super-imposed fibrillatory (Q) waves.
P–R interval:	Not measurable because of the absence of P waves.
QRS:	Of normal duration (0.06 second).
Comment:	Rapid atrial fibrillation substantially reduces cardiac output, and the ventricular rate must be slowed promptly.

Atrial Fibrillation with Normal Ventricular Rate (Figure 10–11)

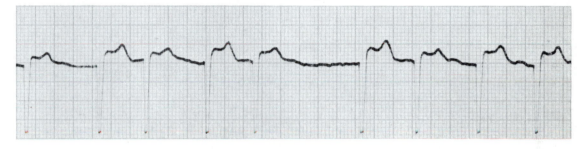

Rate:	The ventricular rate is about 90/minute.
Rhythm:	Grossly irregular.
P waves:	Absent. Fibrillatory waves are shallow in this particular lead.
P–R interval:	Not measurable.
QRS:	Normal (0.08 second).
Comment:	The ST segments are distinctly elevated (2–3 mm) and there are no R waves. These are signs of AMI.

Slow Atrial Fibrillation (Figure 10–12)

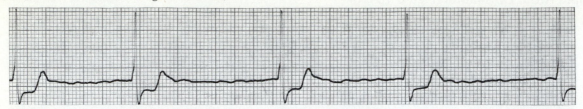

Rate:	The ventricular rate averages about 50/minute.
Rhythm:	Irregular.
P waves:	Shallow, fibrillatory waves are present.
P–R interval:	Not measurable.
QRS:	Normal (0.10 second).
Comment:	The slow ventricular response is caused by advanced AV block, allowing only a few atrial impulses to pass through to the ventricles. AV block may be due to damage to the AV node or to digitalis toxicity. In either case digitalis should not be administered since it increases the degree of AV block and may further slow the heart rate.

Atrial Fibrillation/Flutter (Figure 10–13)

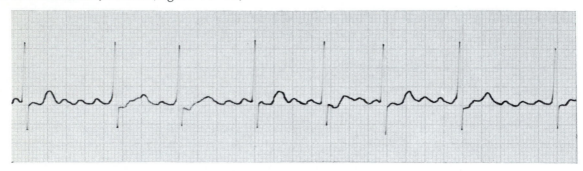

Rate:	The ventricular rate is about 80/minute.
Rhythm:	Irregular.
P waves:	Absent. Replaced by sawtooth F waves of atrial flutter and irregular f waves of atrial fibrillation.
P–R interval:	Not determinable.
QRS:	Normal (0.08 second), indicating that conduction below AV node is normal.
Comment:	The irregular ventricular rhythm indicates atrial fibrillation, but the sawtooth F waves suggest atrial flutter. In this sense the arrhythmia in this case represents a combination of both arrhythmias, and is often called atrial fibrillation/flutter.

Treatment

1. Atrial fibrillation can be treated either with drugs or by electrical means (elective precordial shock). The choice depends on several factors, including the ventricular rate, duration of the arrhythmia, and above all the presence or absence of circulatory insufficiency as manifested by left ventricular failure or angina.
2. If a patient develops left ventricular failure or angina as a direct consequence of rapid atrial fibrillation, the arrhythmia should be terminated without delay and normal sinus rhythm restored by means of synchronized precordial shock (cardioversion).

3. Drug therapy should be the primary method of treating atrial fibrillation that is not accompanied by signs of impaired circulation. Drug treatment of atrial fibrillation is similar to that of atrial flutter. A drug (digitalis, beta-blocker, or calcium-channel blocker) is given to control the rapid ventricular rate by increasing the degree of block at the AV node, but usually does not restore normal sinus rhythm. Chemical cardioversion to sinus rhythm, and interruption of the reentrant circuit is accomplished with a class IA antiarrhythmic agent (eg, quinidine or procainamide).

4. When rapid control of atrial fibrillation is needed, the cardioselective beta-blocker esmolol can be given intravenously. This is a short-acting drug with a half life of 9 minutes and a duration of action of 10 to 20 minutes. It is given as a 0.5 mg/kg bolus followed by a 0.05 mg/kg infusion titrated to provide the desired heart rate.

5. Patients in chronic atrial fibrillation who have had recent heart failure, left atrial enlargement, global left ventricular dysfunction, or a history of hypertension or thromboembolism should be given anticoagulant therapy to reduce the risk of embolization.

6. When atrial fibrillation is of long duration and is not associated with a rapid ventricular rate, attempts to restore normal sinus rhythm are not usually indicated. Although cardioversion can restore sinus rhythm, a patient with longstanding atrial fibrillation will almost always revert to having atrial fibrillation.

Nursing Responsibility

1. If atrial fibrillation develops abruptly or is present and rapid at the time of admission:
   a. Document the arrhythmia with a rhythm strip and notify the physician.
   b. Ascertain whether the arrhythmia is compromising circulatory efficiency and inquire specifically whether the patient has chest pain or dyspnea.
   c. Record the pulse rate, extent of the pulse deficit, and blood pressure.
   d. Prepare for elective cardioversion if the patient is symptomatic.
2. If atrial fibrillation is not rapid or if it existed before the present admission:
   a. Observe the patient's clinical status, particularly with regard to signs of left ventricular failure. Record the pulse rate, apical rate, and blood pressure.
   b. Obtain serial rhythm strips at regular intervals for comparative purposes.
   c. Advise the physician of any significant increase or decrease in the ventricular rate, or of the development of signs or symptoms that suggest left ventricular failure.
3. If digitalis or quinidine is used to treat atrial fibrillation, observe the ECG for signs of drug overdosages (see Chapter 16). If the ventricular rate falls below 60/minute, discuss the need for further administration of these drugs with the physician.
4. The possibility of embolization secondary to atrial fibrillation should always be considered during clinical assessment of the patient with atrial fibrillation.

CASE HISTORY

A 72-year-old man was admitted to the CCU with acute pulmonary edema. He had no history of atrial fibrillation, but the ECG revealed atrial fibrillation with a ventricular response of 136/minute. The nurse initiated a planned treatment program that included morphine (15 mg intravenously), the administration of oxygen, and an intravenous injection of furosemide. Although there was improvement within the next hour, the patient was still very dyspneic. His heart rate was 140/minute and irregular, and rales were heard throughout the entire chest. The decrease in the patient's cardiac output (which caused left ventricular failure) was related in part to the inefficient pumping action associated with his rapid ventricular rate. Accordingly, digoxin was administered intravenously (0.5 mg) in an attempt to slow the ventricular response. After two additional doses of digoxin within the next 12 hours, the ventricular response decreased to 70 to 80/minute. Clinical improvement was clearly evident during this period.

ATRIAL STANDSTILL

Mechanism

Atrial standstill denotes that the SA node and the atria have lost their ability to generate any electrical impulses. As a result, atrial contractions cease (atrial standstill) and the ventricles are stimulated by a lower pacemaker located either in the AV nodal area or in the ventricles. In atrial standstill the pacemaker usually descends progressively: pacemaker failure begins at the SA node, then moves to the atria, and then to the AV nodal area, leaving only an undependable ventricular pacemaker to sustain the heart beat. This sequence of events is called *downward displacement of the pacemaker.* In most cases atrial standstill is a terminal arrhythmia associated with severe left ventricular failure or cardiogenic shock. In patients with AMI atrial standstill is seldom reversible, indicating extensive damage to or severe ischemia of the higher pacemaking centers. Atrial standstill may also occur in the presence of hyperkalemia and is described as atrial paralysis, a reversible condition. Rarely does atrial standstill develop from overdosages of digitalis or quinidine.

Significance

1. Failure of the SA node and the atria to initiate impulses leaves the AV nodal area and ventricles as the only remaining pacemakers. These latter centers are far less dependable than higher pacemakers, and *ventricular standstill* may occur at any time.
2. *Risk:* Downward displacement of the pacemaker usually indicates irreversible damage of the higher pacing centers of the heart, and often heralds death.

Clinical Features

1. Atrial standstill with downward displacement of the pacemaker is seen most often in patients with severe circulatory failure. The arrhythmia itself does not produce specific signs or symptoms.
2. The disappearance of P waves, particularly in patients with advanced circulatory failure, suggests that downward displacement of the pacemaker is occurring because of damage to the SA node and atria.
3. When the pacemaker has descended to the AV-nodal area, the ECG has the same characteristics as in an arrhythmia originating in the AV-nodal area (as described in Chapter 11). However, the differences in clinical circumstances and prognosis in the two kinds of arrhythmia make it important to consider atrial standstill and AV nodal arrhythmias as separate entities.

ECG FEATURES IDENTIFYING ATRIAL STANDSTILL

1. Rate:	Usually slow (40–60/minute), but depends on the site of the pacemaker.
2. Rhythm:	The ventricular rhythm is generally regular, except in the dying heart, in which ventricular ectopic beats may be interspersed.
3. P waves:	P waves are absent and there is essentially a straight line between the QRS complexes.
4. P–R interval:	Absent. There is no electrical activity in the SA node or atria.
5. QRS:	The configuration of the QRS complex depends on the site of the pacemaker If the ventricle is stimulated from the AV-nodal area the QRS complex may be normal. However, if the impulse originates within the ventricle itself, the QRS complex will be widened and distorted.

Atrial Standstill (Figure 10–14)

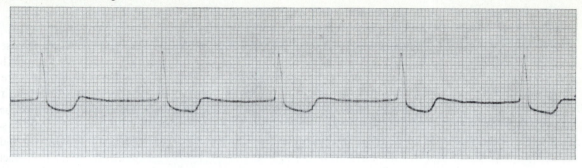

Rate:	About 50/minute.
Rhythm:	Regular.
P waves:	Absent (no atrial activity).
P–R interval:	Not determinable.
QRS:	Normal (0.10 second).
Comment:	The absence of P waves indicates that all atrial activity has ceased and that the pacemaker is in the AV-nodal area.

Treatment

1. When atrial standstill occurs with advanced heart failure or cardiogenic shock, survival is very unlikely. The only hope comes from improving the patient's left ventricular function and tissue oxygenation with intraaortic balloon pumping and vigorous drug therapy.
2. A transvenous pacing catheter should be inserted as soon as there is suspicion that the SA node or atria are failing as pacemakers, and ventricular pacing should be done during the course of treatment for left ventricular failure.
3. If atrial standstill is a result of digitalis toxicity or hyperkalemia (rather than a reflection of progressive ischemia), measures to correct these disorders should be initiated immediately.

Nursing Responsibility

1. The P waves should be examined repeatedly in all patients with advanced left ventricular failure. The abrupt disappearance of the P waves in this situation suggests the onset of atrial standstill.
2. Notify the physician immediately of changes in the P wave pattern and document these patterns with a rhythm strip.
3. Verify the patient's clinical status. Death may occur during downward displacement of the pacemaker even though ventricular complexes are observed on the monitor. In other words, even though electrical activity may be present, the severely ischemic myocardium cannot respond to this activity and its pumping action ceases (a condition called electromechanical dissociation).
4. At the first suggestion of atrial standstill, prepare for the insertion of a transvenous pacemaker.

CASE HISTORY

A 69-year-old man with an acute anteroseptal infarction was admitted to the CCU with obvious signs of left ventricular failure. His response to treatment was poor and he remained in heart failure. The ECG showed normal sinus rhythm with a heart rate of 84/minute. About 8 hours after the patient's admission the nurse noted that his heart rate suddenly slowed to 50/minute and that the P waves had disappeared from his ECG. The physician was notified immediately. Although a temporary pacemaker was inserted, the patient died several hours later. Death was due to severe heart failure with downward displacement of the pacemaker. The ECG change from normal sinus rhythm to atrial standstill is shown in Figure 10–15A and B.

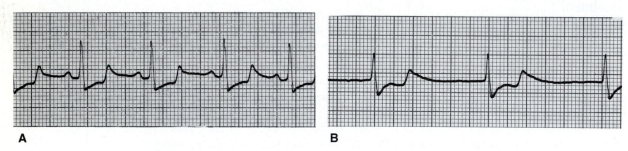

A.   **B.**

Figure 10–15. A. Normal sinus rhythm. **B.** Atrial standstill.

OTHER EXAMPLES OF ARRHYTHMIAS ORIGINATING IN THE ATRIA

Paroxysmal Supraventricular Tachycardia (Figure 10–16)

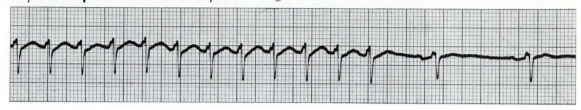

Rate:	185/minute during PSVT.
Rhythm:	Regular.
P waves:	Not identified specifically during PSVT.
P–R interval:	Not measurable.
QRS:	Normal (0.08 second).
Comment:	This example demonstrates the sudden cessation of PSVT and the resumption of normal sinus rhythm.

Paroxysmal Supraventricular Tachycardia with Block (Figure 10–17)

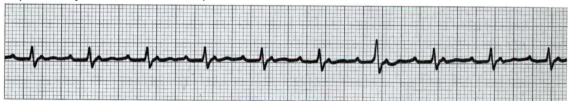

Rate:	The ventricular rate is 100/minute while the atrial rate is 200/minute.
Rhythm:	Regular.
P waves:	There are two P waves between each QRS complex. (One P wave occurs immediately after the QRS complex and below the T wave.)
P–R interval:	The atrial impulses that are conducted to the ventricles have a maximum normal P–R interval (0.20 second).
QRS:	Normal (0.08 second).
Comment:	The atrial rate is 200/minute, typical of atrial tachycardia. The ventricular rate, however, is only 100/minute, indicating that every other atrial impulse is blocked. This arrhythmia, called PSVT with block, is a common manifestation of digitalis toxicity. (The possibility that the arrhythmia is atrial flutter with 2:1 block can be excluded on the basis of the atrial rate, which would be 300 or more per minute in the case of atrial flutter.)

Atrial Flutter with 4:1 Block (Figure 10–18)

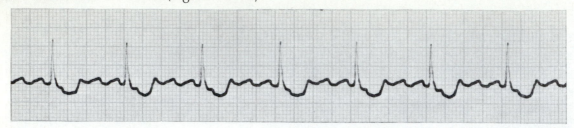

Rate:	The ventricular rate is 75/minute and the atrial rate is 300/minute.
Rhythm:	Regular.
P waves:	Four F waves occur during each R-R interval (4::1).
P–R interval:	Not determinable.
QRS:	Normal (0.08 second).
Comment:	Three of the four flutter waves between each QRS complex are clearly evident. The fourth occurs immediately after the R wave and produces a notch in the ST segment.

Atrial Flutter with 2:1 Block (Figure 10–19)

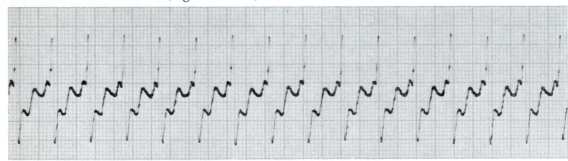

Rate:	Ventricular rate about 150/minute. Atrial rate about 300/minute.
Rhythm:	Regular.
P waves:	There are two flutter waves between QRS complexes, creating a sawtooth appearance.
P–R interval:	Not determinable.
QRS:	Normal.
Comment:	In general, atrial flutter with 2:1 block is more difficult to recognize than atrial flutter with 4:1 block. The reason for this is that flutter waves are often superimposed on other waves when the ventricular rate is fast (as in 2:1 block).

Atrial Fibrillation (Figure 10–20)

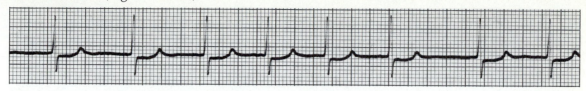

Rate:	About 80/minute.
Rhythm:	Irregular.
P waves:	No identifiable P waves or fibrillatory waves.
P–R interval:	Not measurable.
QRS:	Normal (0.08 second).
Comment:	The diagnosis of atrial fibrillation is evident from: (1) the absence of P waves; and (2) the irregular ventricular rhythm. Although fibrillatory waves can often be identified in atrial fibrillation, none are visible in this particular lead.

Atrial Flutter with Varying AV Block (Figure 10–21)

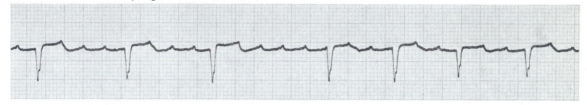

Rate:	Ventricular rate is about 70/minute.
Rhythm:	Irregular.
P waves:	Flutter waves occur regularly at a rate of about 250/minute. Some of the flutter waves are buried in the QRS complexes.
P–R interval:	Not significant.
QRS:	Normal (0.08 second).
Comment:	Unlike typical atrial flutter, which is characterized by a regular ventricular rate, this recording shows atrial flutter with a varying degree of AV block (3:1, 4:1, 5:1), which produces an irregular rhythm. Varying AV block is usually a manifestation of disturbed AV function.

Atrial Fibrillation with High-Degree AV Block (Figure 10–22)

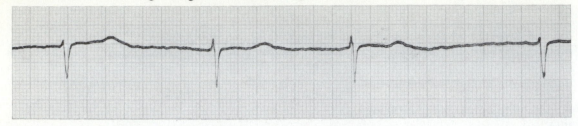

Rate:	The ventricular response is about 80/minute.
Rhythm:	Irregular.
P waves:	None. Very shallow fibrillatory waves are seen occasionally.
P–R interval:	None (since there are no P waves).
QRS:	Normal (0.09 second).
Comment:	Although the atria discharges impulses very rapidly (atrial fibrillation), only a few of these impulses are conducted to the ventricles. The very slow ventricular response (about 40/minute) indicates a high degree of block at the AV node, resulting from either digitalis or AV-nodal disease. In any event, a ventricular rate of only 40/minute is usually hemodynamically ineffective and cannot be tolerated for long.

Atrial Standstill (Figure 10–23)

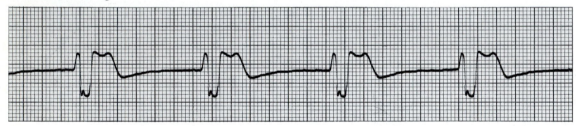

Rate:	About 40/minute.
Rhythm:	Regular.
P waves:	None.
P–R interval:	None.
QRS:	Wide (0.20 second) and distorted, indicating a ventricular origin.
Comment:	There is no evidence of atrial activity (atrial standstill), because the higher impulse-generating centers have been knocked out. A ventricular pacemaker has assumed control. This pattern, in which there is no longer any atrial or junctional activity, and only a ventricular pacemaker remains, occurs in the latter stages of downward displacement of the pacemaker.

Chapter 11

Arrhythmias Originating in the AV Junction

PREMATURE JUNCTIONAL CONTRACTIONS
JUNCTIONAL RHYTHM
PAROXYSMAL JUNCTIONAL TACHYCARDIA
NONPAROXYSMAL JUNCTIONAL TACHYCARDIA
(Accelerated Junctional Rhythm)
Other Examples

Junctional arrhythmias originate at the junction of the AV node and bundle of His. Normally the AV junction discharges impulses only when its inherent rate is faster than that of the SA node or atria. This usually occurs when the higher centers are temporarily suppressed (for one reason or other), allowing the normally slower AV junction to take over as pacemaker, at a rate of 40 to 60/minute. When this happens the resulting arrhythmia is described as a junctional rhythm or junctional escape rhythm (meaning that the pacemaker has "escaped" from the SA node to the AV junction).

On some occasions junctional arrhythmias are caused by impulse formation in the AV junction at a rate that exceeds the discharge rate of the SA node, even though the SA node is not depressed. Two arrhythmias may result from this increased activity in the AV junction: paroxysmal junctional tachycardia (PJT) and nonparoxysmal junctional tachycardia (NPJT, often called accelerated junctional rhythm).

Like the atria and the ventricles, the AV junction can also produce premature beats (premature junctional contractions [PJCs]).

Junctional arrhythmias (except for PJCs) must be regarded as major arrhythmias, and demand prompt attention.

PREMATURE JUNCTIONAL CONTRACTIONS

Mechanism

A PJC is similar to a premature atrial contraction (PAC) except that the impulse arises from an ectopic focus in the AV junctional area rather than in the atria. The impulse is transmitted downward through the His–Purkinje system and produces a normal QRS complex, which occurs earlier than expected in the rhythm cycle. The junctional impulse is also transmitted upward to the atria (retrograde conduction), causing atrial stimulation. Retrograde atrial activation usually results in an inverted P wave that occurs just before or after (or during) the QRS complex, depending on the site of the ectopic focus in the junctional area and the speed of retrograde conduction. After a PJC there is an incomplete compensatory pause until the next sinus impulse arises. PJCs probably reflect irritability of the junctional tissues.

Significance

1. Although it has been suggested that PJCs may give rise to junctional tachycardia in the same sense that atrial premature beats may trigger atrial fibrillation (AF), this sequence of events has not been proven. Consequently, PJCs cannot be regarded as distinct forerunners of junctional tachycardia.
2. Infrequent or isolated PJCs have no significant effect on circulatory efficiency.
3. PJCs are probably a sign of irritability of the junctional tissue, and an increase in the frequency of these ectopic beats may reflect ischemic injury to the nodal or His-bundle areas (eg, during an evolving acute myocardial infarction [AMI]).
4. *Risk:* PJCs are not serious in their own right, and can be classified as a minor arrhythmia.

Clinical Features

1. Although PJCs produce some irregularity of the heartbeat, patients with these contractions seldom experience any symptoms.
2. PJCs cannot be distinguished from other premature beats by clinical examination; the arrhythmia can be identified only by ECG.

ECG FEATURES IDENTIFYING PREMATURE JUNCTIONAL CONTRACTIONS

1. Rate: Normal.

2. Rhythm: Regular except for the premature beat and the pause that follows.

3. P waves: Because the atria are stimulated in a retrograde manner by impulses originating in the junctional tissue, the shape and position of the P waves vary with the conduction time to the atria. Usually the P waves are inverted and occur either immediately before or after the QRS complex. In many instances P waves cannot be identified at all, being buried in the QRS complexes.

4. P–R interval: When a P wave precedes the QRS complex, the P–R interval is usually shortened (less than 0.12 second).

5. QRS: Normal because conduction from the AV-junctional area to the Purkinje network is not disturbed. (Occasionally, however, the impulse may be transmitted abnormally, producing a wide QRS complex. This is called *aberrant conduction.*)

Premature Junctional Contraction (Figure 11–1)

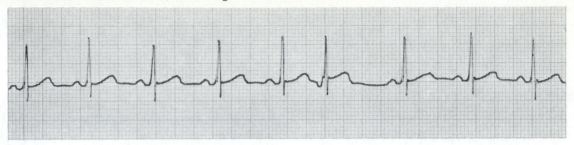

Rate:	About 90/minute.
Rhythm:	Regular except for one PJC.
P waves:	The P wave of the PJC is inverted and occurs immediately before the QRS complex.
P–R interval:	Shortened (0.08 second) in the PJC; other P–R intervals are normal.
QRS:	Normal (0.06 second).
Comment:	An inverted P wave with a very short P–R interval indicates retrograde conduction from the AV junction to the atria.

Premature Junctional Contraction (Figure 11–2)

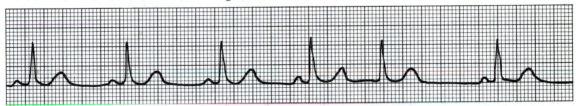

Rate:	About 60/minute.
Rhythm:	A regular rhythm is interrupted by one premature beat and the pause that follows it.
P waves:	The P wave of the PJC is not visible, being hidden in the QRS complex.
P–R interval:	Not measurable.
QRS:	Normal (0.09 second).
Comment:	The P wave of the PJC is hidden in the QRS complex because the atria and ventricles are depolarized simultaneously (ie, the velocities of retrograde and anterograde conduction are the same). If the atria were depolarized first, the P wave would precede the QRS complex. If the atria were depolarized after the ventricles, the P waves would follow the QRS complex.

Treatment

1. If PJCs occur infrequently, treatment is unnecessary.
2. If their frequency increases, PJCs can usually be terminated by administering lidocaine or procainamide intravenously.

Nursing Responsibility

1. Identify PJCs and distinguish them from more serious premature ventricular contractions (PVCs).
2. If the relative frequency of PJCs increases, notify the physician.
3. If PJCs are treated with an intravenous infusion of lidocaine or procainamide, adjust the rate of flow to control these ectopic beats.

CASE HISTORY

A 58-year-old man with an acute inferior myocardial infarction developed infrequent ectopic beats during his second day of hospitalization. From the monitor lead alone, the nurse was unable to decide whether these beats were PJCs or PVCs. When the frequency of these ectopic beats increased gradually over the next 3 hours, a 12-lead ECG was taken to identify their specific origin. The nurse identified them as PJCs and notified the physician. The physician decided that no therapy was necessary, however, since the patient remained asymptomatic.

JUNCTIONAL RHYTHM

Mechanism

If for any reason the SA node fails to initiate impulses or discharges too slowly, the AV junction may assume control of the cardiac rhythm, replacing the SA node as pacemaker. When this occurs, a *junctional rhythm* exists. In other words, a junctional rhythm develops because of default of the primary (SA node) pacemaker, and serves as a safety mechanism to sustain the heartbeat. Because the pacemaker has "escaped" from the SA node to the AV junction, the rhythm is also described as a *junctional escape rhythm.*

In this circumstance the AV junction discharges impulses at its own intrinsic rate of 40 to 60/minute. The impulses travel upward to activate the atria and downward to stimulate the ventricles. Depending on the relative velocities of retrograde and anterograde conduction, the P waves may precede, follow, or be hidden within the QRS complexes. Since ventricular stimulation is not disturbed, the QRS complexes are normal.

The suppression of the SA node, which permits junctional rhythm to develop, is often the result of excessive vagal activity. Other causative factors are ischemic damage to the SA node and digitalis or quinidine toxicity.

Significance

1. Because of the inherently slow rate of junctional impulses (40–60/minute), ectopic foci with more rapid rates may take over the pacemaking function. Such foci may cause either junctional or ventricular tachycardia, especially in the presence of myocardial ischemia.
2. A junctional pacemaker is not dependable and there is a danger of downward displacement of the pacemaker to the ventricle, with the heart rate decreasing even more.
3. As with other slow-rate arrhythmias, cardiac output may decrease significantly in cases of junctional rhythm, leading to myocardial ischemia or heart failure.
4. *Risk:* Although most patients can tolerate a junctional rhythm without difficulty, the arrhythmia is nevertheless dangerous because it indicates that a less dependable pacemaker than the SA node is in command of the heart rate. Also, there is a potential threat of other ectopic rhythms developing, as well as of the adverse hemodynamic consequences of the slow rate and lack of contribution of atrial contraction to the cardiac output.

Clinical Features

1. A junctional rhythm seldom produces symptoms unless the rate is very slow (about 40/minute).
2. At the bedside, junctional rhythm may resemble sinus bradycardia because the QRS complex is the same in both. Both arrhythmias are characterized by a slow, regular heart rate of 40 to 60/minute. An ECG is necessary to distinguish the two arrhythmias.
3. Junctional rhythm is often transient (lasting for only a few beats), after which the SA node regains control.

ECG FEATURES IDENTIFYING JUNCTIONAL RHYTHM

1. Rate: Slow (usually 40–60/minute).

2. Rhythm: Regular.

3. P waves: The P waves may occur: (1) before the QRS complex; (2) after the QRS complex; or (3) may not be visible, being buried within the QRS complex. When present, the P waves are usually inverted because of retrograde conduction through the atria.

4. P–R interval: When the P waves precede the QRS complexes, the P–R interval is shortened to less than 0.12 second, reflecting retrograde stimulation of the atria by a pacemaker in the AV junction.

5. QRS: Normal, indicating that conduction downward through the His-Purkinje system is not disturbed.

Junctional Rhythm (Figure 11–3)

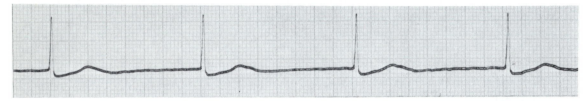

Rate: About 40/minute.
Rhythm: Regular.
P waves: None visible.
P–R interval: Not measurable.
QRS: Normal (0.06 second)
Comment: The presence of this junctional rhythm (at a rate of about 40/minute) indicates that the SA node is no longer discharging or is firing at a rate of less than 40/minute. Junctional rhythm is a safety mechanism for preserving ventricular function.

AV-Junctional Rhythm (Figure 11–4)

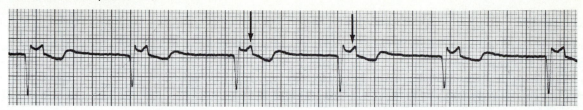

Rate:	54/minute.
Rhythm:	Regular.
P waves:	Occur after QRS complexes, as evident by the notch in the S–T segment (see arrows).
P–R interval:	Indeterminate.
QRS:	Normal (0.06 second).
Comment:	When the P wave follows the QRS complex it indicates that the junctional impulses activated the ventricles before the atria. Put differently, anterograde conduction to the ventricles is faster than retrograde conduction to the atria.

Treatment

1. There is no specific drug therapy for junctional rhythm, but atropine is sometimes successful in increasing the discharge rate of the SA node, allowing it to regain control.
2. If the slow heart rate compromises the circulation, a transvenous pacemaker should be used to increase the ventricular rate (and the cardiac output).
3. If ventricular ectopic beats develop in the presence of a junctional rhythm, they are best controlled by rate acceleration (cardiac pacing or atropine). For some reason lidocaine is less effective in terminating ventricular ectopic beats that develop during slow heart rates than it is in controlling premature ventricular beats that occur during normal or fast heart rates.
4. If the junctional rhythm is secondary to digitalis or quinidine overdosage, the offending drug should be withdrawn.

Nursing Responsibility

1. Identify the arrhythmia as junctional rhythm. Rule out the possibility that the slow heart rate is due to sinus bradycardia or advanced heart block. A 12-lead ECG may be necessary for this.
2. Observe the monitor carefully for premature ventricular beats, which are likely to develop in the presence of a slow heart rate. Notify the physician if such ectopic activity is noted.
3. Be alert for symptoms of heart failure or myocardial ischemia, particularly when the heart rate is below 50/minute.
4. If a junctional rhythm develops suddenly, notify the physician.
5. If the patient is receiving digitalis or quinidine, withhold further dosing and confer with the physician about discontinuing the drug before administering the next dose.

CASE HISTORY

A 56-year-old man was admitted to the CCU with a heart rate of 48/minute. He was in no distress and there was no evidence of left ventricular failure. The nurse noted that the P waves on a rhythm strip were inverted and followed the QRS complexes, from which she concluded that the patient's bradycardia was due to a junctional rhythm. Two hours later the patient developed PVCs at a rate of 4 to 6/minute. When four PVCs occurred consecutively (ventricular tachycardia [VT]), lidocaine was administered. It was not effective in suppressing the ectopic beats. After an unsuccessful attempt at increasing the heart rate with intravenous atropine, a transvenous temporary pacemaker was inserted and the ventricle was paced at a rate of 80/minute. The ectopic beats disappeared promptly.

PAROXYSMAL JUNCTIONAL TACHYCARDIA

Mechanism

Paroxysmal junctional tachycardia (PJT) is the most common form of paroxysmal supraventricular tachycardia (PSVT). It is similar in most respects to other forms of PSVT (ie, to PSVT that originates in the atria). Both arrhythmias begin and end suddenly, and both are characterized by a regular, rapid rate of 140 to 250/minute. As with other tachyarrhythmias, the mechanism is one of reentry in 90% of cases, with the reentrant loop localized to the AV node.

Impulses from the AV junction are conducted normally to the ventricles and in a retrograde manner to the atria. As with other junctional arrhythmias, the P waves occur before, after, or during the QRS complexes, depending on the speed of retrograde conduction.

PJT may result from increased catecholamine secretion and metabolic disturbances, but ischemia of the AV node is probably its most common cause. Digitalis toxicity is occasionally the underlying mechanism of PJT.

Since PJT is the most common form of PSVT and is usually caused by reentry, the mechanism by which it occurs will be explained in detail. In most patients with AV-nodal reentry, the AV node contains two functionally different pathways that can be designated as A and B. Conduction down pathway A is slower than that down pathway B, but the refractory period is shorter. In most instances a stimulus conducted from the atria travels down both pathways, but the impulse down the faster pathway, B, reaches the bundle of His first. By the time the impulse in the slower pathway A gets to the bundle of His, it finds the bundle already depolarized and refractory to further stimulation. Thus the impulse is blocked.

If the patient experiences a premature atrial beat, however, the situation in the pathways changes. The premature beat may find pathway B refractory because of its long refractory period. However, pathway A, with its shorter refractory period, is ready to accept a stimulus. The impulse travels down pathway A, and by the time it reaches the bundle of His finds pathway B repolarized and ready to accept a new stimulus. The impulse now travels up (in a retrograde direction) pathway B and finds pathway A repolarized. A sustained reentrant rhythm is created within the AV node (Figure 11–5).

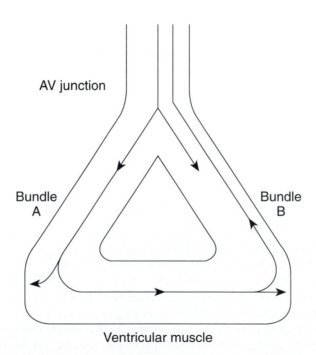

Figure 11–5. Mechanism of reentry established by having a conduction pathway through the AV junction that has a different conduction time than the AV node (a bypass tract).

Significance

1. The rapid ventricular rate in PJT usually results in a decrease in cardiac output and predisposes to left ventricular failure. This threat is directly related to the duration of the tachycardia.
2. PJT increases myocardial oxygen demand and decreases oxygen supply because the coronary arteries have less time to fill in diastole. It may produce angina or additional ischemic damage.
3. *Risk:* PJT is a dangerous arrhythmia from a hemodynamic standpoint, particularly if the episode is prolonged.

Clinical Features

1. The clinical presentation of PJT closely resembles that of paroxysmal atrial tachycardia (PAT), with the sudden onset and termination of a rapid, regular rhythm (140–250/minute).
2. The symptoms are those anticipated with a very fast ventricular rate: dyspnea, apprehension, and angina are common, especially if the tachycardia is sustained.
3. It is often difficult and sometimes impossible to distinguish the ectopic focus of a PSVT electrocardiographically. The rapid rate frequently obscures the position of the P waves.

ECG FEATURES IDENTIFYING PAROXYSMAL JUNCTIONAL TACHYCARDIA

1. Rate:	Usually 140 to 250/minute.
2. Rhythm:	Regular.
3. P waves:	May precede, follow, or be hidden in QRS complexes, depending on the speed of retrograde conduction to the atria.
4. P–R interval:	If P waves precede the QRS complexes, the P–R interval is usually less than 0.12 second.
5. QRS:	Normal, since conduction to the ventricles is not disturbed.

Paroxysmal Junctional Tachycardia (Figure 11–6)

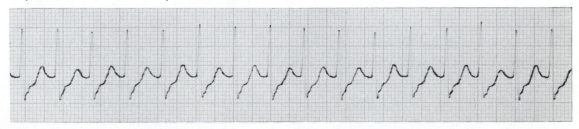

Rate:	160/minute.
Rhythm:	Regular.
P waves:	Follow the QRS complexes, being visible in the S–T segments.
P–R interval:	Not determinable.
QRS:	Near normal. (Although widened, the QRS complexes appear to be 0.10 second in duration.)
Comment:	It is often difficult to distinguish PJT from PAT with a monitor lead alone. A 12-lead ECG may be necessary to identify the position of the P waves.

Paroxysmal Junctional Tachycardia (Figure 11–7)

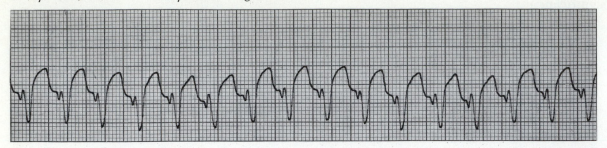

Rate:	About 160/minute.
Rhythm:	Regular.
P waves:	Inverted, and immediately precede the QRS complexes.
P–R interval:	Shortened (0.06 second).
QRS:	Normal (0.08 second).
Comment:	This arrhythmia began abruptly and terminated spontaneously 3 minutes later in typical paroxysmal fashion.

Treatment

1. Vagal stimulation by means of carotid sinus massage may terminate PJT and is usually the first step in its treatment. This increases parasympathetic stimulation to the AV node, decreasing AV conduction and breaking the reentrant circuit.
2. If PJT is sustained and results in angina or signs of left ventricular failure, the arrhythmia should be *terminated immediately* with synchronized precordial shock (cardioversion).
3. If the arrhythmia produces no obvious symptoms and the patient is not in distress, drug therapy can be attempted initially. The most effective pharmacologic therapy is intravenous adenosine. However, this is contraindicated in VT, and therefore the nurse must be quite certain that the rhythm is SVT and not VT. A 12-lead ECG may be required to make this diagnosis.
4. Other drugs useful for treating PJT include the calcium-channel blockers (especially verapamil) and beta-blockers (propranolol), all of which slow conduction and block reentrant circuits in the AV node. Digitalis also slows conduction through the AV node, but is less useful because of its slow onset of action.
5. Even if the paroxysm of junctional tachycardia is of short duration and subsides spontaneously without treatment, antiarrhythmic therapy should nevertheless be instituted in an attempt to prevent recurrent episodes. The choice of drugs for this purpose includes propranolol, quinidine, digitalis, and calcium-channel–blocking agents.

ECG FEATURES IDENTIFYING NONPAROXYSMAL JUNCTIONAL TACHYCARDIA

1. **Rate:** Usually 70 to 130/minute. Rates below 60/minute indicate a junctional escape rhythm. Rates above 140/minute suggest PJT.

2. **Rhythm:** Regular.

3. **P waves:** May occur before or after the QRS complex, or may not be present.

4. **P–R interval:** Retrograde conduction to the atria may or may not occur. When a P–R interval is identifiable, the interval is usually less than 0.12 second. The P–R interval is normal because conduction from the AV junction to the ventricles is not affected.

Nonparoxysmal Junctional Tachycardia (Accelerated Junctional Rhythm) (Figure 11–8)

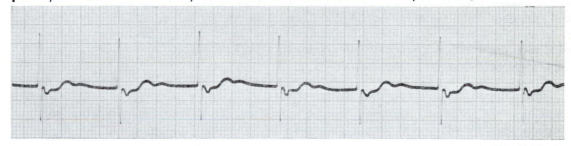

Rate:	About 70/minute.
Rhythm:	Regular.
P waves:	Inverted and occur immediately after QRS complexes.
P–R interval:	Not determinable.
QRS:	Normal (0.06 second).
Comment:	This arrhythmia is often called accelerated junctional rhythm because its rate is faster than the inherent rate of junctional tissue (40–60/minute), yet is much slower than that in PJT (140–220/minute). Since the arrhythmia is not actually a tachycardia (which requires a rate exceeding 100/minute), the term "accelerated junctional rhythm" is used.

Nonparoxysmal Junctional Tachycardia (Accelerated Junctional Rhythm) (Figure 11–9)

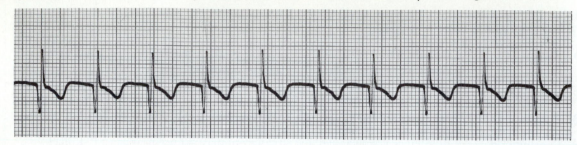

Rate:	About 100/minute.
Rhythm:	Regular.
P waves:	Not visible, probably buried in QRS complexes.
P–R interval:	Not measurable in the absence of P waves.
QRS:	Normal (0.10 second).
Comment:	In contrast to PJT, which develops abruptly, the arrhythmia shown here developed gradually and its rate never exceeded 100/minute.

Treatment

1. There is no specific treatment for NPJT. When circulatory failure is present the treatment plan is aimed at improving left ventricular function, after which the arrhythmia may disappear.
2. Because of the threat of further downward displacement of the pacemaker to the ventricles in NPJT, a transvenous pacemaker may be required.
3. If there is any possibility that NPJT is the result of digitalis toxicity, the drug should be stopped immediately and potassium administered intravenously.
4. If the patient becomes symptomatic because the heart rate is high, quinidine, procainamide, or propranolol can be used to slow the ventricular rate.

Nursing Responsibility

1. Because the NPJT develops gradually and its rate is between 70 and 130/minute, the alarm system of the cardiac monitor will not be activated; therefore, the identification of this arrhythmia depends on careful observation of the monitor.
2. Ascertain that the arrhythmia is NPJT and document it with a rhythm strip.
3. Be especially alert for this arrhythmia among patients with advanced circulatory failure or cardiogenic shock, and notify the physician immediately once identification has been made.
4. Prepare for the insertion of a transvenous pacemaker, which may be utilized in the treatment program for NPJT.
5. Always consider the possibility of digitalis intoxication when NPJT develops in the absence of circulatory failure. If this is the case, digitalis should be immediately stopped.

CASE HISTORY

A 74-year-old man was admitted to the CCU with severe chest pain and signs of marked left ventricular failure. The ECG revealed an acute anterior wall myocardial infarction and sinus tachycardia. The patient was treated with furosemide, dopamine, and nitroprusside but showed little improvement during the next 2 hours. The nurse noted that the heart rate gradually decreased from 130 to 80/minute. Initially the nurse thought that the decrease in heart rate was a positive response to unloading therapy. However, on examining a rhythm strip, the nurse noted a change in the P waves, which were now inverted and followed the QRS complexes. It was apparent that the patient had developed NPJT. The physician was notified immediately, but the CCU team decided to continue treatment without change, since the patient was not symptomatic.

OTHER EXAMPLES OF ARRHYTHMIAS ORIGINATING IN THE AV JUNCTION

Supraventricular Ectopic Beats: Either PJCs or PACs (Figure 11–10)

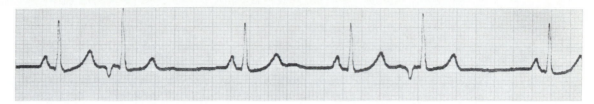

Rate:	About 70/minute.
Rhythm:	Regular except for premature ectopic beats.
P waves:	The fourth P wave occurs prematurely and is inverted.
P–R interval:	The P–R interval of the premature beat is 0.12 second.
QRS:	Normal (0.06 second).
Comment:	Although the P waves of the two ectopic beats are inverted, this does not indicate that they are PJCs. The P waves of atrial ectopic beats may also be inverted. However, the P–R intervals of PJCs should be less than 0.12 seconds, while they can be longer with PACS. In this example (where the P–R interval is 0.12 second) the ectopic beats are best classified as *supraventricular ectopic beats,* meaning that they are either atrial or junctional in origin.

Junctional Rhythm (to Normal Sinus Rhythm) (Figure 11–11)

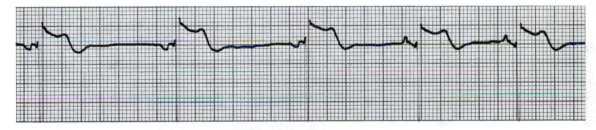

Rate:	During junctional rhythm: 45/minute.
Rhythm:	Regular (but at different rates).
P waves:	Inverted with junctional rhythm; upright with normal sinus rhythm.
P–R interval:	Normal (0.12 second during junctional rhythm).
QRS:	Normal (0.08 second).
Comment:	The first three beats originate in the AV junction at a rate of 45/minute. The SA node, which apparently had been suppressed, suddenly regains control as the pacemaker starting with the fourth beat. Note the faster heart rate during sinus rhythm, which explains why the SA node resumed its control.

Junctional Rhythm (Figure 11–12)

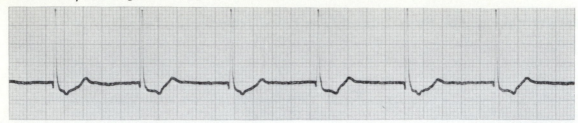

Rate:	About 60/minute.
Rhythm:	Regular.
P waves:	Occur after QRS complexes and appear as downward notches in S–T segments.
P–R interval:	Not determinable.
QRS:	Normal (0.06 second).
Comment:	A junctional rhythm is a protective or escape mechanism which develops when the SA node or atria are suppressed.

Junctional Escape Beat (Figure 11–13)

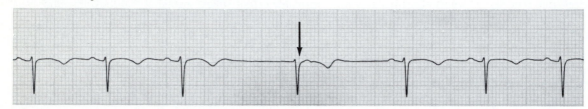

Rate:	About 70/minute.
Rhythm:	Irregular.
P waves:	At approximately three beats, the next anticipated P wave is not visible (junctional escape beat). The P waves occur regularly thereafter.
P–R interval:	Normal except with the junctional escape beat, where the P–R interval is indeterminate.
QRS:	Normal (0.06 second), including the junctional escape beat.
Comment:	After three beats there is a pause (perhaps because of sinus arrest or block, or marked sinus bradycardia). In any event, after 1.2 seconds, no sinus or atrial beat has occurred. As a protective mechanism, the AV junction, which is the next downward pacemaker, discharges an impulse to stimulate the ventricles and prevent cessation of the heartbeat. This junctional beat is called a junctional escape beat. Note that the escape beat does not occur unless the heart rate slows and the R–R interval is prolonged, even if only for one beat.

Paroxysmal Junctional Tachycardia (Figure 11–14)

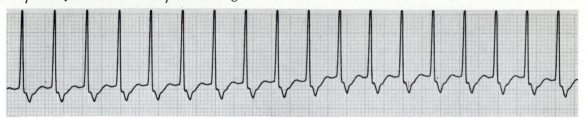

Rate:	About 180/minute.
Rhythm:	Regular.
P waves:	These occur after QRS complexes, producing T waves with a spiked appearance.
P–R interval:	Not determinable.
QRS:	Normal (0.04 second).
Comment:	Sharp, spiked T waves usually indicate that a P wave is superimposed. Hidden P waves, as in this example, can often be located through this T-wave sign.

Supraventricular Tachycardia (Figure 11–15)

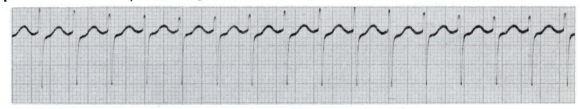

Rate:	160/minute.
Rhythm:	Regular.
P waves:	Not identifiable.
P–R interval:	Not determinable.
QRS:	Normal (0.06 second).
Comment:	This rapid tachycardia is characterized by a regular rhythm with QRS complexes of normal duration. The normal QRS complexes indicate that the arrhythmia originated above the ventricles. However, since P waves cannot be identified, the tachycardia may be either atrial tachycardia (PAT), junctional tachycardia (PJT), or atrial flutter with 2:1 block, and is simply called a supraventricular tachycardia. Only by using additional leads can a definite interpretation be made.

Accelerated Junctional Rhythm (Figure 11–16)

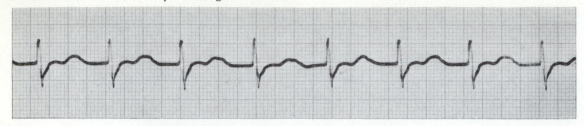

Rate:	About 80/minute.
Rhythm:	Regular.
P waves:	Not identified, probably buried in QRS complexes.
P–R interval:	Not measurable.
QRS:	Normal, at just under 0.12 second.
Comment:	This arrhythmia is called an accelerated junctional rhythm because its rate is faster than the inherent rate of junctional tissue (40–60/minute). On the other hand, it is much slower than PJT (140–220/minute).

Accelerated Junctional Rhythm (Figure 11–17)

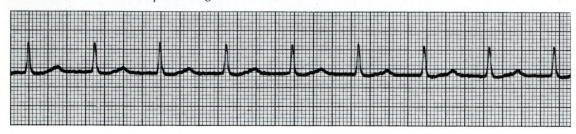

Rate:	About 90/minute.
Rhythm:	Regular.
P waves:	None visible.
P–R interval:	Not determinable.
QRS:	Normal (0.08 second).
Comment:	Since the normal discharge rate of the AV junction is 40 to 60/minute, the arrhythmia represents an accelerated junctional rhythm. Unlike an escape junctional rhythm, which occurs by default and is a protective mechanism, accelerated junctional rhythms (or NPJT) are active rhythms; they may be caused by various drugs.

Chapter 12

Arrhythmias Originating in the Ventricles

PREMATURE VENTRICULAR CONTRACTIONS
VENTRICULAR TACHYCARDIA
ACCELERATED IDIOVENTRICULAR RHYTHM
VENTRICULAR FIBRILLATION

Disturbances in the heartbeat that originate in the SA node, the atria, or the AV-junctional area are classified as *supraventricular* arrhythmias. Disturbances in which the impulse begins in the ventricles, below the level of the AV-nodal area, are termed *ventricular* arrhythmias.

The most common ventricular arrhythmia (in fact, the most common of all arrhythmias) is the premature ventricular contraction (PVC). Premature ventricular beats result from the discharge of an ectopic focus within the ventricular walls (or the conduction pathway) before the expected arrival of the next impulse from a supraventricular center. These ectopic beats usually represent a sign of myocardial irritability secondary to ischemia, and the frequency and type of PVCs is probably a fair index of the degree of ischemic irritation. Practically all patients with acute myocardial infarction (AMI) exhibit PVCs during the first few days after the attack.

There is good evidence that ventricular fibrillation (VF), the most frequent cause of sudden death, is a direct consequence of myocardial irritability, and that this lethal arrhythmia usually begins with a PVC. The scale of myocardial irritability leading to VF can be viewed as follows:

1. Isolated PVCs.
2. Complex PVCs (more than 6/minute), or PVCs originating from more than one ventricular focus (multifocal premature beats) or occurring in pairs (couplets).
3. A series of three or more consecutive premature contractions occurring at a rapid rate (ventricular tachycardia [VT]).
4. VF.

Although the relationship between PVCs and VF is clearly established, it should not be assumed that all ventricular ectopic beats are potentially dangerous. *It is only in the presence of myocardial ischemia that PVCs are likely to provoke VF.* Many normal individuals without evidence of heart disease display premature ventricular beats that pose no threat at all.

VT is an immediate forerunner of VF in many instances. In addition to this extreme threat, VT when sustained seriously endangers the circulation by markedly reducing cardiac output. For these reasons this ventricular arrhythmia must never be allowed to persist.

Accelerated idioventricular rhythm, like VT, consists of a series of consecutive ventricular ectopic beats. However, these beats occur at a rate of only 50 to 100/minute, compared to the much faster (140 to 250/minute) rate of VT. Furthermore, accelerated idioventricular rhythm does not lead to VF, and is a benign arrhythmia in this sense.

VF, by far the main cause of sudden cardiac death, is understandably of supreme importance.

PREMATURE VENTRICULAR CONTRACTIONS

Mechanism

A PVC occurs when an irritable focus in the ventricles discharges before the arrival of the next anticipated impulse from the SA node (or another supraventricular pacemaker). The ectopic focus stimulates the ventricles directly (without an impulse traversing the normal conduction pathway) and produces a wide, distorted QRS complex which is one of the main characteristics of a PVC. The SA node is not usually affected by the PVC and continues to discharge independently and on schedule; however, P waves are seldom visible in the ECG, being hidden in the abnormal QRS complex. Following the PVC there is a *complete compensatory pause* before the next sinus impulse arrives to initiate a normal ventricular beat. (A complete or fully compensatory pause means that the interval between the beat preceding the PVC and the beat following it is exactly equal to two cardiac cycles. When the interval is less than two cardiac cycles, as with premature atrial or junctional contractions, the compensatory pause is described as incomplete.)

PVCs are the most common of all arrhythmias associated with AMI and are thought to represent a sign of ventricular irritability secondary to ischemia. Patients with advanced heart failure also have frequent PVCs because the dilatation (thinning) of the ventricular walls in this condition results in myocardial ischemia.

Significance

1. PVCs reflect myocardial irritability and are of particular importance because they may initiate repetitive ventricular firing in the form of VT or VF. The sequence of PVCs leading to VT and then VF is most apt to arise when:
   a. PVCs occur frequently, especially six or more times per minute.
   b. Every second beat is a PVC (bigeminy).
   c. The PVC strikes on the T wave of the preceding complex (the "R-on-T" pattern).
   d. PVCs originate from more than one irritable focus in the ventricle (multiple PVCs).
   e. There are two consecutive PVCs (couplets or pairs).
2. Since PVCs develop in 90% of all patients with AMI, their mere presence has little significance in its own right. PVCs are of concern if they increase in frequency or occur in one of the five dangerous forms described above.
3. Overdosages of digitalis (digitalis toxicity) frequently cause PVCs. This relationship is suggested especially when PVCs occur as bigeminy.
4. Hypokalemia (insufficient potassium) also predisposes to PVCs. Patients receiving diuretic agents in the emergency room or ICU particularly without potassium replacement, may become suddenly hypokalemic. Serum potassium levels should be measured on admission and should be monitored closely in patients receiving diuretics.
5. PVCs are also increased with caffeine, sympathomimetic drugs, hypoxia, and anxiety.
6. *Risk:* If PVCs appear infrequently, the threat of their provoking serious ventricular arrhythmias is not great. However, if these ectopic beats occur with increasing frequency or are of a dangerous type, they should be considered a serious warning of impending VT or VF. Among patients with AMI, mortality is greater in those who have frequent PVCs (more than 10/minute), couplets (two PVCs in a row), or triplets (three PVCs in a row).

Clinical Features

1. Many patients are aware of PVCs and describe the accompanying sensation as "palpitations" or "skipping of the heart." The greater the frequency of these ectopic beats, the more likely the patient is to notice them.
2. When listening to the heart or taking the pulse, a relatively long pause is noted immediately after the premature beat. This delay (called a complete compensatory pause) is characteristic and practically diagnostic of PVCs.
3. If PVCs are very frequent, cardiac output will decrease and the patient may complain of fatigue or dizziness. Cardiac output decreases because ventricular diastole (filling time) is shorter with PVCs.

ECG FEATURES IDENTIFYING PREMATURE VENTRICULAR CONTRACTIONS

1. Rate: Often normal, but PVCs can occur at any rate.

2. Rhythm: The premature beat and the compensatory pause that follows it create an irregularity in the heart rhythm. Characteristically, the interval between the beat preceding and the beat following a PVC is equal to two normal beats (a complete compensatory pause, as shown in Figure 12–1).

3. P waves: Although the SA node discharges independently of the PVC, the P wave is usually hidden in the QRS complex.

4. P–R interval: A PVC does not have a P–R interval because the ventricle is stimulated directly and there is no conduction from the atrium to the ventricles.

5. QRS: The QRS complex is always widened and distorted in shape because the impulse travels from its ectopic site through the ventricles via slow cell-to-cell connections rather than through the normal rapid-conduction-system pathway. The particular configuration of the QRS complex depends on the ventricular focus from which the PVCs arise. The T wave is usually directed opposite from the QRS complex.

Isolated Premature Ventricular Contraction (Figure 12–1)

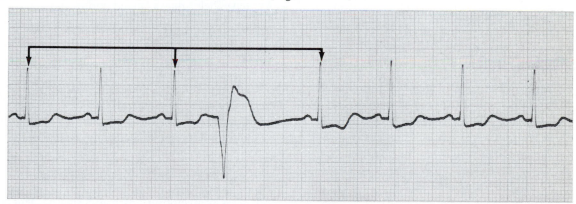

Rate:	About 80/minute.
Rhythm:	Irregular because of PVC.
P waves:	Not seen in the cycle of the PVC; normal in the other cardiac cycles.
P–R interval:	Absent in the PVC because the impulse originates in the ventricle (conduction of the remaining beats is normal.)
QRS:	The ectopic complex is widened and bizarre in configuration, and the T wave is in the direction opposite that of the QRS complex.
Comment:	The interval between the beat preceding the PVC and the beat following the PVC is equal to the period of two normal beats (arrows), and represents a full compensatory pause.

Treatment

1. Lidocaine is the primary agent used to control PVCs. Suppression of the irritable ventricular focus can in most instances be achieved promptly by administering 50 to 100 mg lidocaine via a rapid intravenous injection ("intravenous push"). This should be followed by a continuous infusion of lidocaine at a rate of 2 to 3 mg/minute (20–30 microdrops/minute of a solution containing 3,000 mg lidocaine in 500 mL glucose solution) in order to control further myocardial irritability. If the PVCs are not controlled with this regimen, a second or third intravenous bolus of lidocaine (50–100 mg) can be administered at 15-minute intervals. The total dosage, however, should not exceed 500 mg/hour, since lidocaine toxicity can lead to seizures.

2. If adequate doses of lidocaine fail to suppress PVCs, procainamide (Pronestyl) can be given intravenously as a second-line agent. Although sometimes successful in this situation, procainamide has the disadvantage of producing hypotension, and has a higher incidence of side-effects than lidocaine. (The methods of administration of procainamide are described in Appendix A.)

3. Occasionally neither lidocaine nor procainamide in customary doses is effective in inhibiting PVCs. In this circumstance it is unwise to increase the dosage of either drug beyond its recommended levels, since overdosages of both drugs can produce serious toxic effects. Resistance to drug therapy often indicates a depletion of myocardial potassium, and for this reason it is useful to administer an intravenous infusion of potassium (40 mEq KCl in 500 mL dextrose solution), particularly if there is evidence of hypokalemia.

4. Oral antiarrhythmic agents are often effective in controlling ventricular ectopic activity. However, their action is too slow for acute situations and therefore they are reserved for maintenance therapy. The most commonly used drugs for this purpose are procainamide (500 mg every 4 hours) and quinidine (400 mg every 6 hours). Long-acting procainamide (Procan-SR, given at a dosage of 500–750 mg every 6 hours) is available. Disopyramide and flecainide are sometimes used but should be avoided in patients with heart failure because they depress myocardial function.

5. If PVCs develop during treatment with digitalis or diuretics, the possibility of drug-induced ectopic beats must always be considered. In this circumstance the drugs may have to be discontinued and potassium administered.

6. Patients with recurrent symptomatic PVCs may need to have their drugs assessed during an electrophysiologic study.

Nursing Responsibility

1. Identify PVCs and distinguish them from less serious atrial or junctional premature contractions.

2. Carefully assess the relative frequency of PVCs during successive time intervals so as to ascertain any change in their number. Also identify the type of PVC noted (ie, multifocal, couplet).

3. If PVCs occur in any of the most threatening forms, administer lidocaine immediately (using standing protocols) and notify the physician.

4. When an infusion of lidocaine is used to control PVCs, adjust the rate of flow to suppress ectopic activity with the minimal dosage.

5. If lidocaine is given repeatedly or in large doses, seek signs of overdosage as manifested by petit mal or grand mal seizures or drowsiness. If procainamide is being administered, monitor the patient's blood pressure frequently in order to detect hypotension.

6. In the event that PVCs develop during digitalis therapy, advise the physician before administering the next dose of digitalis.

CASE HISTORY

A 51-year-old woman with an AMI showed evidence of PVCs from the time of her admission to the CCU. These ectopic beats occurred at a rate of 1 to 2/minute. During the next several hours the nurse noted that the PVCs gradually increased in frequency and that bigeminy had developed. Lidocaine in a dose of 75 mg was given as an intravenous push, and the nurse notified the physician of the bigeminy. The PVCs disappeared within a minute of the injection. An intravenous infusion of lidocaine was then started. Two hours later the PVCs reappeared and the nurse increased the rate of lidocaine infusion from 1 mg to 2 mg/minute, after which the PVCs disappeared.

FIVE DANGEROUS FORMS OF PREMATURE VENTRICULAR CONTRACTIONS

Frequent PVCs Occurring More Often Than 6/Minute (Figure 12–2)

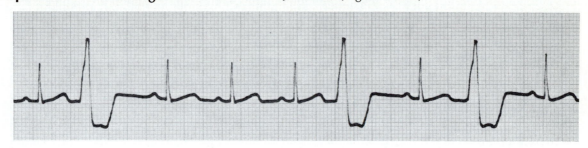

Rate:	About 90/minute.
Rhythm:	Irregular, as the result of PVCs.
P waves:	Not identified in ectopic beats.
P–R interval:	Absent in PVCs. The remaining beats are conducted normally from the SA node.
QRS:	The PVCs are very wide (0.16 second) and distorted in shape, indicating their ventricular origin.
Comment:	There are three PVCs in this 6-second strip. At this frequency, about 30 PVCs would occur per minute, constituting a serious sign of ventricular irritability.

Bigeminy (Alternate PVCs or Coupled Rhythm) (Figure 12–3)

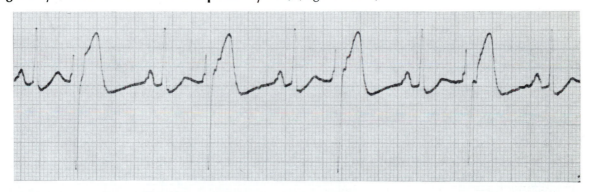

Rate:	About 90/minute.
Rhythm:	Irregular due to bigeminy (coupled beats).
P waves:	Not seen in the PVCs.
P–R interval:	There is no P–R interval in the ectopic beats. The ventricles are stimulated directly by an ectopic focus.
QRS:	Grossly distorted in PVCs and obviously different from the beats originating in the SA node.
Comment:	Bigeminy may warn of more dangerous ventricular arrhythmias. It is often a forerunner of VT.

The R-on-T Pattern (Figure 12–4)

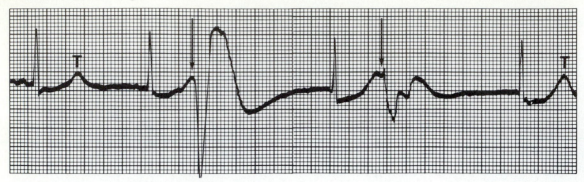

Rate:	About 60/minute.
Rhythm:	The ectopic beats create an irregularity in the basic sinus rhythm.
P waves:	Not seen in the PVCs.
P–R interval:	Absent. The ectopic beats arise in the ventricle. There is no conduction from the atrium and hence no P–R interval.
QRS:	The two ectopic beats are distorted and have different configurations. The difference in their shape indicates that more than one irritable focus is present in the ventricle (multifocal PVCs).
Comment:	Both PVCs strike directly on the T waves of the preceding complexes (arrows). When a PVC occurs at the time of the T wave (the R-on-T pattern), there is a high risk of precipitating VF.

Onset of Ventricular Fibrillation (Figure 12–5)

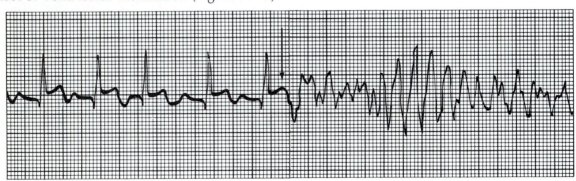

Rate:	About 100/minute prior to VF.
Rhythm:	Regular until onset of chaotic pattern of VF.
P waves:	Precede each QRS until VF, then not identified.
P–R interval:	0.20 sec until onset of VF. In VF there is no conduction from the atrium and no P–R interval.
QRS:	Not identified in VF.
Comment:	Note the onset of VF when an isolated PVC (arrow) strikes the T wave of the preceding beat.

Multifocal PVCs (Figure 12–6)

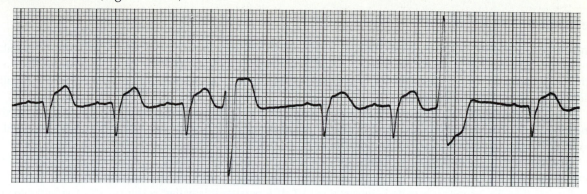

Rate:	About 80/minute.
Rhythm:	Irregular.
P waves:	No P waves are visible with the two PVCs.
P–R interval:	Not determinable with PVCs.
QRS:	The two PVCs show characteristically widened and distorted QRS complexes. However, the configuration (and direction) of the two contractions is distinctly different, indicating that they originated from different foci in the ventricle (multifocal PVCs).
Comment:	Multifocal PVCs usually reflect advanced ventricular ectopic activity and are considered more serious than PVCs that originate from a single focus (unifocal PVCs).

Consecutive PVCs (Figure 12–7)

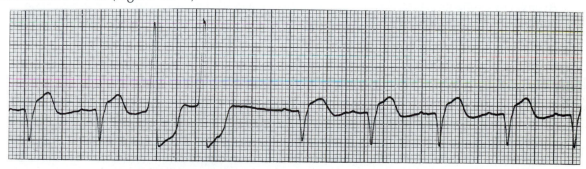

Rate:	About 90/minute.
Rhythm:	Irregular.
P waves:	Not visible in pair of PVCs.
P–R interval:	Not determinable in PVCs; otherwise P–R intervals are normal (0.18 second).
QRS:	Typically widened and distorted. PVCs occur consecutively for two beats.
Comment:	Two consecutive PVCs (usually called couplets or pairs) often lead to repetitive ventricular firing in the form of VT or VF.

VENTRICULAR TACHYCARDIA

Mechanism

Ventricular tachycardia (VT) can be considered as a series of three or more *consecutive* premature ventricular contractions occurring at a rapid rate (usually 140–250/minute). The electrophysiologic mechanism of their occurrence is unclear, but evidence exists for both enhanced automaticity and reentry. The occurrence of VT usually reflects marked myocardial irritability.

The QRS complexes are wide and bizarre, as is typical of PVCs. Although the ventricular focus serves as the dominant pacemaker, the atria continue to discharge independently. As a result, the P waves (which are usually obscured) bear no relationship to the QRS complexes.

Occasionally, VT may develop without any warning signs, but most often the arrhythmia is preceded by frequent or dangerous types of PVCs. VT may terminate spontaneously, after only a few beats (a short run). If it lasts for less than 30 seconds it is called *nonsustained VT*. If it persists it is called *sustained VT*. The latter condition is ominous, since it produces serious hemodynamic effects and can degenerate into ventricular fibrillation (VF).

Significance

1. The seriousness of VT depends primarily on its duration. Short runs of VT, lasting for only a few seconds, are seldom dangerous in their own right. However, they represent a warning of sustained VT and the possible development of VF.
2. In contrast, when VT persists and becomes an established rhythm, serious hemodynamic consequences can be expected. These are manifested by a marked reduction in cardiac output, which leads to left ventricular failure, cardiogenic shock, and myocardial and cerebral ischemia. The hemodynamic deficit may be so great that sudden death can occur during ventricular tachycardia.
3. At any time during its course, VT may suddenly change into VF. For this reason VT must be considered to be in the same life-threatening category as VF.
4. *Risk:* When sustained, VT is an extremely dangerous arrhythmia constituting a true emergency.

Clinical Features

1. Most patients with VT are immediately aware of the sudden onset of rapid cardiac activity and describe dyspnea, palpitations, and lightheadedness. When angina accompanies these symptoms, as it usually does, the patient senses that a catastrophe has occurred, and marked apprehension is evident.
2. The blood pressure falls soon after the onset of VT (often to hypotensive levels), and signs of left ventricular failure may develop with surprising rapidity if the tachycardia continues. These adverse hemodynamic effects are due to a reduction in cardiac output resulting from a decreased ventricular filling time.
3. On many occasions VT occurs as short runs lasting for only a few seconds before terminating spontaneously. These brief episodes may not produce any signs or symptoms.

ECG FEATURES IDENTIFYING VENTRICULAR TACHYCARDIA

1. Rate: Usually 140 to 220/minute, but may be faster.

2. Rhythm: The ventricular rhythm is essentially regular, but there may be a slight irregularity.

3. P waves: The SA node continues to discharge independently during VT, but the P waves bear no relationship to the QRS complexes. (The P waves can seldom be identified specifically, being buried in the QRS complexes.)

4. P–R interval: There is no conduction from the atria to the ventricles, and therefore no P–R interval.

5. QRS: Wide, slurred complexes, typical of repetitive PVCs.

Sustained Ventricular Tachycardia (Figure 12–8)

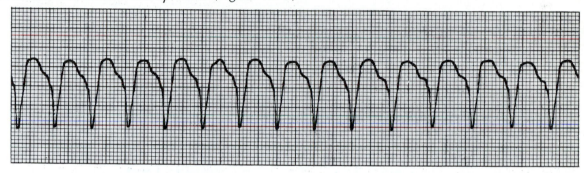

Rate: About 150/minute.
Rhythm: Regular.
P waves: Not identified.
P–R interval: Absent.
QRS: Successive PVCs with a widened, bizarre configuration.
Comment: Sustained VT is likely to degenerate into VF. The arrhythmia must be terminated without delay.

Ventricular Tachycardia Stopping Spontaneously (Figure 12–9)

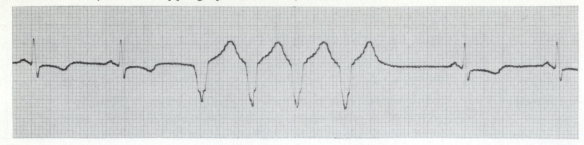

Rate:	About 130/minute (during the brief burst of VT).
Rhythm:	Slightly irregular during VT.
P waves:	Not identified during VT.
P–R interval:	Normal before and after salvo of VT.
QRS:	The four consecutive PVCs (comprising the short run of VT) are wide and distorted. They contrast sharply with the beats of sinus origin.
Comment:	This brief episode of VT stopped spontaneously without treatment and was followed by normal sinus rhythm. Short bursts of this type are the most common form of VT.

Rapid Ventricular Tachycardia (Figure 12–10)

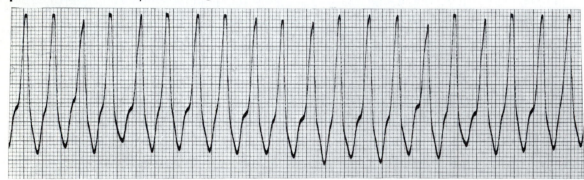

Rate:	About 200/minute.
Rhythm:	Slightly irregular.
P waves:	Not identified.
P–R interval:	Absent. The ventricles are stimulated directly by an ectopic focus at a rate of 200/minute. There is no atrioventricular conduction.
QRS:	The complexes are widened and distorted in shape.
Comment:	This very rapid ventricular rate is extremely detrimental to the pumping efficiency of the heart, and must be terminated immediately.

Extreme Ventricular Tachycardia (Figure 12–11)

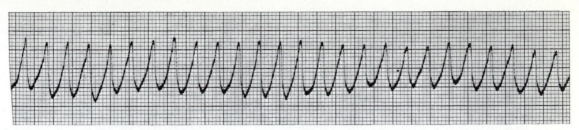

Rate:	About 200/minute.
Rhythm:	Slightly irregular.
P waves:	Not visible.
P–R interval:	Absent.
QRS:	The very rapidly occurring complexes resemble a helix (similar to a stretched, coiled spring).
Comment:	This is an extreme form of ventricular tachycardia that will most certainly be accompanied by severe symptoms. In many instances it is an immediate forerunner of ventricular fibrillation and must be treated with the same urgency as ventricular fibrillation—by means of precordial shock (defibrillation).

Torsade de Pointes ("Twisting of the Points") (Figure 12–12)

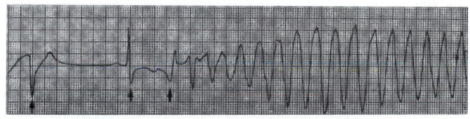

A

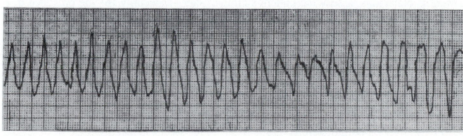

B

Rate:	300/minute
Rhythm:	Slightly irregular
P waves:	Not visible.
PR interval:	Absent.
QRS:	The very rapid complexes have varying amplitudes, which gives the pattern an undulating appearance.
Comment:	This form of VT occurs in conditions causing a prolonged QT interval (eg, quinidine or electrolyte disturbances [particularly hypocalcemia or hypokalemia]). Treatment is aimed at shortening the QT interval by overdrive pacing. A transcutaneous pacemaker can be used while preparations are made to insert a transvenous pacemaker. Isoproterenol (2–10 mg/minute) or magnesium sulfate (1–2 g) can also be given intravenously.

Treatment

1. VT must be terminated promptly and never allowed to persist. The first step in terminating it is to administer 100 mg lidocaine intravenously as a bolus injection. If this is successful, additional lidocaine should be given in the form of a continuous intravenous infusion at a rate of 2 to 4 mg/minute, so as to prevent recurrent episodes of VT.
2. Failure to convert VT to normal sinus rhythm with a bolus injection of lidocaine should be considered an indication for *immediate electrical cardioversion*, particularly if the patient experiences angina or shows evidence of hypotension or heart failure. Further attempts at cardioversion with injections of lidocaine (or other drugs) are ill-advised in this situation. As a general rule, if VT persists after the bolus injection of lidocaine is completed, the next step should be electrical cardioversion.
3. At least 50% of all episodes of VT are of short duration and stop spontaneously without treatment (nonsustained VT). The transiency of these attacks, although momentarily reassuring, should not afford great comfort since there is a high risk of additional episodes of VT or the sudden onset of VF. Consequently, vigorous antiarrhythmic treatment is indicated even when VT occurs as a short run. An infusion of 3,000 mg lidocaine in 500 mL glucose solution should be started promptly. The flow should be set initially at 2 mg/minute and adjusted subsequently (2–4 mg/minute) to suppress ventricular ectopic activity.
4. In some instances VT is refractory to lidocaine (and other conventional drugs) or recurs soon after cardioversion. In this circumstance procainamide is administered intravenously at a rate of 20 to 30 mg/minute to a maximum total of 17 mg/kg. If this fails to terminate or prevent recurrent attacks, bretylium tosylate is administered at 5 to 10 mg/kg over a period of 8 minutes, to a maximum total of 30 mg/kg over a 24-hour period.
5. Automatic implantable defibrillators are increasingly used to manage symptomatic or sustained episodes of VT.

Nursing Responsibility

1. When the high-rate alarm of the cardiac monitor sounds and VT is identified, an emergency situation exists. A planned treatment program must be initiated at once.
2. Go to the bedside and examine the patient. If the patient is unconscious, proceed immediately with precordial shock.
3. If the patient is conscious, assess the patient's clinical state, especially for the presence of dyspnea, angina, and hypotension.
4. Call the physician immediately.
5. Prepare a syringe containing 100 mg lidocaine and administer the drug intravenously as a bolus injection.
6. If the injection of lidocaine is successful in terminating the arrhythmia, an infusion of lidocaine should be started with a flow of 2 to 4 mg/minute.
7. If the bolus injection of lidocaine is unsuccessful and the patient is *not* in distress, a second bolus injection (100 mg) may be administered.
8. Bring the defibrillator to the bedside. *Remember that VF may develop at any time.*
9. If VT occurs as a short run and terminates spontaneously, start an intravenous infusion of lidocaine (2–4 mg/minute) to prevent recurrent episodes.

CASE HISTORY

A 47-year-old man with an AMI was admitted to the CCU in no distress. Just after the monitor electrodes had been attached and an intravenous infusion of dextrose solution started, the high-rate alarm sounded. The nurse recognized immediately that VT had developed and examined the patient. The patient experienced both dyspnea and chest pain. In accordance with the standing orders of the unit, the nurse prepared a syringe containing 100 mg lidocaine and injected it rapidly into the existing intravenous line. The VT stopped within 30 seconds. The physician was notified of this event and the patient was placed on a continuous intravenous lidocaine infusion at a rate of 4 mg/minute.

ACCELERATED IDIOVENTRICULAR RHYTHM

Mechanism

Like VT, accelerated idioventricular rhythm is characterized by a series of consecutive ventricular ectopic beats. However, the ventricular rate is only 50 to 100/minute, in contrast to the rapid rate (140–250/minute) of VT. Also, accelerated idioventricular rhythm begins and ends gradually, unlike VT. Because of these latter characteristics the arrhythmia has been called slow ventricular tachycardia or nonparoxysmal ventricular tachycardia. Neither of these terms is appropriate, and the arrhythmia is best described as accelerated idioventricular rhythm.

Accelerated idioventricular rhythm denotes that the ventricles initiate impulses on their own (idioventricular), without stimulation from a higher center, but that instead of discharging at the inherent rate of ventricular tissue (25–40/minute), the pacemaker fires at an accelerated rate of 50 to 100/minute. The ventricular pacemaker takes command only if its rate exceeds the sinus rate. This occurs most often as the result of momentary slowing of discharge of the SA node. As soon as the sinus rate increases the ventricular focus is subdued. Probably the most common cause of accelerated idioventricular rhythm is ischemia of the SA node after myocardial infarction. The arrhythmia may also be a manifestation of digitalis toxicity.

Significance

1. Accelerated idioventricular rhythm develops in about 20% of patients with AMI. It is a transient arrhythmia, lasting from only a few seconds to a minute (usually 3–30 beats), and produces no hemodynamic effects.
2. In the great majority of cases, accelerated idioventricular rhythm is uncomplicated and does not lead to more serious ventricular arrhythmias.
3. Only rarely is accelerated idioventricular rhythm associated with VT. In these instances the ventricular rate increases suddenly after a few idioventricular beats.
4. *Risk:* Accelerated idioventricular rhythm is a benign arrhythmia. It has no serious consequences and does not affect prognosis except in rare instances in which it occurs together with VT.

Clinical Features

1. Because the heart rate is usually normal and there is no hemodynamic deficit, accelerated idioventricular rhythm produces no symptoms.
2. Although both accelerated idioventricular rhythm and VT consist of a repetitive series of ventricular ectopic beats, the two arrhythmias are readily distinguishable on the basis of their ventricular rates.

ECG FEATURES IDENTIFYING ACCELERATED IDIOVENTRICULAR RHYTHM

1. **Rate:** 50 to 100/minute.

2. **Rhythm:** Regular (or nearly regular).

3. **P waves:** The atria are stimulated independently by the SA node or by retrograde conduction from the ventricles. However, P waves are seldom visible, being buried in the QRS complexes.

4. **P–R interval:** Not measurable during accelerated idioventricular rhythm.

5. **QRS:** Wide and distorted, as is typical of ventricular ectopic beats.

Accelerated Idioventricular Rhythm (Figure 12–13)

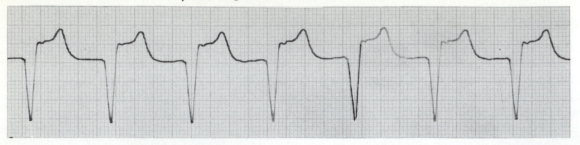

Rate:	About 70/minute.
Rhythm:	Regular.
P waves:	Not identified specifically.
P–R interval:	Not measurable.
QRS:	Wide (0.16 second) and distorted.
Comment:	Accelerated idioventricular rhythm resembles VT but is readily distinguishable from the latter by the slower rate (less than 100/minute).

Accelerated Idioventricular Rhythm (Figure 12–14)

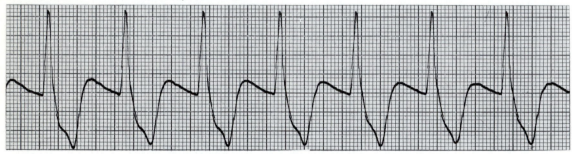

Rate:	About 70/minute.
Rhythm:	Regular.
P waves:	None visible.
P–R interval:	Not measurable.
QRS:	Very wide, distorted, and bizarre in shape.
Comment:	Accelerated idioventricular rhythm begins when the SA node slows or fails to discharge, and ends when normal sinus rhythm returns. The arrhythmia usually lasts for only a few beats.

Treatment

1. Accelerated idioventricular rhythm seldom requires treatment; it is usually a self-limiting arrhythmia.
2. If episodes of accelerated idioventricular rhythm occur frequently or are associated with independent premature ventricular beats, atropine (1 mg) may be administered intravenously to accelerate the rate of discharge of the SA node and allow it to regain control of the heart rate.
3. In the event that accelerated idioventricular rhythm leads to VT, 100 mg lidocaine should be injected intravenously at once (as described previously).
4. Digitalis therapy should be discontinued if there is any suspicion that the arrhythmia is digitalis-induced.

Nursing Responsibility

1. The detection of accelerated idioventricular rhythm requires careful cardiac monitoring. Without close observation the arrhythmia may go unnoticed, since it usually lasts for only a few seconds and does not trigger the low- or high-rate alarms of the monitor.
2. Document the arrhythmia, determine the ventricular rate, and distinguish the arrhythmia from VT.
3. Observe the monitor closely for additional episodes of accelerated idioventricular rhythm and for the possible development of VT.
4. If the patient is being treated with digitalis, consult the physician before administering the next dose.

CASE HISTORY

Sixteen hours after admission to the CCU, a 52-year-old man with an acute inferior myocardial infarction developed a series of eight consecutive ventricular ectopic beats. At first glance the nurse thought these ectopic beats represented VT, but a rhythm strip showed that their rate was 76/minute. Recognizing that the arrhythmia was accelerated idioventricular rhythm, the nurse did not administer lidocaine (as indicated for VT). The rhythm spontaneously resolved to sinus rhythm.

VENTRICULAR FIBRILLATION: A FATAL ARRHYTHMIA

Ventricular fibrillation (VF) is the most common cause of sudden death in patients with coronary heart disease. As noted, this lethal arrhythmia is most often triggered by PVCs or VT. However, VF can also arise spontaneously without preceding signs of ventricular irritability, and therefore always poses the threat of sudden death in patients with myocardial ischemia (eg, AMI or advanced heart failure). Once VF develops, the only hope for survival is the instant application of resuscitative techniques.

Within the CCU the program for resuscitating the patient with cardiac arrest caused by VF is distinctly different from that utilized elsewhere in the hospital. *In the CCU the first step in resuscitation is to terminate VF by precordial shock (defibrillation).* This means that external cardiac compression, mouth-to-mouth ventilation, the administration of oxygen, and other cardiopulmonary resuscitative measures are deliberately bypassed in favor of immediate defibrillation. It is sometimes difficult for nurses and physicians to realize that no reason exists for initiating external cardiac compression and mouth-to-mouth ventilation when VF occurs in the CCU. These techniques are only interim measures used in other settings to sustain the circulation until VF can be terminated electrically. In the CCU, where everything is in readiness to immediately halt this arrhythmia, supportive measures have little importance and in fact do no more than waste precious time. *When a patient develops VF in the CCU, precordial shock must be given without delay by the first person reaching the bedside, and should precede any and all other steps!*

This reversal of the customary management of cardiac arrest (as practiced in the CCU) in no way minimizes the value of cardiopulmonary resuscitation (CPR) as a lifesaving measure. The ability to sustain an adequate circulation by means of external cardiac compression and mouth-to-mouth ventilation has been of inestimable help in combating sudden death outside the prepared setting of a specialized unit. The purpose of these methods is to sustain the perfusion of vital organs until resuscitative equipment can be brought to the patient. All medical and paramedical personnel should be thoroughly competent in performing CPR.

Mechanism

The individual muscle fibers that jointly constitute the ventricular wall are normally stimulated simultaneously and contract in unison. The fibers then recover together and rest until the next impulse causes another contraction. In VF an electrical force arising within the ventricle repeatedly stimulates these muscles at a rate so extremely rapid that the recovery period disappears and the individual muscle fibers merely twitch continuously rather than contracting. Since the muscular twitching (VF) is completely ineffective in propelling blood from the ventricles, the circulation stops abruptly and *death follows within minutes.* Immediately after the onset of VF, the patient becomes unconscious because of inadequate cerebral oxygenation.

The exact mechanism that triggers VF is unknown. It is thought to result from multiple small waves of reentry. Although VF may develop spontaneously, there is usually evidence of myocardial irritability in the form of PVCs before the onset of this catastrophic arrhythmia. It is generally believed that following myocardial infarction the injured myocardium is sensitized, so that a minimal electrical stimulus can initiate VF. The electrical stimulus responsible for this chain reaction is often a PVC that strikes during the vulnerable phase of the cardiac cycle (at the time of the T wave).

VF can develop in patients with AMI who have no obvious complications at the time. It also is the cause of death in 50% of patients with advanced left ventricular failure. The likelihood of successfully resuscitating someone with VF depends on both the underlying disease state of the heart and on the amount of time that elapses between the beginning of VF and defibrillation.

Significance

1. Death occurs within a few minutes after the onset of VF unless the arrhythmia is terminated. The exact duration of life with primary VF depends on several factors, probably the most important of which is the patient's age. For example, an 80-year-old man may die less than a minute after the onset of VF, whereas a much younger patient may survive 4 minutes or more before death becomes irreversible. For this reason the precise time available for successful resuscitation cannot be defined. *The average time is probably 3 minutes.*
2. Although VF can still be terminated after the crucial period for resuscitation, irreversible brain damage may have developed.
3. *Risk: SUPREME DANGER! Death is inevitable unless resuscitation is accomplished immediately.*

Clinical Features

1. The patient loses consciousness almost instantly after the onset of VF. *It is safe to assume that a conscious patient does not have VF.*
2. Peripheral pulses cannot be detected, no heart sounds are audible, and the blood pressure is unobtainable. All are signs of circulatory collapse.
3. The pupils dilate rapidly.
4. Cyanosis develops quickly and total cessation of circulation is evident.

ECG FEATURES IDENTIFYING VENTRICULAR FIBRILLATION

The ECG pattern in VF is characterized by a rapid, repetitive series of chaotic waves originating in the ventricles; the waves have no uniformity and are bizarre in configuration. PQRST waves cannot specifically be identified. The complexes differ from each other and occur in completely irregular fashion. A typical example of VF is seen in Figure 12–15.

The grossly irregular, bizarre waves of VF can hardly be mistaken as representing any other arrhythmia. The only other possibility for such gross distortion is a malfunction of the cardiac monitor (or electrocardiograph machine) or a loose electrode.

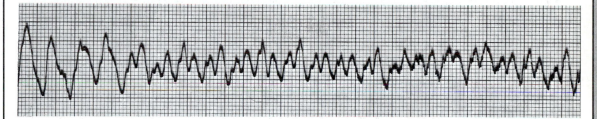

Onset of Ventricular Fibrillation (R-on-T Pattern) (Figure 12–16)

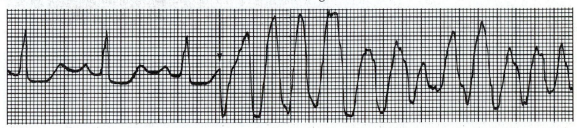

Comment: A premature ventricular contraction striking the T wave of the preceding complex (arrow) precipitates VF.

Treatment

The treatment program for primary VF consists of four phases.

1. *Recognition.* The first step in treating VF is to identify the arrhythmia immediately. VF instantly activates the alarm system of the cardiac monitor, alerting the CCU staff. The electrocardiographic pattern of VF is unmistakable: a series of chaotic waves that lack any uniformity and have a bizarre configuration (Figure 12–17). If the arrhythmia cannot be identified immediately (eg, because of the possibility of artifact from a loose electrode), no time should be wasted in further observing the monitor. Instead, the nurse should proceed at once to the bedside and determine if the patient is unconscious as the result of VF. If the patient is found to be unconscious and peripheral pulses are not detectable, the planned treatment program for terminating VF should be initiated instantly.

2. While the defibrillator is being attached, the patient's airway and breathing should be assessed. If the patient is not breathing, two slow breaths should be delivered and cardiopulmonary resuscitation (CPR) should be begun.

3. *Termination of VF.* Defibrillation (precordial shock) is the first and only means for terminating VF and restoring an effective heartbeat. The shock should be delivered by the first person to reach the bedside, whether a nurse or a physician. The sooner the shock is administered, the greater the chance for recovery. In any case, defibrillation must be accomplished within 2 minutes or the procedure may be ineffective, particularly in elderly patients. Also, any delay in reestablishing an effective heartbeat may result in permanent brain damage secondary to prolonged cerebral ischemia.

   The technique of precordial shock is standardized. Current practice is to give three sequential shocks at energy settings of 200 J, 200 to 300 J, and up to 360 J. Defibrillation with higher energies (eg, 400 to 500 joules) is probably no more efficacious and may in fact be dangerous, causing cardiac damage.

4. Epinephrine in a dose of 1 mg is given intravenously every 3 to 5 minutes. If VF continues, the following drugs are given: (1) lidocaine at 1.5 mg/kg by intravenous push every 3 to 5 minutes to a total loading dose of 3 mg/kg; (2) bretylium at 5 mg/kg by intravenous push, repeated in 5 minutes at a dose of 10 mg/kg; (3) magnesium sulfate at 1 to 2 g by intravenous push; (4) procainamide at 30 mg/minute to a maximum total of 17 mg/kg.

5. *Correction of acidosis.* Metabolic acidosis is hazardous, since it reduces the threshold for recurrent VF. Consequently, sodium bicarbonate should be administered immediately after VF has been terminated. However, recent studies indicate that large doses of sodium bicarbonate (as used in the past) are not necessary and may in fact provoke alkalosis. The currently recommended dose of sodium bicarbonate is 1 mEq/kg initially, followed by half this dose every 10 minutes, if necessary. Serial blood gas determinations should be performed until acid-base balance is assured.

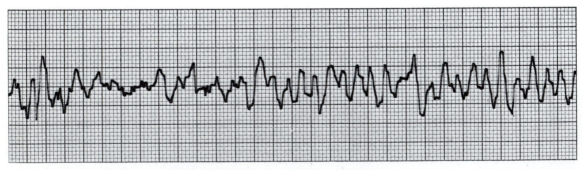

Figure 12–17. Ventricular fibrillation.

6. *Prevention of recurrence of VF.* The myocardial irritability that leads to VF in the first place may produce subsequent episodes of this lethal arrhythmia. In other words, the cause of the original electrical instability of the myocardium continues to exist and must be treated vigorously if further episodes of VF are to be prevented. The main approach to preventing recurrence of VF involves a continuous infusion of lidocaine administered at 2 to 4 mg/minute. Bretylium tosylate may be used for recurrent resistant episodes of VF. This drug raises the threshold for VF and at the same time makes defibrillation easier to accomplish.

Nursing Responsibility

1. VF will trigger the alarm system of the cardiac monitor. (Either the high- or low-rate alarm may sound.)
2. Identify the bizarre, irregular electrocardiographic pattern of VF. Even if in doubt do not waste time with further observation of the monitor. Allow the electrocardiographic record to run continuously to document the event.
3. Go to the bedside and examine the patient. If the patient is conscious and responds to your call, VF is *not* the problem. If the patient is unconscious, ascertain for the absence of breathing and assess the circulation (peripheral pulse and heart sounds).
4. If assistance is available, ask that the emergency system call be sounded. If the patient is not breathing, deliver two slow breaths.
5. Turn on the power switch of the defibrillator and, depending on the type of equipment, set the energy dial at 200 J. Make certain that the synchronizer switch of the defibrillator (used for elective cardioversion) is in the "Off" position.
6. *Perform defibrillation immediately. Do not wait for the arrival of a physician or other personnel before proceeding.* Remember that survival after VF depends directly on the rapidity with which the shock is delivered.
   The steps in defibrillation are as follows:
   a. Make certain the defibrillator is turned on; that the delivered energy level is 200 J; and that the synchronizer is turned off.
   b. Apply a generous amount of electrode paste to the defibrillator paddles and spread it evenly by approximating the surfaces of the paddles and rubbing them together.
   c. Hold the paddles tightly against the patient's chest wall. The exact position of the paddles is not important as long as the current will traverse the axis of the heart.
   d. Make sure that no personnel are in physical contact with the bed or the patient.
   e. Trigger the discharge mechanism of the defibrillator.
7. Immediately after the shock is delivered, observe the monitor to see if the fibrillation has terminated.
8. If VF persists after the initial attempt, a second or third shock should be given promptly.
9. If precordial shock has not been successful after three attempts (an unlikely situation with the use of proper technique), additional shocks are probably unwarranted at this time. Instead, continue CPR and intubate the patient at once. During the period of CPR, epinephrine 1 mg should be injected rapidly and then defibrillation attempted again. Lidocaine or bretylium tosylate may also be utilized in this situation.

CASE HISTORY

Note: The following case history describes the first instance of lifesaving defibrillation performed by a nurse in the absence of a physician. This event took place in 1963 and became the precedent for the now established practice of defibrillation by nurses.

A 72-year-old male was admitted to the CCU of the Presbyterian–University of Pennsylvania Medical Center with a history of chest pain that had subsided by the time of his arrival. He had no complaints and in fact, wanted to go home. An ECG showed an AMI. The findings upon physical examination were normal and there was no evidence of complications. The patient remained in normal sinus rhythm, with a heart rate ranging from 60 to 74/minute. Occasional premature ventricular beats were noted.

Some 60 hours after admission, in the middle of the night, the patient's cardiac monitor alarm sounded. The nurse instantly recognized VF on the monitor and ran to the bedside, where she found the patient to be unconscious. The nurse immediately called the physician and set a timing device for 2 minutes. She turned on the defibrillator, set the energy level at 200 J and applied electrode paste to the defibrillator paddles. The nurse defibrillated the patient without further delay. Normal sinus rhythm was established almost immediately (Figure 12–18). The patient survived and was still alive 10 years later.

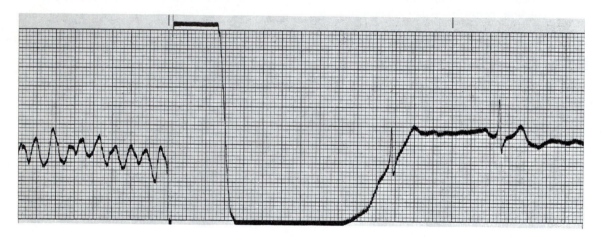

Figure 12–18. Ventricular fibrillation is converted to normal sinus rhythm with defibrillation.

OTHER EXAMPLES OF ARRHYTHMIAS ORIGINATING IN THE VENTRICLES

Ventricular Trigeminy (Figure 12–19)

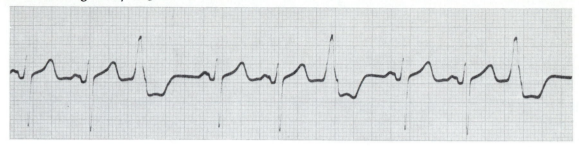

Rate:	About 90/minute.
Rhythm:	Irregular.
P waves:	Not identified with PVCs.
P–R interval:	Not measurable with PVCs.
QRS:	Every third beat is a PVC with widened, distorted QRS complexes.
Comment:	The occurrence of a PVC at every third beat is described as ventricular trigeminy. (When PVCs occur with every other beat, the arrhythmia is called ventricular bigeminy.)

Consecutive PVCs: Multifocal Couplet (Figure 12–20)

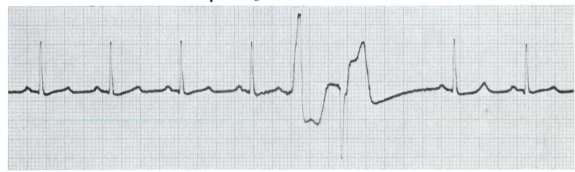

Rate:	About 80/minute.
Rhythm:	Irregular.
P waves:	Not identified with PVCs; otherwise normal.
P–R interval:	Not measurable with PVCs.
QRS:	Two PVCs with grossly different configurations (multifocal) occur consecutively to produce a couplet.
Comment:	Multifocal couplets of this type represent high-grade ventricular ectopic activity and warn of VT or VF.

Ventricular Tachycardia Beginning with R-on-T PVC (Figure 12–21)

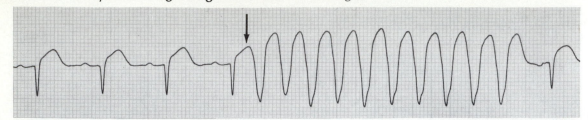

Rate:	About 200/minute during VT.
Rhythm:	Regular during episode of VT.
P waves:	Not visible during the burst of VT.
P–R interval:	Indeterminate.
QRS:	After four normal sinus beats a PVC suddenly strikes the apex of the preceding T wave (R-on-T pattern) and precipitates an episode of VT.
Comment:	This episode of VT lasted for 10 beats before ending spontaneously.

PVCs Occurring as Couplets (Figure 12–22)

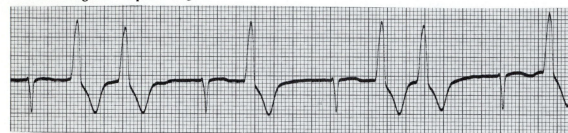

Rate:	About 100/minute.
Rhythm:	Irregular.
P waves:	Not identified in PVCs (or in other beats, perhaps because of lead placement).
P–R interval:	Not measurable.
QRS:	There are six wide, bizarre complexes typical of PVCs.
Comment:	The high frequency of PVCs and the presence of two sets of couplets (pairs) in this brief 6-second strip should be considered a distinct warning of the possible development of a life-threatening ventricular arrhythmia.

Ventricular Tachycardia (Figure 12–23)

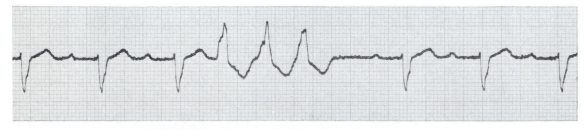

Rate:	About 90/minute.
Rhythm:	Irregular
P waves:	Not visible in PVCs, but otherwise normal.
P–R interval:	Prolonged (0.28 second) in sinus beats. Not measurable in PVCs.
QRS:	About 0.12 second in sinus beats. Wide and distorted in PVCs.
Comment:	Three consecutive PVCs in rapid succession fulfill the criterion for the diagnosis of VT. The first-degree heart block (PR interval of 0.28 second) and widened QRS complexes (0.12 second) observed in this tracing are unrelated to the episode of VT.

Ventricular Tachycardia: Sustained (Figure 12–24)

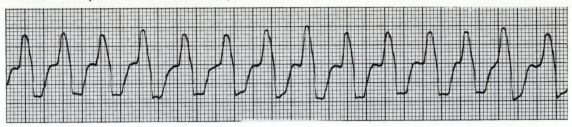

Rate:	About 140/minute.
Rhythm:	Regular.
P waves:	None identifiable.
P–R interval:	Not measurable.
QRS:	Consecutive PVCs that are wide (0.20 second) and distorted.
Comment:	Sustained VT must be terminated as soon as possible because of its adverse hemodynamic effects and the threat of VF.

Accelerated Idioventricular Rhythm (Figure 12–25)

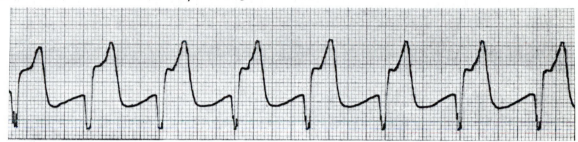

Rate:	About 80/minute.
Rhythm:	Regular.
P waves:	None visible.
P–R interval:	Not determinable.
QRS:	Wide and distorted.
Comment:	The series of eight consecutive ventricular ectopic beats seen in this example should not be classified as VT because they occur at a rate of only 80/minute. The preferred terminology for such an arrhythmia is accelerated idioventricular rhythm, meaning that the beats originate in the ventricle but at a normal (nontachycardiac) rate.

Ventricular Fibrillation: Onset (Figure 12–26)

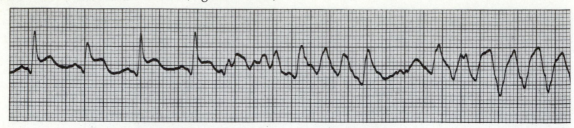

Rate:	Before the onset of VF the heart rate is 110/minute.
Rhythm:	Chaotic beating with no rhythm once VF begins.
P waves:	Normal prior to VF.
P–R interval:	Normal until onset of VF.
QRS:	When VF begins, the QRS complexes are replaced by a series of chaotic waves that have no uniformity and are bizarre in configuration.
Comment:	VF may begin without any previous warnings, but antecedent PVCs are usually the case.

Artifact Mimicking Ventricular Fibrillation (Figure 12–27)

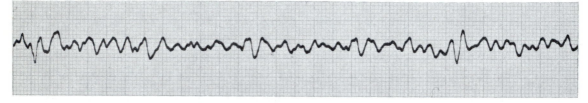

Comment:	This strip seems to demonstrate ECG findings typical of VF. However, the bizarre pattern was in fact due to a loose electrode! Similar patterns can occur when patients brush their teeth. Remember: Go to the bedside immediately and examine the patient when VF appears on the monitor.

Chapter 13

Disorders of Conduction and Ventricular Asystole

FIRST-DEGREE ATRIOVENTRICULAR HEART BLOCK
SECOND-DEGREE ATRIOVENTRICULAR HEART BLOCK
Mobitz Type I (Wenckebach) Block
Mobitz Type II Block
THIRD-DEGREE (COMPLETE) ATRIOVENTRICULAR HEART BLOCK
INTRAVENTRICULAR BLOCKS
Bundle-Branch Blocks
VENTRICULAR ASYSTOLE

As described previously, impulses normally arise in the sinoatrial (SA) node; travel by way of the internodal tracts to the atrioventricular (AV) node; pass through the AV node to the bundle of His, the left and right bundle branches and their divisions (fascicles) to the Purkinje network; and terminate in the myocardial cells. Any interference or abnormal delay in the passage of impulses from the SA node through the Purkinje–myocardial junction is described as a *heart block.* Heart blocks can occur at any level of the conduction system, and it is customary to categorize these disorders into three groups according to the main anatomic sites of involvement (Figure 13–1), as follows:

1. Blocks in the SA node or atria.
2. Blocks in the AV node or the surrounding junctional area (AV or junctional blocks).
3. Blocks in the His–Purkinje system (intraventricular blocks, hemiblocks, or fascicular blocks).

BLOCKS IN THE SA NODE OR ATRIA

When an impulse is blocked within the SA node or in the internodal tracts, the electrical stimulus does not reach the atria or the ventricles. As a result, the entire PQRST complex is absent. Blocks in the SA node or internodal tracts cannot be specifically distinguished electrocardiographically or clinically from SA arrest, a disorder of impulse formation discussed previously (see Chapter 9). Therefore blocks involving the SA node are not considered separately in this section.

ATRIOVENTRICULAR (JUNCTIONAL) BLOCKS

Blocks interfering with conduction of impulses between the atria and ventricles usually develop because of ischemic injury to the AV node or AV-junctional tissue. Less commonly, increased parasym-

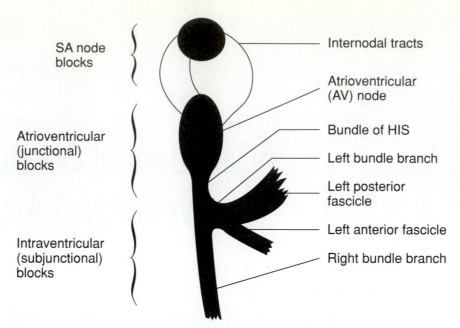

Figure 13–1. Anatomy of the AV junction.

pathetic (vagal) activity or drugs (especially digitalis) produce these disturbances.

AV blocks are categorized into first-degree, second-degree, and third-degree (complete) blocks, a classification based on the extent of the conduction defect between the atria and the ventricles. In first-degree block, the AV node merely delays impulses before they enter the intraventricular conduction system, but each impulse is conducted to the ventricles. In second-degree AV block, in which nodal involvement is greater, some atrial impulses are actually blocked in the AV node or AV junction and are not conducted beyond this point. In third-degree (complete) AV block, the more seriously affected AV node prevents transmission of all impulses from the atria to the ventricles. (In this circumstance the inherent automaticity of the ventricles produces ventricular contractions in the absence of stimulation from supraventricular centers.) These three forms of AV block are discussed individually in this chapter.

INTRAVENTRICULAR BLOCKS

Disturbances in conduction occurring *below* the level of bifurcation of the bundle of His are categorized as intraventricular blocks.

When these blocks develop during the acute phase of acute myocardial infarction (AMI) they generally reflect ischemic damage to the conduction pathways (particularly in the interventricular septal area). However, intraventricular blocks may exist be-

fore AMI. In this circumstance the block is a consequence of chronic degeneration or fibrotic scarring of the bundle branches and intraventricular network.

Until recently it was believed that the bundle of His consisted of two branches, the left bundle branch and the right bundle branch. Histologic studies have shown, however, that the left bundle branch consists of two parts, an anterior and a posterior fascicle. For this reason the bundle of His is considered to have three branches (or fascicles), any of which can be blocked individually or in combination. Several types of intraventricular block may develop in this trifascicular system, as shown schematically in Figure 13–2 and listed below.

1. Block of the right bundle branch (RBBB).
2. Block of the *main* left bundle branch (LBBB).
3. Block of the *anterior fascicle* of the left bundle branch (called left anterior hemiblock or LAH).
4. Block of the *posterior fascicle* of the left bundle branch (called left posterior hemiblock or LPH).
5. Block involving the right bundle branch and one of the fascicles of the left bundle branch (called bifascicular block, since two of the three branches of the bundle of His are involved).
6. Blocks involving all three branches of the bundle of His (called trifascicular blocks).

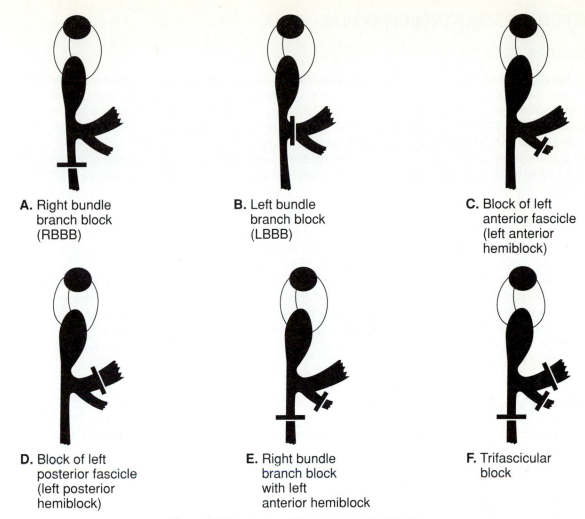

A. Right bundle branch block (RBBB)

B. Left bundle branch block (LBBB)

C. Block of left anterior fascicle (left anterior hemiblock)

D. Block of left posterior fascicle (left posterior hemiblock)

E. Right bundle branch block with left anterior hemiblock

F. Trifascicular block

Figure 13–2. Types of intraventricular blocks.

The diagnosis and differentiation of all of these various forms of intraventricular block require a 12-lead ECG (and sometimes even more sophisticated studies of electrical conduction, called His-bundle electrograms). It certainly is not possible to ascertain the precise type of an intraventricular block from a single monitor lead used in the CCU. However, intraventricular blocks are characterized by wide QRS complexes (exceeding 0.12 second); this one electrocardiographic finding, readily detectable on a cardiac monitor, should indicate that a bundle branch block is present. Intraventricular blocks developing as the result of AMI are more dangerous than AV blocks, particularly when more than one fascicle is involved. Bi-fascicular or trifascicular blocks often lead to complete heart block and ventricular standstill. Moreover, acute intraventricular blocks generally reflect extensive myocardial infarction involving the interventricular septum, and require immediate use of an artificial pacemaker.

Treatment of Heart Blocks

1. Observe the patient and cardiac monitor.
2. Administer atropine.
3. Administer isoproterenol (Isuprel).
4. Apply pacemaking with a transcutaneous, transvenous temporary, or permanent pacemaker.

FIRST-DEGREE ATRIOVENTRICULAR HEART BLOCK

Mechanism

First-degree AV block denotes that conduction from the SA node to the ventricles is abnormally delayed. The block may be due to a prolongation of conduction in any of the structures between the SA node and the bundle of His. Most commonly, when the QRS duration is normal, a long P–R interval is due to a delay within the AV node or junctional area. The delay is caused by ischemic, degenerative (aging-related), or inflammatory changes in the AV conduction systems. Each sinus impulse reaches the ventricles and causes a ventricular response (ie, each P wave is followed by a QRS complex). The delay in conduction usually results from ischemia of the AV node, but digitalis, antiarrhythmic agents, and increased vagal activity can also produce this type of AV block.

Significance

1. First-degree AV block is not a serious arrhythmia in its own right. It does not reduce hemodynamic efficiency nor does it affect the rate or rhythm of the heart.
2. The arrhythmia is important because it usually indicates injury to the AV-nodal area and may warn of impending second- or third-degree heart blocks. The latter blocks, which reflect *advanced* stages of AV nodal involvement, are far more dangerous and may lead to ventricular standstill.
3. First-degree AV block is more commonly seen in acute inferior myocardial infarctions.
4. *Risk:* First-degree AV block is often an early warning of more advanced heart block, but is not a dangerous arrhythmia in itself.

Clinical Features

1. Prolonged AV conduction produces no symptoms or physical findings, except that the first heart sound (S_1) becomes softer.
2. The diagnosis of first-degree AV block can be made only by ECG.

ECG FEATURES IDENTIFYING FIRST-DEGREE ATRIOVENTRICULAR HEART BLOCK

1. **Rate:**   Usually normal.

2. **Rhythm:**   Regular.

3. **P waves:**   Normal, originating in the SA node.

4. **P–R interval:**   Prolonged beyond 0.20 second. This prolongation is due to a delay in the passage of impulses through the AV node.

5. **QRS:**   Normal. Intraventricular conduction is not disturbed.

First-Degree AV Heart Block (Figure 13–3)

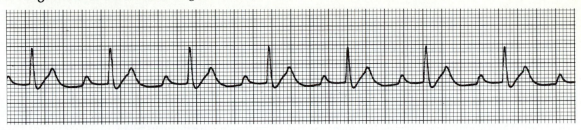

Rate:	About 70/minute.
Rhythm:	Regular.
P waves:	Normal.
P–R interval:	Prolonged (0.26 second).
QRS:	Normal (0.08 second).
Comment:	The prolongation of the P–R interval indicates a delay in conduction between the SA node and ventricle, usually in the AV node.

First-Degree AV Block (Figure 13–4)

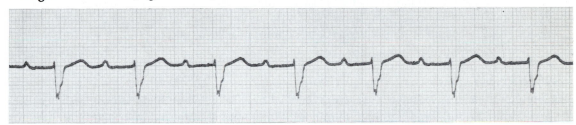

Rate:	About 70/minute.
Rhythm:	Regular.
P waves:	Normal.
P–R interval:	Prolonged to 0.32 second.
QRS:	Slightly widened, but normal (just less than 0.12 second).
Comment:	Conduction through the AV node can often be accelerated by intravenous atropine, as evidenced by shortening of the P–R interval.

Treatment

1. If there is only a slight delay in AV conduction (P–R interval of 0.21 to 0.28 second) and the block does not increase, no treatment is necessary.
2. If the P–R interval is longer than 0.28 second or, more significantly, if it shows progressive lengthening, atropine (0.5–1.0 mg intravenously) may be used in an attempt to accelerate conduction through the AV node.
3. If drug therapy is unsuccessful in controlling a progressive first-degree block, or if the block is extreme (more than 0.5 second), insertion of a temporary transvenous pacing catheter may be indicated. This prophylactic approach reduces the risk of sudden complete heart block or asystole.
4. If first-degree heart block develops during the course of treatment with digitalis or any antiarrhythmic agent, the further use of these drugs should be carefully considered in view of their known ability to depress AV-nodal conduction.

Nursing Responsibility

1. When first-degree heart block is identified, record a rhythm strip and carefully measure the P–R interval. If the P–R interval is greater than 0.26 second or if it shows progressive lengthening, advise the physician.
2. Carefully observe the monitor for the appearance of second- or third-degree block. If these advanced forms of heart block develop, notify the physician immediately.
3. In patients with evidence of first-degree block who are receiving digitalis or other antiarrhythmic agents, discuss the further administration of these drugs with the physician.

CASE HISTORY

The day after his admission to the CCU, a 64-year-old man with an inferior myocardial infarction developed a first-degree heart block. The P–R interval was 0.24 second at first, and then increased to 0.30 second. The nurse notified the physician about the progressive P–R prolongation, and atropine (0.5 mg intravenously) was ordered. The P–R interval then decreased to 0.26 second and remained stable thereafter.

SECOND-DEGREE ATRIOVENTRICULAR HEART BLOCK
Mobitz Type I (Wenckebach) Block

Mechanism

In second-degree AV block, some impulses from the SA node do not reach the ventricles because they are blocked within (or sometimes below) the AV node. When this happens a P wave is *not* followed by a QRS complex and a ventricular beat is absent (dropped).

Mobitz Type I second-degree AV block (also called Wenckebach block) is characterized by progressive lengthening of the P–R intervals preceding the blocked beat. Conduction through the AV node becomes more difficult with each successive impulse until finally an atrial impulse is completely blocked in the AV node and a QRS complex fails to appear. The pause resulting from the dropped beat allows the conduction system to recover momentarily, after which the entire sequence of progressive P–R prolongation is repeated.

The most common cause of Mobitz Type I second-degree block is ischemic damage to the AV node. In most instances this process is temporary. Digitalis, propranolol, and increased vagal tone can also produce it.

Significance

1. Mobitz Type I (Wenckebach) block is usually caused by ischemic injury to the AV node and therefore may progress to third-degree (complete) AV block. However, it rarely leads to ventricular standstill or sudden death because a pacemaker in the junctional area assumes command and stimulates the ventricles.
2. The block is most often a temporary disorder of conduction associated with inferior myocardial infarction because of vagal stimulation; it generally subsides spontaneously within 72 to 96 hours.
3. Unless the ventricular rate is very slow, circulatory efficiency is seldom affected and the block is generally well tolerated.
4. *Risk:* Mobitz Type I second-degree AV block is usually a temporary disorder of conduction that may lead to third-degree (complete) heart block but rarely to ventricular standstill and sudden death.

Clinical Features

1. Symptoms of Mobitz Type I (Wenckebach) block depend primarily on the frequency of blocked beats and the resulting ventricular rate. Unless the rate is markedly slow (below 50/minute), the patient is usually unaware of the presence of this conduction disorder.
2. Although Mobitz Type I block produces an irregular rhythm (when ventricular beats are dropped), the diagnosis can be established only by ECG findings, not by physical examination.
3. If vagal tone is increased (eg, by digitalis or propranolol), the heart rate may become very slow and the patient will experience lightheadedness, syncope, or fatigue.

ECG FEATURES IDENTIFYING SECOND-DEGREE ATRIOVENTRICULAR (MOBITZ TYPE I OR WENCKEBACH) BLOCK

1. Rate: The ventricular rate is usually slow, but may be normal.

2. Rhythm: Irregular because of dropped beats.

3. P waves: Because some sinus impulses are blocked in the AV node, the number of P waves always exceeds the number of QRS complexes.

4. P–R interval: There is progressive prolongation of the P–R interval until a sinus impulse is blocked and a QRS complex fails to appear (a dropped beat). Following the dropped beat, the P–R interval shortens and the entire sequence is then repeated. (The sequence is called a Wenckebach period.)

5. QRS: Normal.

Mobitz Type I Second-Degree AV Block (Figure 13–5)

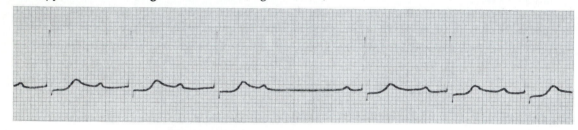

Rate:	The ventricular rate is about 60/minute.
Rhythm:	Irregular because of blocked beat.
P waves:	Normal in configuration and occur at regular intervals. The number of P waves exceeds the number of QRS complexes.
P–R interval:	The P–R interval increases during the first three beats. After this a P wave is blocked and a QRS complex does not occur. The first P–R interval after the blocked beat is much shorter than the intervals before it, after which lengthening of the P–R interval begins once again.
QRS:	Normal.
Comment:	The sequence of progressive lengthening of the P–R interval until a ventricular beat is dropped is the key diagnostic feature of Mobitz Type I or Wenckebach block.

Mobitz Type I Second-Degree AV Block (Figure 13–6)

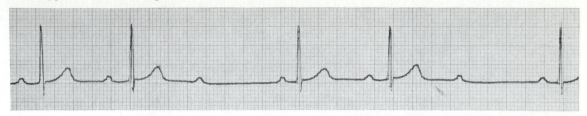

Rate: The ventricular rate is about 50/minute, while the atrial rate is about 70/minute.
Rhythm: Irregular.
P waves: Normal configuration. The third and sixth P waves are blocked in the AV node.
P–R interval: On two occasions, progressive lengthening of the P–R interval occurs for two beats
                     before a P wave is blocked.
QRS: Normal (0.06 second).
Comment: There are two Wenckebach cycles in this 6-second strip. As a result of the noncon-
                     ducted beats, the ventricular rate is reduced to about 50/minute.

Treatment

1. Since Mobitz Type I (Wenckebach) blocks seldom progress to ventricular standstill, many physicians believe that they require no therapy. Others, however, adopt a more cautious attitude and prefer to insert a temporary transvenous pacemaker when the conduction disorder is identified, particularly if it is associated with a slow ventricular rate.
2. If the ventricular rate is less than 50/minute, isoproterenol (Isuprel) can be used in an attempt to increase conduction through the AV node. An intravenous infusion of this drug (1 mg in 250 mL 5% glucose solution) may be administered. Atropine (1 mg intravenously) sometimes decreases the degree of AV block but is less dependable than isoproterenol.
3. If Wenckebach block persists for more than 3 or 4 days, temporary pacemaker insertion may be indicated.
4. If there is any suspicion that digitalis or propranolol is implicated, these drugs should be stopped promptly.

Nursing Responsibility

1. When second-degree heart block is identified, determine whether it is a Mobitz Type I (Wenckebach) or Mobitz Type II block. The two types of block can be distinguished by analyzing the P–R intervals preceding the dropped beats: the P–R intervals lengthen progressively with Type I block, while with Type II block (as described in the following pages) they are of constant duration.
2. Determine the heart rate and the frequency of dropped beats. Symptoms (angina, dyspnea, lightheadedness) may occur with slow ventricular rates.
3. Notify the physician of your findings.
4. If the plan of care is to observe the patient without any treatment, monitor the heart rate carefully and watch for signs of third-degree (complete) AV heart block.
5. Obtain standing orders for medications to be given if the heart rate falls below 50/minute or if the patient becomes symptomatic. If the ventricular rate is 50 or less per minute, atropine or isoproterenol may be given. Document the response to therapy.
6. Prepare for insertion of a temporary pacemaker if there is no response to drug treatment or if the patient is symptomatic.
7. Withhold digitalis, quinidine, procainamide, or propranolol until the physician has been consulted.

CASE HISTORY

Eighteen hours after admission to the CCU, a 48-year-old man with an inferior myocardial infarction developed a Mobitz Type I (Wenckebach) second-degree heart block. There were no signs of left ventricular failure and the patient had no complaints. The nurse advised the attending physician of this development, and the physician requested a cardiology consultation to determine the need for a temporary transvenous pacemaker. The consultant felt that a temporary pacemaker was not required since the ventricular rate was 72/minute and there were no other complications. The consultant advised that atropine be administered if the ventricular rate dropped below 60/minute. The clinical course was uneventful and the heart block disappeared after 48 hours.

SECOND-DEGREE ATRIOVENTRICULAR HEART BLOCK
Mobitz Type II Block

Mechanism

Like Mobitz Type I (Wenckebach) block, Mobitz Type II block is characterized by failure of some sinus impulses to conduct to the ventricles. However, in contrast to Type I (Wenckebach) block, the P–R intervals in Type II block do not lengthen progressively before the dropped beats. In other words, in Type II block the P–R intervals of the preceding beats are of *constant* duration, with sudden blockade of a sinus P wave.

Impulses may be blocked occasionally or at regular intervals. When the dropped beats occur regularly, such as, after every second, third, or fourth P wave, the conduction defect is called, respectively, a 2:1, 3:1 or 4:1 second-degree AV block.

Mobitz Type II block is much less common than Type I (Wenckebach) block, but is far more serious. It results from injury to the conduction system *below* the AV junction, involving the bundle branches and Purkinje system.

Significance

1. Mobitz Type II block may progress abruptly to complete heart block or ventricular standstill. Since the block is below the AV junction, a junctional pacemaker cannot take over in the event of a long series of blocked sinus beats. Only the inherent automaticity of the ventricles (at a rate of 30–40/minute) is left to sustain the heart beat.
2. When impulses are blocked regularly during Mobitz Type II block (eg, 2:1 AV block), the heart rate may be too slow to maintain effective circulation, and angina, syncope, or heart failure can develop.
3. Mobitz Type II block is usually (but not always) associated with anterior or anteroseptal infarction, and because of extensive ventricular damage, left ventricular failure may complicate the clinical course.
4. *Risk:* Mobitz Type II block is a very serious disorder of conduction that often presages complete heart block or ventricular asystole.

Clinical Features

1. Symptoms are related to the ventricular rate. With rates under 50/minute, patients may experience angina, dyspnea, or cerebral insufficiency.
2. Mobitz Type II block can only be identified (and distinguished from Type I block) by ECG.

ECG FEATURES IDENTIFYING SECOND-DEGREE ATRIOVENTRICULAR (MOBITZ) TYPE II HEART BLOCK

1. Rate:	The ventricular rate is usually slow, but depends on the frequency of blocked beats.
2. Rhythm:	When the block occurs at regular intervals (eg, 2:1 AV block), the rhythm is regular. If occasional, blocked beats occur and the rhythm at the time is irregular.
3. P waves:	More numerous than QRS complexes, but normal in configuration.
4. P–R interval:	The P–R intervals of the beats preceding a blocked beat are of constant duration.
5. QRS:	Usually widened, indicating that the block is below the AV junction.

Mobitz Type II Second-Degree AV Block (Figure 13–7)

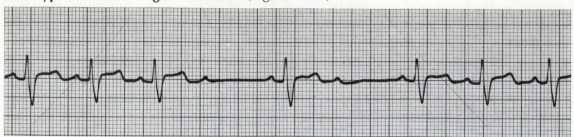

Rate:	The ventricular rate is about 70/minute. The atrial rate is about 90/minute.
Rhythm:	Irregular because of two blocked beats.
P waves:	Normal in shape and occurring regularly. The fourth and sixth P waves are blocked and not conducted to the ventricles.
P–R interval:	The P–R intervals are of constant duration and do not lengthen before the blocked beats.
QRS:	Widened (0.14 second), indicating that an intraventricular conduction defect is present (a common finding in Mobitz Type II blocks).
Comment:	The distinguishing characteristic of a Mobitz Type II block is a constant P–R interval before and after the blocked beats, unlike the changing P–R intervals of a Mobitz Type I second-degree AV block.

Mobitz Type II Second-Degree AV Block (2:1 Type) (Figure 13–8)

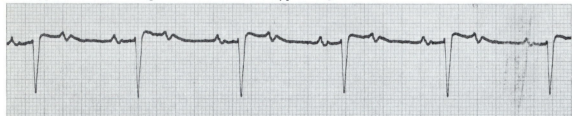

Rate:	The ventricular rate is 56/minute. The atrial rate is 112/minute.
Rhythm:	Regular.
P waves:	There are two P waves in each R–R interval. The first of these P waves (which occurs just before the T waves) is blocked.
P–R interval:	Mildly prolonged (0.22 second). The P–R intervals are constant.
QRS:	Normal (0.08 second). No QRS complex follows the blocked P wave.
Comment:	The ventricular rate is one-half the atrial rate because every other P wave is blocked (2:1 block).

Treatment

1. Because of the unpredictable course of Type II block and the ever-present threat of sudden complete heart block or ventricular standstill, a temporary transvenous pacemaker should be inserted when this conduction disorder is identified.
2. Isoproterenol may be administered before pacemaker insertion can be accomplished, particularly if the ventricular rate is slow.
3. Atropine is seldom useful in Type II block, and can be detrimental. Although it usually increases the atrial rate, it does not decrease the degree of block. As a result, more P waves may be blocked, causing a further reduction in the ventricular rate.
4. Digitalis and antiarrhythmic drugs should be discontinued in the presence of Type II block.

Nursing Responsibility

1. Distinguish Mobitz Type II from Type I (Wenckebach) second-degree AV block by measuring the P–R intervals preceding the dropped beats.
2. Notify the physician promptly.
3. Withhold digitalis and antiarrhythmic agents.
4. Prepare for the insertion of a temporary pacemaker.
5. Give intravenous isoproterenol (Isuprel) per standing order (usually 1 mg in 250 mL glucose solution, infused slowly) if the patient bcomes symptomatic and a pacemaker cannot be inserted immedately.
6. Observe the cardiac monitor carefully for the sudden appearance of complete heart block or ventricular asystole.

CASE HISTORY

A 64-year-old man was admitted to the CCU because of an acute myocardial infarction of the anterior wall. The original rhythm strip revealed normal sinus rhythm, but the P–R interval was 0.24 second (first-degree AV block). About 1 hour later the slow-rate alarm of the cardiac monitor sounded, and the nurse noted that the patient's heart rate had suddenly decreased from 90 to 45/minute. On examining the rhythm strip, it was apparent that there were two P waves for each QRS complex and that a 2:1 Mobitz Type II second-degree heart block had developed. It was also noted that the QRS complex was widened (0.12 second). The nurse advised the physician of these findings, and it was decided that a temporary transvenous pacemaker should be inserted, particularly in light of the widened QRS complexes and the potential threat of progression to complete heart block (or ventricular standstill).

THIRD-DEGREE (COMPLETE) ATRIOVENTRICULAR HEART BLOCK

Mechanism

In third-degree AV block, all impulses from the atria are blocked and none reach the ventricles. The block may occur above or below the bifurcation of the bundle of His. Regardless of the site of the block, the atria and ventricles beat independently, each being controlled by a separate pacemaker. The SA node serves as the pacemaker for the atria, while the ventricles are governed by a ventricular focus at an inherent rate of 30 to 40/minute. (If the block is *above* the bifurcation of the His bundle, the ventricles may be stimulated by a junctional escape pacemaker at a rate of 40–60/minute.) In either case there is no relationship between P waves and QRS complexes—a condition called *atrioventricular dissociation.* In patients with AMI, complete heart block is almost invariably due to ischemic injury to either the AV-junctional area or the conduction system below it. Only rarely is digitalis toxicity responsible for the block.

Significance

1. An *independent* ventricular pacemaker is not dependable and may fail abruptly, causing ventricular standstill. Also, the slow ventricular rate in third-degree AV block predisposes to ventricular tachycardia (VT) or ventricular fibrillation (VF) by allowing more rapid foci in the ventricles to gain control of the heart rate.
2. Complete heart block almost always causes a marked reduction in cardiac output because the ventricular rate is constant at 30 to 40/minute and cannot increase to meet circulatory demands. Consequently, left ventricular failure and myocardial ischemia are common hemodynamic complications of complete block.
3. A gross reduction in blood flow to the brain, resulting from the very slow heart rate and low cardiac output, may cause episodes of syncope with or without convulsion. Lesser degrees of cerebral ischemia are manifested by confusion and lightheadedness.
4. As a general rule, complete heart block occurring within or about the AV node is less dangerous than blocks below the AV junction. With blocks at the AV-nodal level, a junctional escape pacemaker may maintain the ventricular rate at 40 to 60/minute.
5. *Risk:* Complete heart block, especially below the junctional level, is an *extremely dangerous* arrhythmia. It represents a clear warning of impending ventricular standstill or VF.

Clinical Features

1. Complete heart block can be suspected on the basis of clinical examination. The key finding is a very slow, regular heart rate (usually less than 40/minute) that remains constant and does not fluctuate with activity (a fixed heart rate).
2. Signs of cerebral ischemia, ranging from confusion and lightheadedness to syncope and convulsions, are common during complete heart block.
3. Symptoms and signs of left ventricular failure are usually present, as is hypotension.

ECG FEATURES IDENTIFYING THIRD-DEGREE (COMPLETE) ATRIOVENTRICULAR HEART BLOCK

1. Rate: The ventricular rate is usually 30 to 40/minute (but can be 40–60/minute with a junctional escape pacemaker). The atrial rate, which is independent of the ventricular rate, is always faster.

2. Rhythm: Both atrial and ventricular rhythms are regular, but are independent of each other.

3. P waves: There are more P waves than QRS complexes. Because atrial stimulation is unaffected, the size and shape of the P waves are normal.

4. P–R interval: Because the atria and ventricles have separate pacemakers, there is no relationship between P waves and QRS complexes (atrioventricular dissociation). Therefore, the P–R interval is inconstant.

5. QRS: The configuration of the QRS complex depends on the site of the block and location of the ectopic ventricular pacemaker. If the block and ectopic pacemaker are near the AV node, the QRS complex may be normal. In contrast, when the block and pacemaker are below the AV junction the QRS complexes are widened and distorted.

Complete Heart Block with Wide QRS Complexes (Figure 13–9)

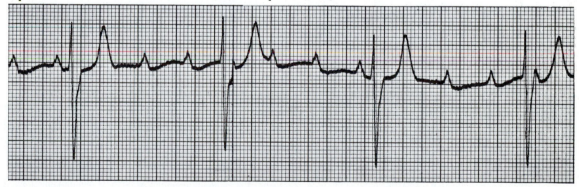

Rate:	The ventricular rate is about 40/minute. The atrial rate is about 130/minute.
Rhythm:	Regular.
P waves:	Occur at regular intervals, independent of QRS complexes, at a rate of 130/minute.
P–R interval:	There is no relationship between P waves and QRS complexes; therefore the P–R intervals are inconstant.
QRS:	Wide and distorted, indicating their ventricular origin.
Comment:	No impulses from the SA node or AV junction reach the ventricles (complete heart block), and the only remaining pacemaker is ventricular (at a rate of about 40/minute).

Complete Heart Block with Normal QRS Complexes (Figure 13–10)

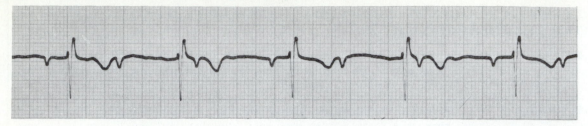

Rate:	The ventricular rate is about 50/minute. The atrial rate is about 80/minute.
Rhythm:	Regular.
P waves:	Occur at regular intervals, but none are conducted to the ventricles. The P waves are inverted in this particular lead.
P–R interval:	Inconstant, reflecting independent atria and ventricular rhythms.
QRS:	Normal (0.10 second).
Comment:	The heart rate (about 50/minute) and the normal QRS complexes (lasting 0.10 second) indicate that a pacemaker just below the AV junction has assumed control. Compare this example with the one above, in which a ventricular pacemaker is in command.

Complete Heart Block Leading to Ventricular Tachycardia and Ventricular Fibrillation (Figure 13–11)

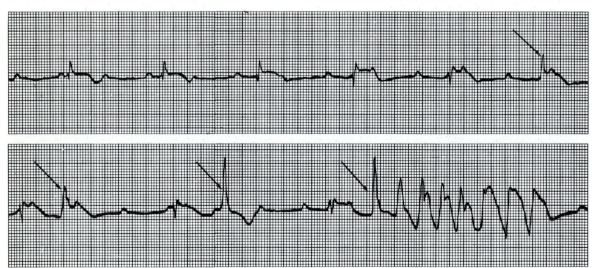

Comment:	The electrocardiographic sequence seen in Figure 13–11 demonstrates one of the greatest dangers of complete heart block: the development of ventricular fibrillation (VF). In the presence of the very slow ventricular rate associated with complete heart block, PVCs developed (arrows). These ectopic beats caused repetitive ventricular firing and VF (lower strip). *Note:* This rhythm strip was continuous but has been divided and reduced in scale for purposes of full reproduction.

Treatment

1. The only dependable method of treating complete heart block is transvenous cardiac pacing. This procedure should be undertaken as soon as third-degree block is identified.
2. While preparing for insertion of the pacemaker, an intravenous infusion of isoproterenol (Isuprel), 1 mg in 250 mL glucose solution, should be given slowly. Occasionally, isoproterenol may reduce the degree of AV block and increase the heart rate. Despite the apparent effectiveness of drug therapy, complete block often suddenly recurs, and therefore it is wise to insert a transvenous pacemaker in all patients who develop complete heart block.
3. Cardiac pacing should be continued until normal sinus rhythm returns, and the pacing catheter should remain in place for at least 5 days thereafter.
4. Rarely, complete heart block persists because of irreversible damage to the conduction system. In this circumstance a permanent pacemaker is required.
5. Because complete heart block is often preceded by lesser degrees of AV block, the treatment of this arrhythmia should begin ideally when progressive heart block is first identified (as explained in the description of second-degree block).

Nursing Responsibility

1. Identify the slow-rate arrhythmia of complete AV block and distinguish it from marked sinus brady-cardia, junctional rhythm, and second-degree AV block. Document the disorder with a rhythm strip.
2. Notify the physician immediately after this arrhythmia is recognized.
3. Prepare an infusion containing 1 mg isoproterenol in 250 mL dextrose solution and give it according to standing order.
4. Because of the threat of VF developing in the presence of the slow ventricular rate that results from complete heart block, a defibrillator should be brought to the patient's bedside and made ready for use.
5. Keep a syringe containing 100 mg lidocaine at the bedside.
6. Prepare for the insertion of a transvenous pacemaker (see Chapter 14).
7. Assess the patient's clinical condition repeatedly, with particular emphasis on signs or symptoms that indicate left ventricular failure.
8. Diligently observe the monitor for premature ventricular contractions (PVCs); these ectopic beats may forewarn of VT or VF.
9. If a transvenous pacemaker has previously been inserted for prophylactic reasons (because of second-degree AV block or block in the His-Purkinje system), verify that the pacemaker is functioning properly.
10. If ventricular standstill develops, initiate cardiopulmonary resuscitation (CPR) immediately. Sound an emergency alarm.

CASE HISTORY

A 56-year-old man was admitted to the CCU in acute distress. He complained of substernal pain, short-ness of breath, and a feeling of faintness. On examining the patient the nurse found that his blood pres-sure was 96/68 mm Hg, and that his pulse rate was only 36/minute. A rhythm strip confirmed the nurse's clinical suspicion of complete heart block. The physician was notified promptly of these findings, and it was decided that a temporary transvenous pacemaker should be inserted without delay to increase the heart rate. The physician requested that an intravenous infusion of isoproterenol be given while prepara-tions were being made to insert a pacing catheter. When the heart was paced at a rate of 75/minute, there was marked clinical improvement, reflecting increased cardiac output. A rhythm strip recorded during the course of cardiac pacing is shown in Figure 13–12.

Although the complete heart block continued to exist (as evidenced by the random position of the P waves) the ventricular rate was now controlled by the pacemaker. The pacing stimuli were delivered at a rate of 75/minute, creating a ventricular response at this rate.

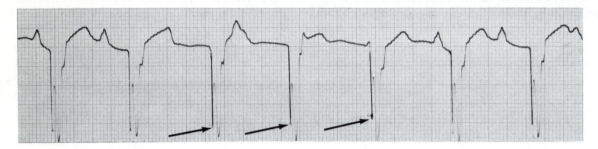

Figure 13–12. Rhythm strip with 100% cardiac pacing. The arrows show the pacing spikes.

INTRAVENTRICULAR BLOCKS (BUNDLE-BRANCH BLOCKS)

Mechanism

All blocks occurring below the bifurcation of the bundle of His are categorized as intraventricular (or subjunctional) blocks. The term *bundle-branch block* refers to an obstruction or delay in conduction through one of the main branches of the His bundle.

Normally, sinus impulses, after traversing the AV node and bundle of His, are conducted down the left and right bundle branches and stimulate the respective ventricles simultaneously. The total time for depolarization of both ventricles, as represented by the width of the QRS complex, is less than 0.12 second.

When one of the bundle branches is blocked, impulses travel through the intact branch and stimulate the ventricle it supplies on schedule. The ventricle affected by the bundle-branch block is activated indirectly by impulses crossing through the interventricular septum from the unaffected side in a cell-to-cell fashion. The delay caused by this circuitous route for complete ventricular activation (ie, activation of both ventricles) is manifested electrocardiographically by widening of the QRS complex beyond 0.12 second, which constitutes the characteristic feature of a bundle-branch block.

The most common cause of bundle-branch block is chronic degeneration or fibrotic scarring of the intraventricular conduction system. Consequently, bundle-branch blocks are often present before AMI, particularly in elderly patients, and have no relation to the attack itself. Bundle-branch blocks that develop as a complication of acute infarction usually reflect extensive myocardial damage involving the interventricular septum and the bundle branches.

Significance

1. Intraventricular blocks that develop *acutely* as a result of myocardial infarction are associated with a high mortality because they usually are the result of an extensive infarction. Death may be due to electrical failure (ventricular standstill) or circulatory (power) failure.
2. There is a high risk of sudden electrical failure when more than one of the three intraventricular pathways are blocked. For example, a right bundle-branch block in conjunction with a block of the anterior fascicle of the left bundle branch (collectively called a bilateral bundle-branch block) may progress abruptly to complete heart block or ventricular standstill. (In this circumstance the only remaining conduction pathway to the ventricle is the posterior fascicle of the left bundle branch.)
3. *Risk:* Bundle-branch block is a very serious disorder when the block develops as a consequence of AMI and involves more than one bundle branch. In the elderly, right bundle-branch block is common and relatively benign.

Clinical Features

1. Bundle-branch block causes no symptoms because the heart rate and rhythm are not affected.
2. The presence of a bundle-branch block can be recognized by very wide QRS complexes on a single cardiac monitoring lead. However, the location of the block (ie, right or left bundle branch or fascicular) can be determined only by means of a 12-lead ECG.
3. A left bundle-branch block obscures the characteristic electrocardiographic signs of AMI; therefore the diagnosis of acute infarction in this situation depends primarily on enzyme studies and clinical history. A right bundle-branch block does not affect the ECG signs of infarction.

ECG FEATURES IDENTIFYING BUNDLE-BRANCH BLOCK

1. Rate: Usually normal, but sometimes bundle-branch block is rate-related, appearing and disappearing with changes in the heart rate.

2. Rhythm: Regular.

3. P waves: Normal.

4. P–R interval: Normal, because impulses reach the uninvolved ventricle without delay.

5. QRS: Always widened to at least 0.12 second, and having a distorted configuration. After the uninvolved ventricle is stimulated, the impulses must be transmitted through the interventricular septum to activate the blocked side. This delay in activation causes the QRS complexes to be wide and notched.

Bundle-Branch Block (Figure 13–13)

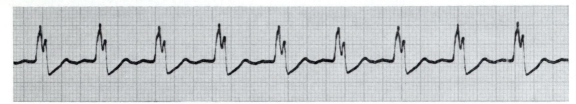

Rate:	About 90/minute.
Rhythm:	Regular.
P waves:	Normal.
P–R interval:	Normal (0.18 second). The impulse from the SA node passes through the uninvolved bundle without delay and activates one ventricle in a normal manner.
QRS:	The complex is abnormally widened (to more than 0.12 second), indicating that the time for total ventricular activation is prolonged. (The impulse must pass through the interventricular septum to stimulate the blocked ventricle.)
Comment:	With a single monitor lead it is usually not possible to distinguish which of the bundle branches is blocked. This localization, which has prognostic importance, is made with a 12-lead ECG, from which the respective patterns can be readily identified. The monitor lead indicates only that an intraventricular conduction defect is present.

Bundle-Branch Blocks (Figure 13–14)

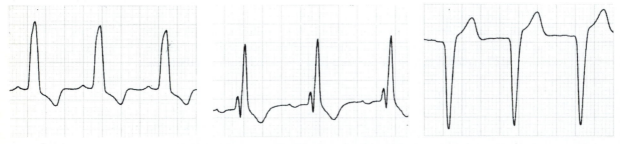

Comment: The three different ventricular complexes shown above are more than 0.12 second in duration, indicating an intraventricular conduction defect in each example. The configuration of the QRS complexes varies with the type of block and the lead locations.

Treatment

1. A temporary transvenous pacemaker should be inserted prophylactically when a bundle-branch block develops acutely after myocardial infarction, in an attempt to combat sudden complete heart block or ventricular standstill.
2. Chronic bundle-branch blocks that are present before AMI generally require no treatment. However, some clinicians believe that a temporary pacemaker should be inserted for chronic blocks that involve more than one bundle branch (bilateral bundle-branch block).
3. There is no drug treatment for intraventricular blocks.
4. Infrequently, overdosages of antiarrhythmic drugs, particularly quinidine, may produce intraventricular blocks. In this circumstance the block may disappear after the drug is discontinued.

Nursing Responsibility

1. If an intraventricular block (manifested on the monitor by a widened QRS complex) develops acutely, document the conduction disturbance with an ECG strip and notify the physician of this change.
2. Obtain a 12-lead ECG at this time to localize the site of the block and the number of fascicles involved. (As noted, these factors cannot be ascertained from the monitor strip alone.)
3. Because it is likely that a temporary transvenous pacemaker will be inserted, prepare for this procedure.
4. Carefully observe the patient's clinical condition. This observation is particularly important because intraventricular blocks are usually associated with extensive infarctions, and the risk of multiple complications is great.
5. If the patient develops an intraventricular block during the course of drug therapy, discuss the problem with the physician before the next dose is administered.

CASE HISTORY

A 70-year-old woman was admitted to the CCU with a history of severe substernal pain of 2 hours' duration. The nurse noted a widened QRS complex on the initial rhythm strip. A 12-lead ECG demonstrated a left bundle-branch block. The admitting physician stated that this pattern had been present for at least 3 years. Because of the LBBB, the diagnosis of AMI could not be made definitely at the time. Despite this uncertainty, the patient was treated as if an acute infarction had occurred. The question was resolved within a few days when enzyme studies confirmed the diagnosis of AMI.

VENTRICULAR ASYSTOLE: A FATAL ARRHYTHMIA

Ventricular contraction depends on an effective electrical stimulus. If for some reason electrical stimuli to the ventricles are of inadequate intensity, or if they cease entirely, the ventricles stop contracting. This state is designated **ventricular standstill** or **ventricular asystole** (meaning "without contraction"). There is some confusion about the proper terminology for this catastrophic event. The terms "ventricular standstill," "ventricular asystole," and "cardiac arrest" are used interchangeably to designate the cessation of cardiac action. At the bedside, one cannot, without an ECG, distinguish ventricular asystole from VF, since both arrhythmias are characterized by the absence of audible heart sounds. It is common practice, therefore, to classify cessation of the circulation as cardiac arrest, even though VF is the usual cause for this. In the CCU, where the lethal arrhythmia can be specifically identified, it is poor practice to use the general term "cardiac arrest" when the arrhythmia is in fact either ventricular asystole or VF. The net effect of ventricular asystole is the same as with VF: sudden death.

Like VF, ventricular asystole may develop as a primary electrical disorder or as a terminal arrhythmia during advanced heart failure. The latter mechanism is far more common.

In ventricular asystole, sinus (or atrial) impulses are discharged normally and produce P waves. Suddenly, however, all of these impulses are blocked and none reach the ventricles. Despite the seeming suddenness of ventricular asystole, the catastrophe is preceded in practically all instances by some form of intraventricular heart block, usually a bifascicular block. Because an inherent ventricular pacemaker does not come to the rescue, ventricular activation stops and all QRS complexes disappear on the ECG (while P waves continue). When ventricular stimulation ceases, unconsciousness develops immediately and death occurs within a very brief period unless effective ventricular action can be restored by CPR. On some occasions, ventricular asystole is a transient phenomenon with conduction and ventricular stimulation returning spontaneously within seconds. These intermittent episodes are characterized by syncope.

In contrast, ventricular asystole associated with circulatory failure is a terminal event in patients dying of cardiogenic shock or advanced left ventricular failure. In these conditions inadequate tissue perfusion results in hypoxia, acidosis, and electrolyte imbalance, all of which depress electrical conductivity. At a critical point, the heart's electrical activity becomes insufficient to stimulate the myocardium, and ventricular asystole develops. This secondary type of asystole seldom yields to resuscitative techniques (including cardiac pacing) because the oxygen-deprived myocardium is unable to respond to any stimulation. Death from ventricular asystole may be sudden or gradual. In the latter case electrical activity may continue, but muscle contractions are weak and ineffective in propelling blood from the ventricles. In the dying heart, the electrical impulses may be unrelated to the weak contractions. This state is described as electro-mechanical dissociation.

Mechanism

Ventricular asystole develops when all impulses from the SA node or atria fail to reach the ventricles and an inherent ventricular focus fails to take over as an escape pacemaker, leading to the cessation of ventricular stimulation and circulation. Ventricular asystole may be the result of a conduction disorder, usually involving two or three fascicles of the bundle branches, or may be caused by hypoxia, which depresses impulse formation, conduction, and myocardial responsiveness to stimulation.

Significance

1. Ventricular asystole results in sudden death unless an effective heartbeat can be restored immediately by resuscitative measures and a pacemaker. This fatal arrhythmia is, however, relatively rare compared to primary VF.
2. Ventricular asystole in the case of advanced heart failure is almost inevitably fatal with currently available means of treatment. It seldom responds to resuscitation (including cardiac pacing) because the severely ischemic myocardium is unable to respond to any stimulation.
3. *Risk: Ventricular asystole is the most dreaded and dangerous of all arrhythmias.* The results of resuscitation are distressingly poor (in sharp contrast to the effectiveness of resuscitation in VF). Consequently, prevention of ventricular asystole is of supreme importance.
4. Many patients waiting for a heart transplant die of ventricular asystole.

Clinical Features

1. Ventricular asystole usually develops as a sudden, complete cessation of circulation. No heartbeat can be heard, no pulses can be felt, the blood pressure cannot be obtained, and the patient loses consciousness immediately. *Death occurs within minutes.* The clinical picture is therefore identical to that in VF; however, the two lethal arrhythmias can be readily distinguished electrocardiographically.

2. Death from ventricular asystole may also occur gradually during the course of cardiogenic shock or left ventricular failure. Electrical activity often continues (in the form of wide QRS complexes) but the ventricles do not respond. Thus the circulation stops even though QRS complexes are still evident on the ECG. This condition is called *electromechanical dissociation.*

ECG FEATURES IDENTIFYING PRIMARY VENTRICULAR ASYSTOLE

1. Rate: At the onset of ventricular asystole the ventricles cease to contract and there is no heartbeat.

2. Rhythm: No ventricular beats.

3. P waves: Usually normal; they continue independently despite the cessation of ventricular activity.

4. P–R interval: Atrial activity may persist, but the impulses are not conducted to the ventricle and there is no P–R interval.

5. QRS: None.

Primary Ventricular Asystole (Figure 13–15)

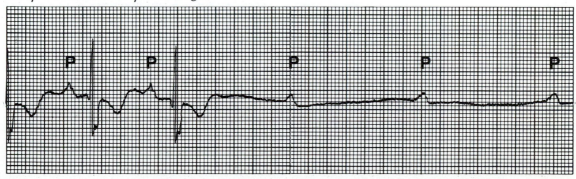

Rate:	After the third QRS complex, ventricular activation ceases and there is no heartbeat.
Rhythm:	There is no cardiac rhythm because of total cessation of ventricular contractions.
P waves:	Atrial activity continues after ventricular asystole.
P–R interval:	Although the atria are stimulated, no impulses reach the ventricles.
QRS:	Absent when the ventricular stimulation ceases.
Comment:	In this case, ventricular asystole developed in the presence of an intraventricular conduction defect. A 12-lead ECG showed a right bundle-branch block as well as a block of the anterior subdivision of the left bundle-branch (bundle-branch block). A first-degree heart block is also apparent in the single-lead tracing shown above.

ECG FEATURES IDENTIFYING SECONDARY VENTRICULAR ASYSTOLE

1. Rate: Electrical activity in the ventricles may continue, producing infrequent QRS complexes (at a rate of 10–30/minute).

2. Rhythm: The isolated electrical activity in the ventricles is insufficient to stimulate ventricular contraction, and consequently there is no heartbeat or peripheral pulse.

3. P waves: Absent, since atrial death has occurred (downward displacement of the pacemaker).

4. P–R interval: No P–R interval. The QRS complexes arise from the ventricles.

5. QRS: Wide, slurred complexes occur at a very slow rate.

Secondary Ventricular Asystole (Figure 13–16)

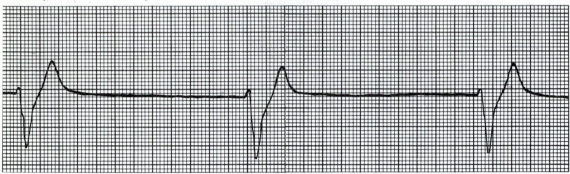

Rate: Isolated ventricular electrical activity at a rate of less than 30/minute.

Rhythm: The occasional ventricular complexes do not actually constitute a cardiac rhythm. They represent isolated electrical activity, but are not associated with effective ventricular contractions.

P waves: Absent.

P–R interval: Absent. There is no conduction through the heart.

QRS: Very wide and distorted.

Comment: Cardiac pacing is seldom effective in secondary ventricular asystole; the myocardium is unable to respond to the electrical stimulus because of hypoxia.

Dying Heart (Figure 13–17)

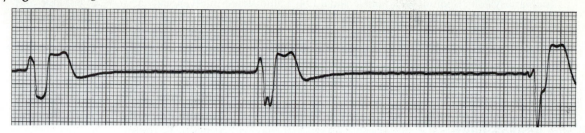

Comment: Although there is occasional electrical activity in the ventricles, true stimulation of the myocardium does not occur. The bizarre, distorted ventricular complexes may continue for several minutes even though the patient is clinically dead. This ECG pattern is common among patients dying of advanced left ventricular failure, and is described as a "dying heart" pattern.

Treatment

The treatment and resuscitation program for ventricular asystole has four phases:

1. *Recognition.* When primary ventricular asystole occurs, the low-rate alarm of the monitoring system is activated. The electrocardiographic pattern is characterized by the absence of ventricular (QRS) complexes, while atrial activity (P waves) persists (Figure 13–18). If the ECG pattern cannot be identified instantly, no further time should be spent observing the monitor. The nurse should immediately determine if the patient is unconscious.

2. *Termination of ventricular asystole.* If the patient is unconscious and there is no evidence of circulation, the nurse or physician who reaches the bedside first should strike the patient's chest with a forceful blow directly over the sternum. Occasionally this simple step, if performed within seconds of the onset of ventricular asystole, will cause resumption of the heartbeat.

    If the blow to the chest is ineffective, external cardiac compression and mouth-to-mouth ventilation should be initiated instantly and continued while the following measures are taken.

    a. An emergency alarm should be sounded to summon other CCU personnel to assist in the resuscitative attempt.

    b. After an airway has been established to administer oxygen, and while effective external cardiac compression is being performed in an effort to maintain cerebral circulation, transcutaneous cardiac pacing should be attempted. The technique of cardiac pacing is described in Chapter 14.

    c. Epinephrine (1 mg IV push every 3 to 5 min) and atropine (1 mg IV every 3 to 5 min) should be given in an effort to stimulate electrical activity.

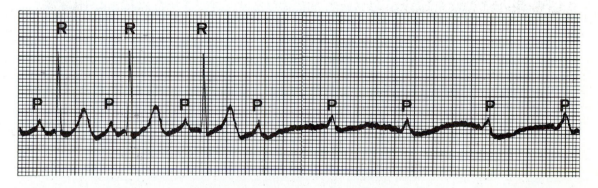

Figure 13–18. Ventricular asystole.

3. *Correction of lactic acidosis.* Lactic acidosis must be anticipated in every patient who develops ventricular asystole. Sodium bicarbonate should be administered intravenously as soon as possible and its administration repeated as necessary (depending on blood-gas values) while CPR is in progress. Unless the acidosis is corrected, the heart will not respond to pacing or other measures.

4. *Prevention of recurrence.* If resuscitation is successful, cardiac pacing should be continued until signs of heart block or bradycardia have disappeared. A transvenous pacemaker should be left in place for at least 1 week after sinus rhythm has been reestablished.

Nursing Responsibility

When a transvenous pacemaker has *not* been inserted prophylactically:

1. Sounding of the low-rate alarm should prompt an attempt to identify the ECG pattern on the monitor to determine whether the arrhythmia is VF or ventricular asystole.
2. The patient should be examined immediately. If the patient is awake and conscious it is quite certain that a false alarm has occurred.
3. If the patient is unconscious and has no peripheral pulses or heartbeat, sound the emergency alarm system.
4. Deliver a sharp blow to the chest wall directly over the sternum. This simple procedure may sometimes reestablish the heartbeat and is always worth trying.
5. If the heartbeat does not return immediately after the blow to the chest, begin CPR.
6. Continue external cardiac compression and mouth-to-mouth ventilation until other personnel provide assistance.
7. While CPR is in progress, one member of the team should prepare three syringes containing 1 mg atropine, 1 mg epinephrine, and 1 mEq/kg sodium bicarbonate for immediate intravenous injection.
8. Bring all necessary equipment for cardiac pacing to the bedside for immediate use.

The development of ventricular asystole cannot actually be considered as unexpected: only its onset is sudden. By recognizing the warning conduction disorder and inserting a transvenous pacemaker prophylactically, it should be possible, at least in some instances, to prevent the occurrence of primary ventricular asystole.

1. When a transvenous demand pacemaker has been inserted prophylactically, it will automatically begin to discharge impulses as soon as a QRS complex fails to appear, and will stimulate the ventricles to contract.
2. The nursing role in cardiac pacing is described in Chapter 15.

CASE HISTORY

A 78 year-old man was admitted to the CCU with signs of advanced left ventricular failure. The ECG revealed an acute anteroseptal myocardial infarction, and a rhythm strip showed sinus tachycardia with a rate of 124/minute. The patient was treated with furosemide (Lasix), nitroprusside, dobutamine, morphine, rotating tourniquets, and 100% oxygen through a face mask with a nonrebreathing bag. A pulmonary artery catheter was placed. The cardiac index was 1.4 L/minute/m^2 and the systemic vascular resistance was 2,200 dynes/cm^2. The response to therapy was poor and the patient continued to exhibit marked dyspnea. During the course of treatment the heart rate slowed abruptly to 58/minute and a junctional rhythm was recognized on a monitor strip. A transvenous pacemaker was inserted, but pacing was ineffective and the ventricles did not respond to stimulation (because of severe hypoxia). About 5 minutes later the patient lost consciousness. The nurse was unable to record a blood pressure, and no peripheral pulses were palpable. The monitor showed isolated, broad, distorted QRS complexes occurring at a rate of about 10 /minute. Resuscitation attempts were unsuccessful. The cause of the patient's death was advanced left ventricular failure. The terminal rhythm was ventricular asystole.

OTHER EXAMPLES OF DISORDERS OF CONDUCTION

Prolonged P–R Interval (First-Degree AV Heart Block) with Intraventricular Conduction Defect (Figure 13–19)

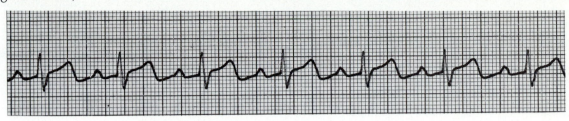

Rate:	About 70/minute.
Rhythm:	Regular.
P waves:	Normal.
P–R interval:	Prolonged (0.24 second).
QRS:	Widened (0.14 second).
Comment:	This example demonstrates a first-degree AV heart block (P–R interval of 0.24 second) as well as an intraventricular conduction defect (QRS interval greater than 0.12 second). The presence of more than one conduction disorder usually indicates diffuse disease of the conduction system.

Short P–R Interval: Lown-Ganong-Levine Syndrome (Figure 13–20)

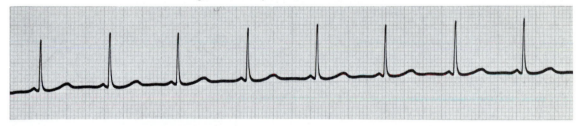

Rate:	About 80/minute.
Rhythm:	Regular
P waves:	Occur regularly and precede each QRS complex.
P–R interval:	Less than 0.10 second (0.08 second).
QRS:	Normal.
Comment:	The very short P–R interval (0.08 second) seen in this example is a manifestation of *accelerated conduction* from the SA node to the ventricle, usually through an anomalous (shorter than normal) pathway. Early stimulation of the ventricles resulting from accelerated conduction is often described as *preexcitation syndrome*. In Lown-Ganong-Levine syndrome the accessory pathway is anatomically close to the AV node.

Short P–R Interval: Wolff-Parkinson-White Syndrome (Figure 13–21)

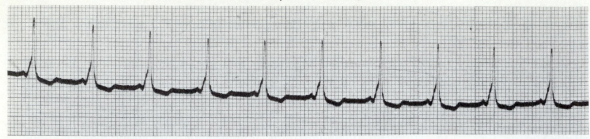

Rate:	About 100/minute.
Rhythm:	Regular.
P waves:	Normal and precede each QRS complex.
P–R interval:	Shortened (0.06 second).
QRS:	Widened (0.14 second), with slurring and notching of the upstroke of the R wave (called a delta wave).
Comment:	The combination of a short P–R interval in conjunction with a widened QRS complex and initial slurring of the R wave (delta wave) is called the Wolff-Parkinson-White syndrome. It is one form of preexcitation syndrome (see above) and is associated with a high incidence of paroxysmal tachycardias. In Wolff-Parkinson-White syndrome the accessory conduction pathway is distant from the AV node but connects the atrium with ventricle.

Mobitz Type I (Wenckebach) Second-Degree AV Block (Figure 13–22)

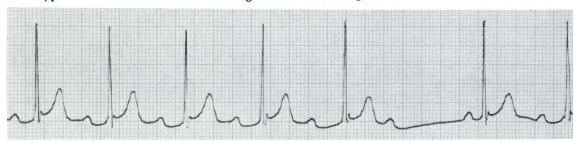

Rhythm:	Irregular as the result of a blocked beat.
P waves:	Normal, and precede each QRS complex.
P–R interval:	The P–R intervals lengthen progressively for five beats until a P wave is blocked. After the blocked beat the cycle starts again.
QRS:	Normal (0.08 second).
Comment:	Progressive lengthening of the P–R intervals until finally a beat is dropped. Mobitz Type I (Wenckebach) second-degree AV block is usually the result of transient injury to the AV node. This type of second-degree block is far less serious than Mobitz Type II second-degree block, which usually occurs below the AV node and may lead to ventricular asystole.

Mobitz Type I (Wenckebach) Second-Degree AV Block (Figure 13–23)

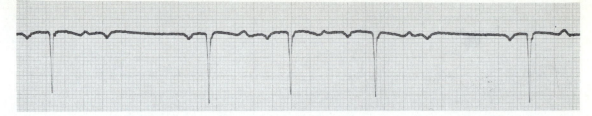

Rate: About 50/minute.

Rhythm: Irregular.

P waves: Normal (inverted in this lead) and occurring at regular intervals.

P–R interval: Vary from 0.20 second to 0.32 second, depending on various stages of the Wenckenbach cycle.

QRS: Normal (0.06 second). Two QRS complexes are absent because the corresponding impulses were blocked in the AV node.

Comment: The key to the interpretation of this conduction disorder is the gradual prolongation of the P–R intervals in the three beats in the center of the strip. Without this important observation, the disturbance might be classified incorrectly as a Mobitz Type II block. (The inverted waves in this example are due to lead placement.)

Mobitz Type II Second-Degree AV Heart Block—2:1 Type (Figure 13–24)

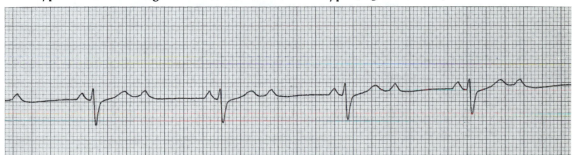

Rate: The ventricular rate is 44/minute. The atrial rate is 88/minute.

Rhythm: Regular.

P waves: Normal and occur at regular intervals. However, every other P wave is blocked.

P–R interval: Constant at 0.16 second.

QRS: Normal (0.10 second).

Comment: That every other P wave is blocked indicates that this is a 2:1 second-degree AV block. (The atrial rate is twice the ventricular rate.) The P–R intervals are constant. The normal width of the QRS complexes suggests that the block is junctional rather than below the junction.

Third-Degree (Complete) AV Heart Block (Figure 13–25)

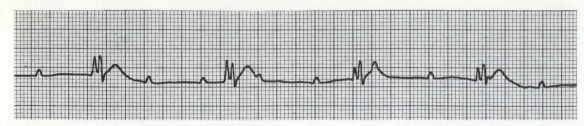

Rate:	The ventricular rate is 44/minute. The atrial rate is 100/minute.
Rhythm:	Regular.
P waves:	Normal, and occur regularly.
P–R interval:	Variable because of dissociation between atria and ventricles.
QRS:	Widened (0.14 second), indicating that the QRS complexes originate in the ventricles.
Comment:	The sinus node continues to discharge normally (at a rate of 100/minute), but all of the impulses from it are blocked. The ventricles discharge independently at a rate of 44/minute. The two rhythms are dissociated (AV dissociation) and bear no relation to each other.

Intraventricular Conduction Defect (Figure 13–26)

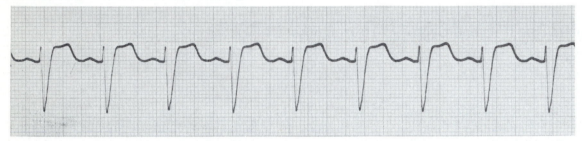

Rate:	About 90/minute.
Rhythm:	Regular.
P waves:	Normal and precede each QRS complex.
P–R interval:	Normal (0.20 second).
QRS:	Widened (0.16 second).
Comment:	The broad QRS complexes preceded by normal P waves indicate an intraventricular conduction defect. However, it cannot be determined from this single lead whether the disorder is a right or left bundle-branch block; a 12-lead ECG is necessary for determining this.

Ventricular Asystole (Figure 13–27)

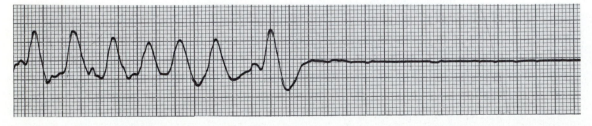

Comment:	This example shows the sudden cessation of all ventricular activity (ventricular asystole) during an episode of VT. Just before this terminal arrhythmia occurred there was evidence of a complete heart block, which allowed the VT to develop.

Chapter 14

Electrocardiographic Diagnosis of Myocardial Infarction, Injury, and Ischemia

Besides its use in interpreting arrhythmias, electrocardiography serves an equally important role in establishing the diagnosis of acute myocardial infarction (AMI), myocardial injury, and myocardial ischemia. The electrocardiogram (ECG), although by no means infallible, remains an indispensable means of verifying these particular manifestations of coronary heart disease (CHD), and deserves top rank among diagnostic tests for such disease even when compared with newer, more sophisticated techniques such as positron emission tomography (PET; used to measure cellular metabolism) or thallium scans (used to measure the extent of myocardial perfusion). It is relatively inexpensive (compared to all other tests of myocardial ischemia and heart rhythm) and without risk.

The ECG has assumed even more importance with the availability of thrombolytic therapy, since thrombolysis is initiated only when it is clear that the patient is experiencing an AMI. Since nurses manage patients receiving thrombolytic drugs, it is important that they understand the electrocardiographic changes that occur with AMI. The purpose of this chapter is to briefly explain the application of electrocardiography in the diagnosis of CHD, focusing primarily on the identification and location of AMI.

THE 12-LEAD ELECTROCARDIOGRAM

Unlike arrhythmias, which often can be identified from a single (monitoring) lead, AMI (and other myocardial abnormalities) can be detected and localized only with a complete 12-lead ECG. Myocardial ischemia, injury, and necrosis are reflected electrocardiographically by disturbances in depolarization and repolarization, which appear in the QRS, S–T segment, and T-wave portions of the ECG. Since disorders of depolarization and repolarization may be confined to only one segment of the myocardium, multiple leads are necessary to provide a comprehensive view of these electrical events throughout the heart.

A complete (12-lead) ECG consists of three standard (limb) leads (leads I, II, and III), three augmented leads (leads aVR, aVL, and aVF), and six chest (precordial) leads (leads V1 through V6). These have been described in Chapter 8 and are shown in Figure 14–1. A complete electrocardiogram depicting these 12 leads is shown in Figure 14–2.

DIAGNOSIS OF ACUTE MYOCARDIAL INFARCTION

An acute transmural myocardial infarction consists of three zones: (1) a central zone of necrosis or dead tissue; (2) a zone of injury surrounding the necrotic area; and (3) a zone of ischemia peripheral to the zone of injury (Figure 14–3). Although not anatomically discrete entities, each of the three zones is reflected differently in the ECG.

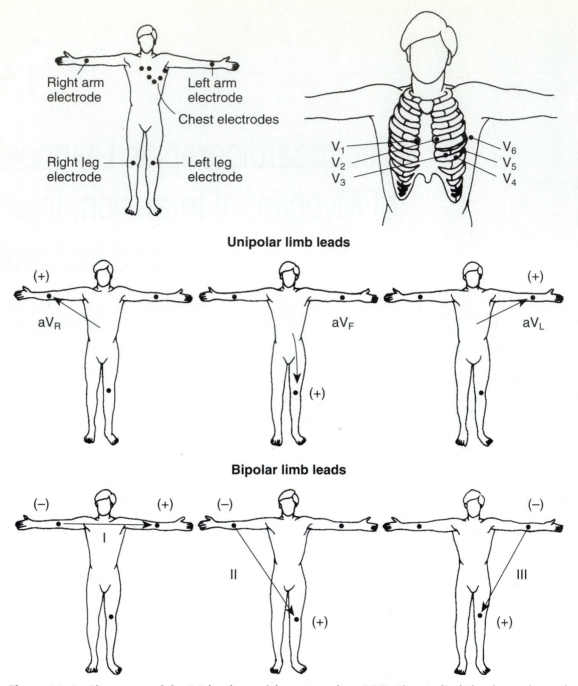

Unipolar limb leads

Bipolar limb leads

Figure 14–1. Placement of the 12 leads used for a complete ECG. The six limb leads are formed from the electrodes placed on the arms and left leg. Each bipolar lead has a specific (–) and (+) electrode. Each unipolar lead has a designated (+) electrode and a neutral electrode that is an average of the other electrodes.

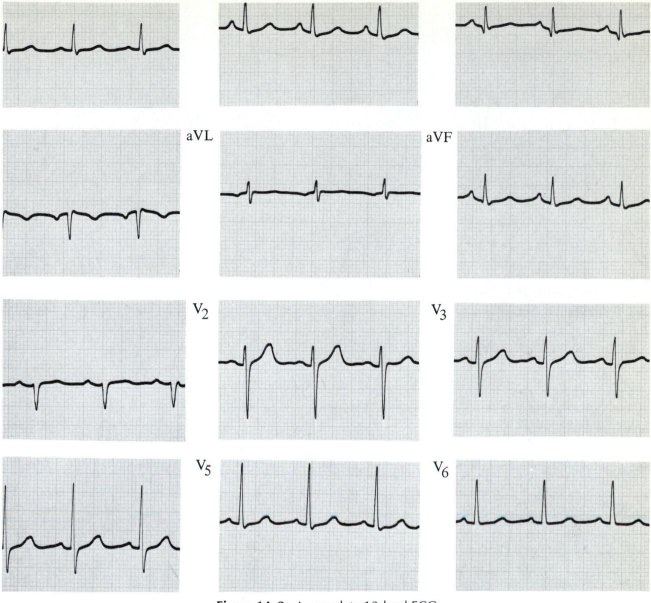

aVL   aVF

V₂   V₃

V₅   V₆

Figure 14–2. A complete 12-lead ECG.

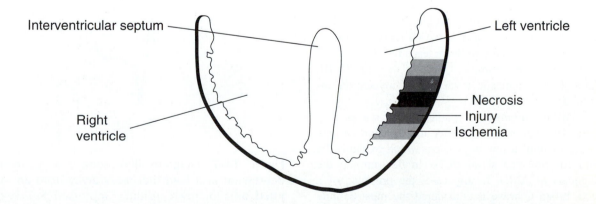

Interventricular septum

Left ventricle

Necrosis

Injury

Ischemia

Right ventricle

Figure 14–3. A cross-sectional diagram of the heart, showing the three zones of acute myocardial infarction (necrosis, injury, ischemia).

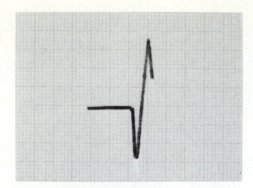

Figure 14–4. Diagram of pathologic Q wave of acute myocardial infarction. This wide, deep Q wave differs from small, normal Q waves.

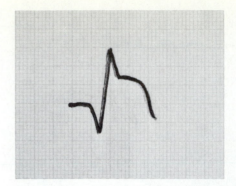

Figure 14–5. Diagram showing S–T-segment elevation resulting from myocardial injury.

Electrocardiographic Signs of Myocardial Necrosis

Myocardial necrosis is reflected by the development of *deep, wide Q waves.* These pathologic waves differ from the normal, small Q waves created by depolarization in the interventricular septum (usually seen in leads I, aVL, and V6). Septal Q waves are of short duration (<0.04 second or one small box on the ECG) and low magnitude (<25% of the total height of the QRS complex).

The Q waves in myocardial necrosis originate as follows: Necrotic tissue is electrically inert and generates no electrical forces. Electrically, the dead area can be considered a hole or "window" in the myocardial wall. Thus, an exploring electrode placed over the zone of dead tissue will in effect look through the hole and record electrical activity (depolarization) from the healthy tissue on the opposite side of the ventricle or interventricular septum. The initial electrical forces (during depolarization) move away from the necrotic zone and the electrode therefore records a broad negative deflection called the Q wave of AMI (Figure 14–4). Q waves are seen only in those leads that face the infarcted area. For example, Q waves in leads II, III, and aVF are diagnostic of an inferior myocardial infarction.

The development of pathologic Q waves may occur within an hour or so after an infarction, or may not occur until a few days later (which explains the need for repeated serial ECGs in determining the diagnosis of AMI). In any case, the presence of a deep, broad Q wave is considered the most definite evidence of an acute transmural myocardial infarction.

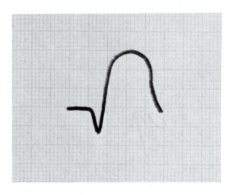

Figure 14–6. Diagram showing elevated S–T segment with a coved configuration.

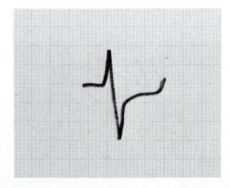

Figure 14–7. Diagram illustrating S–T segment depression in a lead that faces away from an injured area of myocardium. Depressed S–T segments represent a mirror image of the elevated S–T segments and are called reciprocal changes.

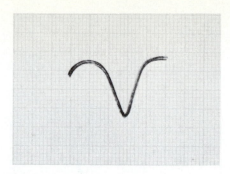

Figure 14–8. Diagram depicting typically inverted T wave of myocardial ischemia. Note that the inverted T wave is sharply pointed and resembles an arrowhead.

Electrocardiographic Signs of Myocardial Injury

Myocardial injury, often the earliest ECG manifestation of AMI, is reflected in changes in the S–T segments. The S–T segments may become elevated or depressed, depending on the site of the infarcted area and the lead in which it is recorded. Leads that face the injured area show *elevated* S–T segments (Figure 14–5). These elevated segments usually develop a convex shape and are described as *coved* S–T segments (Figure 14–6). In contrast, electrodes that face away from the infarction record depression of the S–T segments. The depressed segments (recorded from the opposite side of the injured area) represent a mirror image of the injured region and are categorized as *reciprocal changes* (Figure 14–7). In all, the distinctive ECG manifestation of myocardial injury is elevated, coved S–T segments in leads facing the injured area. Reciprocal changes, which are not diagnostic in their own right, may not occur.

Electrocardiographic Signs of Myocardial Ischemia

The third (and least dependable) electrocardiographic indication of AMI is evidence of myocardial ischemia. The classic sign of myocardial ischemia is *inverted and sharp (i.e., pointed) T waves* that are symmetrical in shape, as shown in Figure 14–8. T-wave inversion of this type indicates an abnormality in myocardial repolarization. However, an inverted T wave is a nonspecific finding and may result from many causes unrelated to myocardial ischemia.

The Combined ECG Signs of Acute Myocardial Infarction

With a typical acute transmural myocardial infarction, signs of myocardial necrosis, injury, and ischemia may all be evident in certain leads. In other words, a deep, wide Q wave (myocardial necrosis), an elevated S–T segment (myocardial injury), and an inverted, sharply pointed T wave (myocardial ischemia) may be noted on recordings from some leads. This combination of findings represents the classic pattern of AMI. It is important to recognize that not all of these ECG signs must be present to diagnose AMI. In fact, with small transmural ("trans" = across and "mural" = wall) infarctions or non-Q-wave infarctions, Q waves or changes in the S–T segment may never develop, and the only ECG evidence of myocardial infarction is nonspecific T-wave inversions. In these circumstances, enzyme studies may help confirm the clinical impression of acute infarction.

LOCALIZATION OF MYOCARDIAL INFARCTION

The location of a myocardial infarction influences the clinical course and outcome of the attack. For instance, the death rate is substantially higher among patients with anterior myocardial infarction than with inferior myocardial infarction, because anterior wall damage usually involves a larger muscle mass

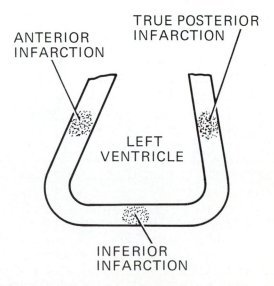

Figure 14–9. Main anatomic sites of acute myocardial infarction.

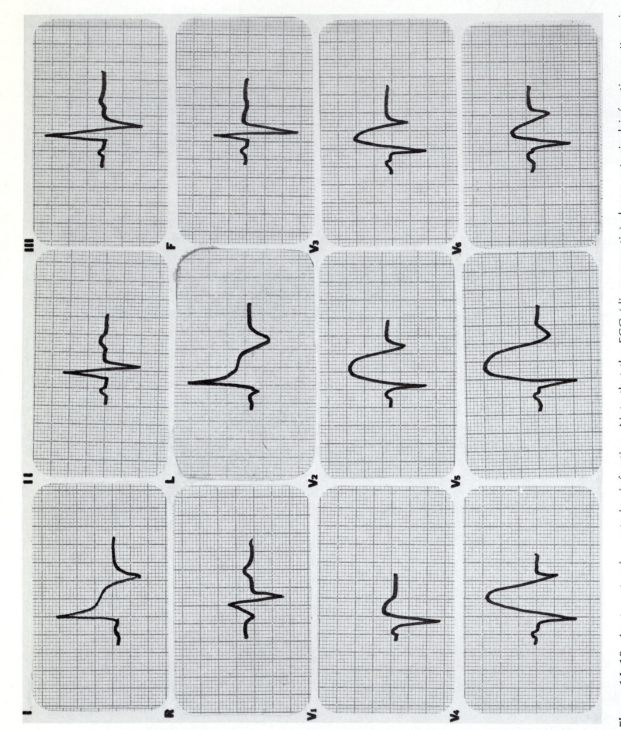

Figure 14–10. Acute extensive anterior infarction. Note that the ECG (diagrammatic) shows a typical infarction pattern in leads I, aVL, and all of the precordial leads (V1–V6).

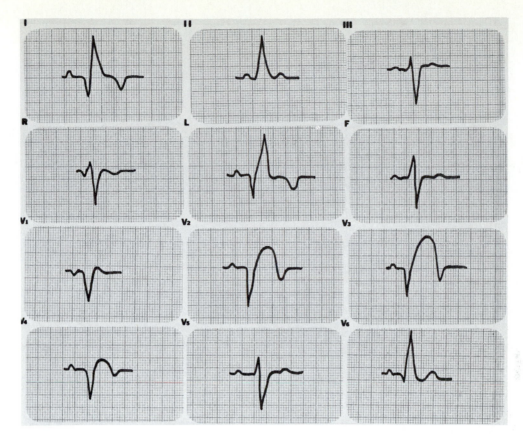

Figure 14–11. Acute anteroseptal infarction. The electrocardiographic features of an acute anteroseptal infarction, as shown in this diagram, are found in leads I, aVL, and V1 through V6.

and therefore leads to pump failure more often. On the other hand, patients with inferior myocardial infarction are more likely to develop AV heart block because this type of infarction frequently involves the AV node itself. Consequently, it is important to know the site of an infarction when anticipating complications and planning a treatment program. Although the anatomic location of an infarction cannot be determined precisely by electrocardiography, the correlation is close enough that the ECG can be regarded as a reliable means of localization for clinical purposes.

Myocardial infarction occurs most often in the anterior and inferior walls of the left ventricle (Figure 14–9). Infarctions involving the posterior left ventricular wall, usually called true posterior infarctions, are rare by comparison and are simply mentioned here. Right ventricular infarction, although more common than was once recognized, does not produce a typical ECG pattern that specifically localizes the infarction to the right ventricle. Accordingly, the ECG of right ventricular infarction is not considered in this discussion.

Anterior Myocardial Infarction

An anterior infarction is revealed by the presence of a characteristic infarction pattern (Q waves, elevated S–T segments, and inverted T waves) in the *precordial (V) leads* that face the infarction. Similar changes usually occur in leads aVL and lead I.

It is customary to classify anterior infarctions into three subgroups, according to the particular ECG findings in each.

An *extensive anterior infarction* is manifested by an infarction pattern in *all* of the precordial leads, as well as in leads I and aVL (Figure 14–10). An *anteroseptal infarction,* involving the anterior wall at the septal area, is reflected by typical ECG signs in leads I, aVL, and V1 to V4 (in contrast to the signs in leads V1–V6 that occur with an extensive anterior infarction). The ECG findings typical of an acute anteroseptal infarction are shown in Figure 14–11. An *anterolateral infarction* is revealed by an infarction pattern in leads V4 to V6 (the outer precordial leads), and leads I and aVL (Figure 14–12).

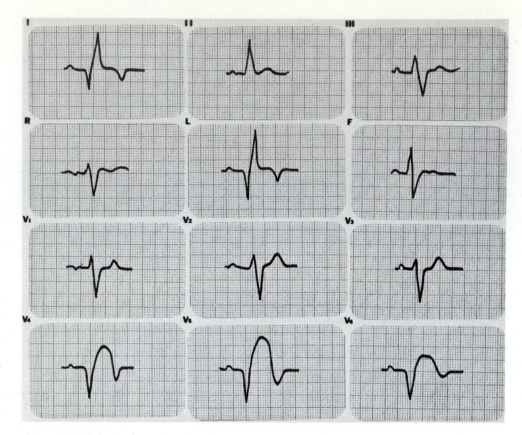

Figure 14–12. Acute anterolateral infarction. The electrocardiographic features of an acute anterolateral infarction, as shown in this diagram, are found in leads I, aVL, and V4 through V6.

Examples of 12-lead ECGs demonstrating acute anterior transmural myocardial infarctions are depicted in Figures 14–13 to 14–16.

Inferior Myocardial Infarction

Myocardial infarction involving the inferior wall of the left ventricle is characterized by an infarction pattern, comprising deep Q waves, elevated S–T segments, and sharply inverted T waves, in *leads II, III, and aVF* (Figure 14–17). Unlike anterior infarctions, the precordial leads in inferior infarctions do not demonstrate an infarction pattern and are often normal. However, on some occasions, S–T segment depression is noted in the precordial leads, reflecting a *reciprocal* change (in which the precordial leads show a mirror image of the S–T-segment elevation found in leads II, III, and aVF). Also, inferior infarctions may be accompanied by infarction of the lateral ventricular wall (an *inferolateral* myocardial infarction). In this circumstance, in addition to signs of an acute inferior infarction, the outer precordial leads (V5 and V6) and leads I and aVL may reveal charac-

teristic S–T-segment and T-wave changes. An example of an acute inferior myocardial infarction is shown in Figure 14–8 and an acute inferolateral infarction in Figure 14–19.

STAGES OF MYOCARDIAL INFARCTION

Besides identifying and localizing AMI, the ECG also provides valuable information about the stages of healing and general age of an infarction. Clinically, myocardial infarction can be divided into three sequential phases: acute, recent, and old. These phases are recognized by the ECG patterns that evolve at different periods after an attack.

The ECG pattern reflecting the *acute* stage of myocardial infarction consists of deep Q waves, elevated S–T segments, and inverted T waves, as described previously. After a few days the raised S–T segments begin to return to the baseline and usually become normal within 1 to 4 weeks. The inverted T waves often show further deepening for several days, but then gradually resume a normal configuration.

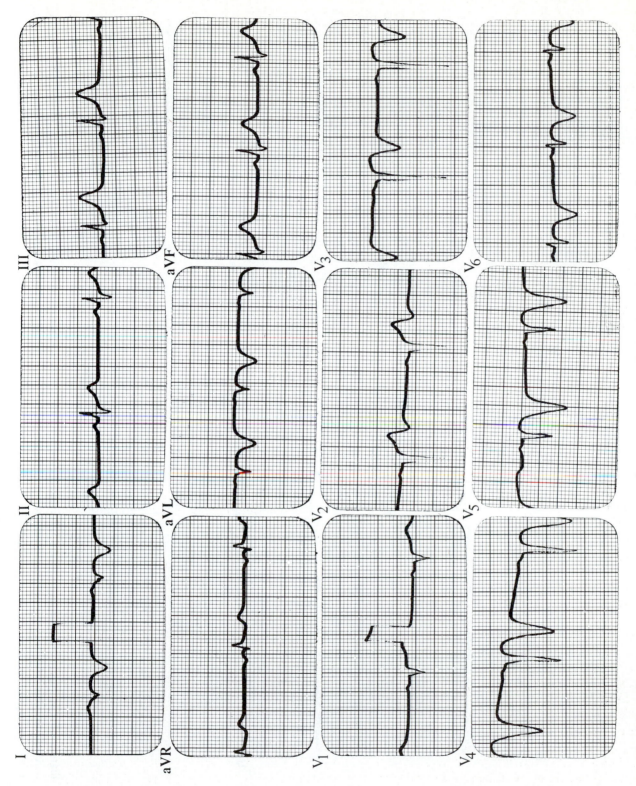

Figure 14–13. Acute extensive anterior infarction. Q waves are evident in leads I, aVL, and V1 through V5. Also, deep, symmetrical T-wave inversions are seen in all of the precordial leads (V1–V6, I, and aVL). (The rectangular wave in lead I represents an ECG standardization mark 10 mm in height.)

259

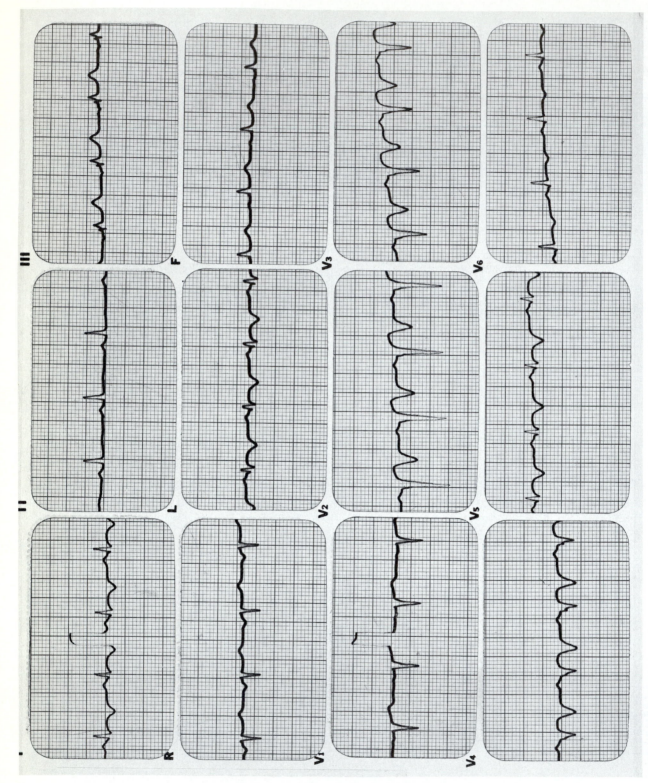

Figure 14-14. Acute anterior myocardial infarction. The precordial leads show deep Q waves in leads V1 through V4, and small Q waves in leads I, aVL and V5 and V6. Symmetrical T-wave inversion is noted in all of the anterior leads (leads I, aVL, and V1–V6). These findings indicate extensive anterior wall damage.

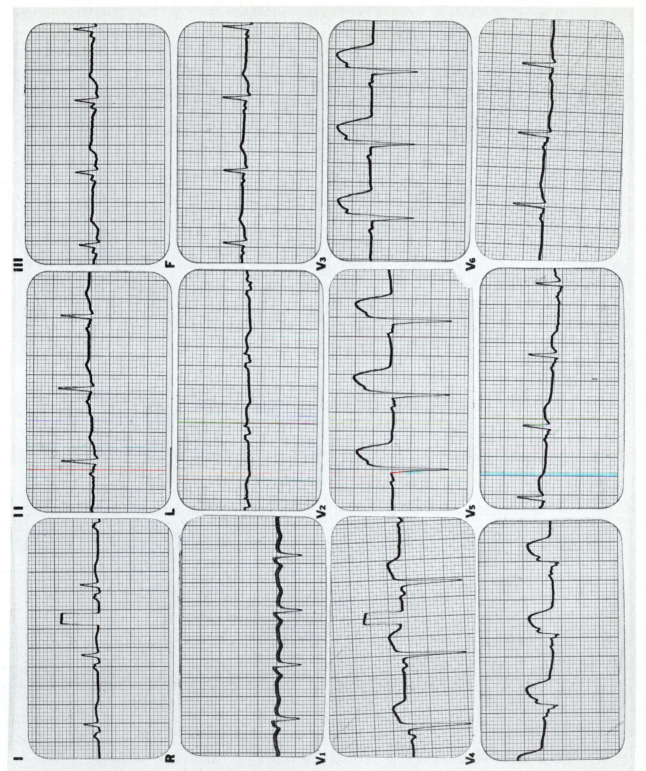

Figure 14–15. Acute anteroseptal myocardial infarction. There is marked S–T-segment elevation in leads V2, V3, and V4, which localizes the infarction to the anteroseptal area. Q waves have already developed in these leads, but T-wave inversion has not occurred at this early stage of infarction.

261

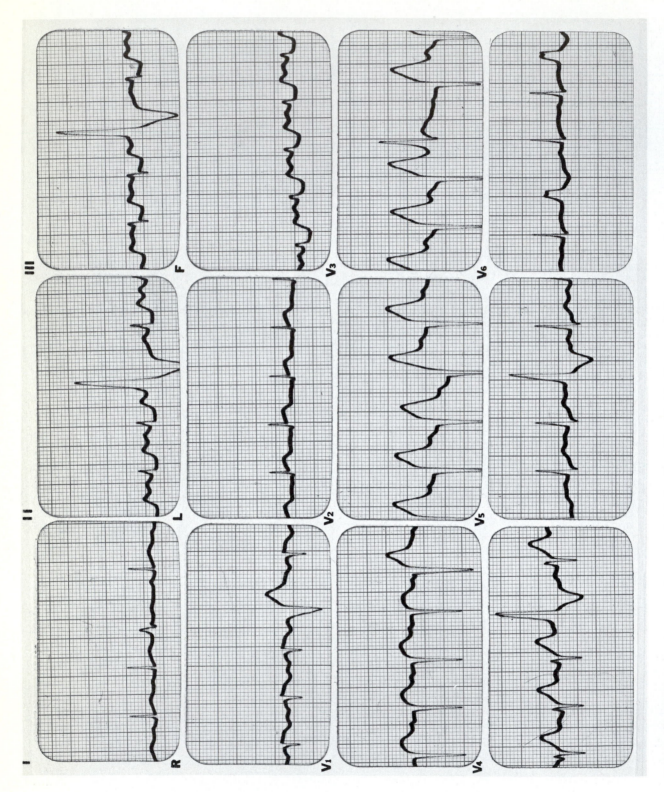

Figure 14–16. Acute anteroseptal myocardial infarction. The key findings are S–T-segment elevations in lead aVL, and V1 through V3, along with significant Q waves in V1 through V3. Note that the S–T segments are markedly depressed in leads II, III, and aVF, reflecting reciprocal changes in these inferior leads. Frequent PVCs are also present.

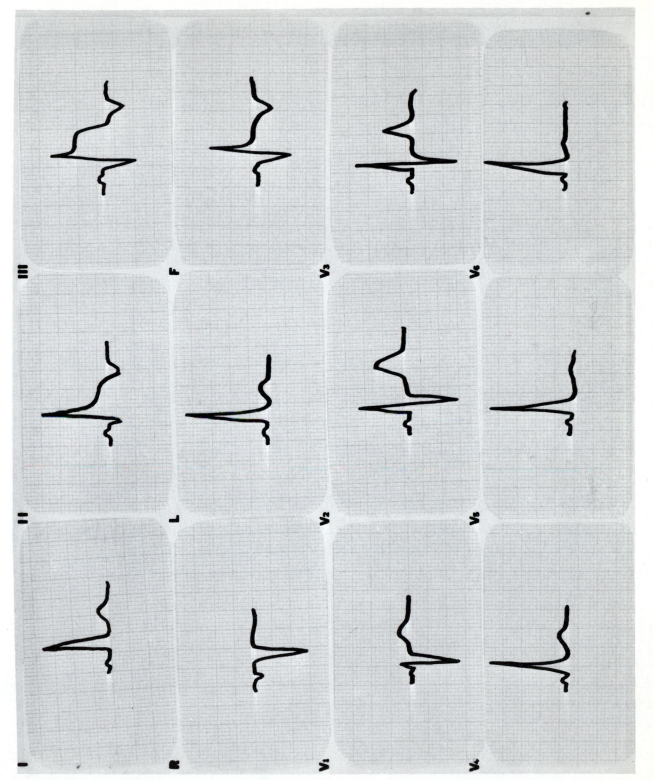

Figure 14–17. Acute inferior infarction. In this diagrammatic representation a typical infarction pattern, consisting of Q waves, elevated S–T segments, and inverted T waves, is noted in leads II, III, and aVF.

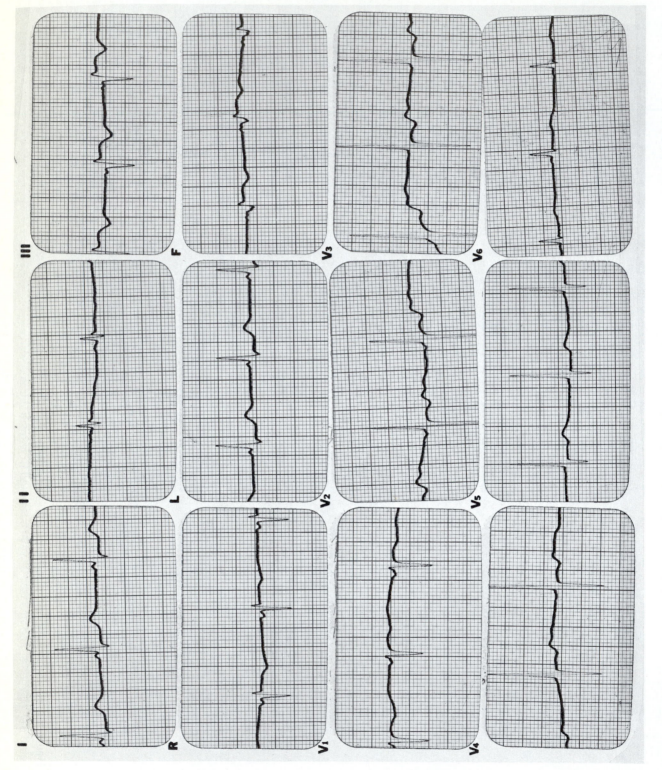

Figure 14–18. Acute inferior infarction. Note the typical Q waves and S–T-segment elevations in leads III and aVF. Reciprocal changes (S–T-segment depression) are seen in the anterior leads I and aVL.

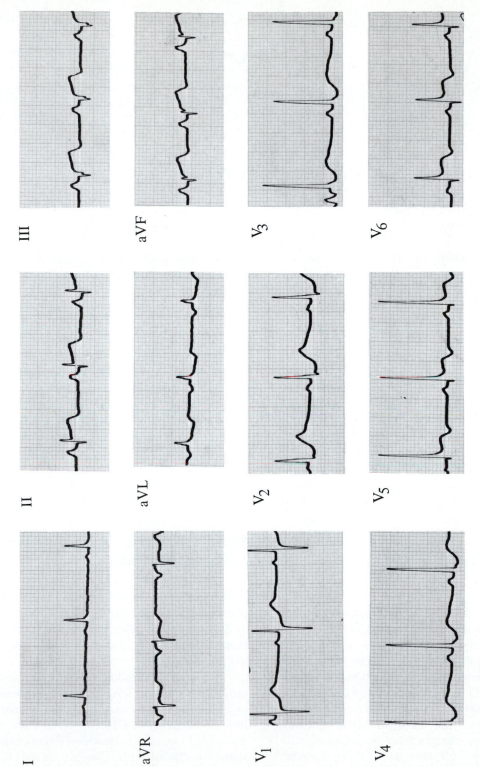

Figure 14–19. Acute inferolateral myocardial infarction. A characteristic infarction pattern is evident in the inferior leads (II, III, aVF) as well as in the lateral leads (V5 and V6).

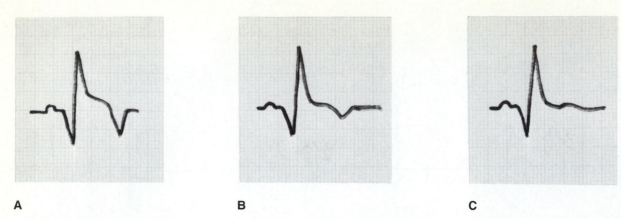

A   **B**   **C**

Figure 14–20. Diagram illustrating ECG patterns of acute **(A)**, recent **(B)**, and old **(C)** myocardial infarction. Note the difference in the configuration of the S–T segment and T wave in an acute infarction as compared with an old infarction.

When the abnormalities of the S–T segments and T waves finally disappear (or at least remain stable), the infarction may be classified as a *recent* myocardial infarction (in contrast to an acute myocardial infarction). Unlike the S–T segments and T waves, the Q waves of AMI persist permanently and are the only diagnostic signs of an *old* myocardial infarction. (It is important to realize that small Q waves may be present normally in some leads, and do not indicate an old myocardial infarction.) Pathologic Q waves are wide (more than 0.04 second) and deep (more than 4 mm in depth). The ECG patterns of acute, recent, and old myocardial infarction are shown diagramatically in Figure 14–20. Complete 12-lead ECGs of an old anterior and an old inferior myocardial infarction are presented in Figures 14–21 and 14–22.

NON–Q-WAVE MYOCARDIAL INFARCTION

Infarctions that do not extend completely through the myocardium are called *nontransmural* or *non-Q-wave infarctions*. These infarctions are small and are associated with only patchy areas of necrosis. For this reason, nontransmural infarctions do not produce pathologic Q waves, and the sole ECG evidence of their occurrence are elevated S–T segments and, especially, symmetrical, deeply inverted T waves. The S–T segment changes may be transient, with the result that by the time an ECG is recorded, the only remaining abnormality is T-wave inversion. Since T waves may invert from dozens of causes other than myocardial ischemia, and their occurrence is therefore a nonspecific ECG sign, it is essential to correlate this ECG evidence with the

patient's history and enzyme studies before concluding that a nontransmural infarction has actually occurred.

Acute nontransmural myocardial infarction may be detected electrocardiographically in the anterior and inferior wall of the left ventricle. An anterior nontransmural infarction, like an anterior transmural infarction, produces S–T segment and T-wave changes in leads I and aVL and the precordial leads, as shown in Figure 14–23. An inferior nontransmural infarction is determined by leads II, III, and aVF (Figure 14–24). Q waves never develop with nontransmural infarction, and consequently there is no definite way to identify an old nontransmural infarction.

TRANSIENT MYOCARDIAL ISCHEMIA (ANGINA PECTORIS)

Aside from its role in the diagnosis of myocardial infarction, electrocardiography is utilized extensively to detect or verify other manifestations of coronary heart disease (CHD), particularly *transient myocardial ischemia.*

Transient myocardial ischemia, the underlying cause of *angina pectoris,* can occur spontaneously or may be induced by exercise (stress) testing to confirm the diagnosis of CHD. In either case, transient myocardial ischemia is identified electrocardiographically by characteristic changes in the S–T segments and, to a lesser degree, by changes in the T waves.

The most reliable ECG sign of transient myocardial ischemia is *S–T-segment depression.* The reason for the S–T segment depression (rather than

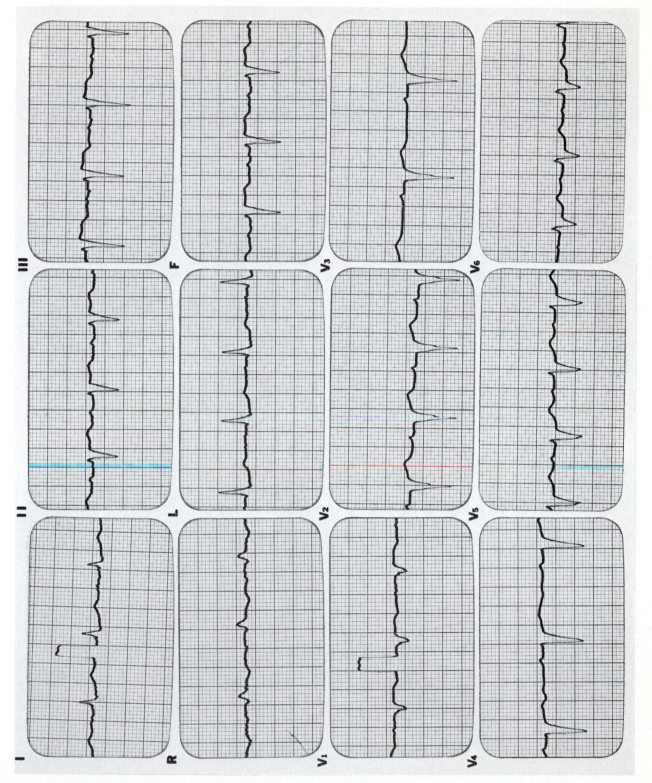

Figure 14-21. Old anterior myocardial infarction. The Q waves in leads V1 through V4, without S–T-segment or T-wave changes, indicate an old infarction.

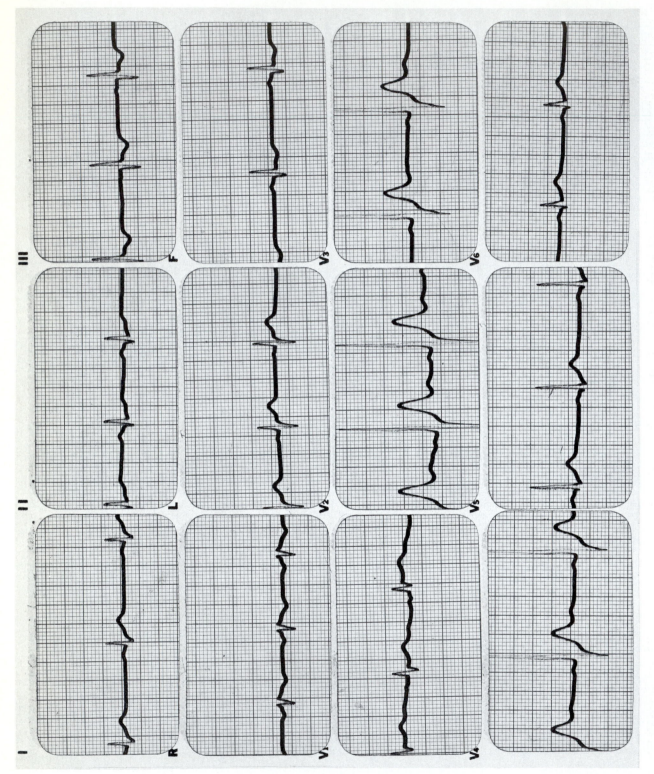

Figure 14–22. Old inferior myocardial infarction. The Q waves in leads II, III, and aVF reflect a previous infarction of the inferior wall of the myocardium.

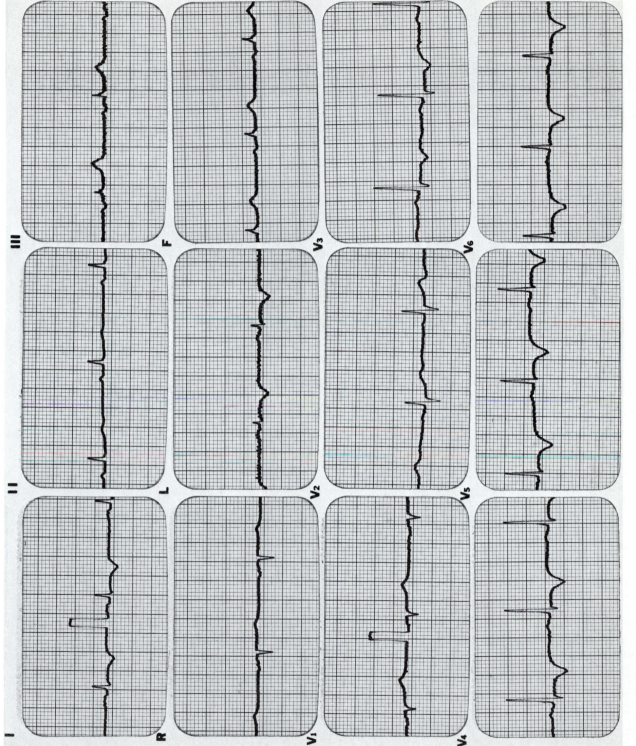

Figure 14–23. Non-Q-wave anterior myocardial infarction. The T waves are sharply inverted in leads I, aVL, and V3 through V6, but the absence of Q waves indicates that the infarction is not transmural.

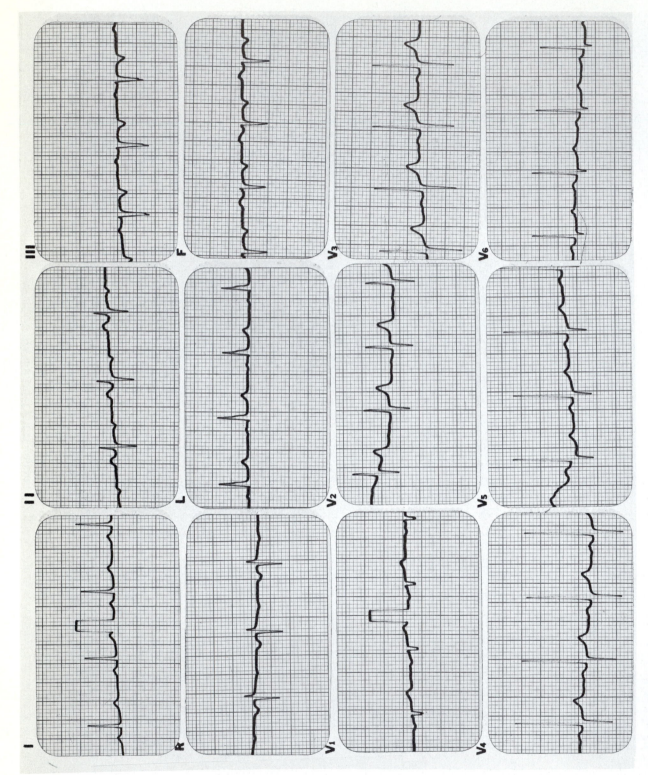

Figure 14–24. Non-Q-wave inferior myocardial infarction. T-wave inversion is evident only in the inferior leads II, III, and aVF. Note the absence of Q waves.

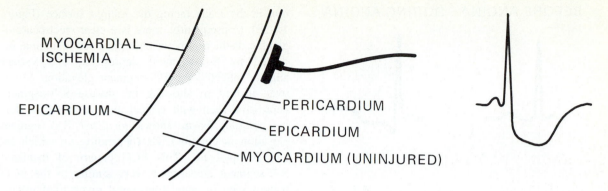

Figure 14–25. Illustration of subendocardial location of myocardial ischemia during angina pectoris. Note that the chest electrode faces away from the area of ischemia, causing downward depression of S–T segments.

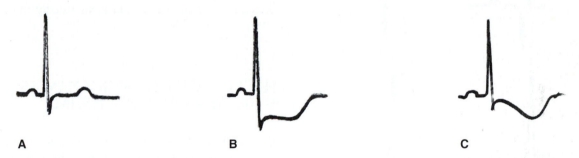

A   B   C

Figure 14–26. Diagrammatic illustrations comparing a normal S–T segment **(A)**, horizontal depression of the S–T segment **(B)**, and downsloping of the S–T segment **(C)**. Myocardial ischemia is manifested either by horizontal or downsloping S–T segments.

S–T-segment elevation, as would be expected with acute myocardial injury) is that the ischemic area of the myocardium associated with angina pectoris involves the *subendocardial* portion of the ventricles, as depicted in Figure 14–25. Note particularly that the chest electrodes do not face the subendocardium, but rather face away from this area. As discussed in Chapter 8, a lead facing an injured area reveals S–T-segment elevation, while a lead facing away from the injury will show depressed (or reciprocal) changes. Since the subendocardial area of ischemia faces away from the chest electrodes, the S–T segments are depressed in these leads during an episode of angina pectoris. The depressed S–T segments are typically horizontal or downsloping in shape (Figure 14–26), which distinguishes them from depressed S–T segments of nonischemic origin. An illustration of the ECG changes associated with angina pectoris is shown in Figure 14–27.

In addition to S–T-segment depression, myocardial ischemia also produces T-wave changes. These T-wave changes, however, are not as dependable or diagnostically significant as the S–T-segment changes just described (because many conditions other than myocardial ischemia can cause similar T-wave abnormalities). Nevertheless, the development of inverted T waves that are sharply pointed and symmetrically shaped is frequently noted during myocardial ischemia (Figure 14–28).

VARIANT (PRINZMETAL'S) ANGINA

As discussed in Chapter 4, variant angina pectoris (also called Prinzmetal's angina) is characterized by chest pain occurring at rest rather than with activity. Also (unlike typical angina), variant angina is caused by coronary artery spasm, which diminishes blood flow through large and medium-sized vessels. Because the coronary arteries lie on the epicardial surface of the ventricles, the effect of arterial spasm is to produce *subepicardial* ischemia (in contrast to the subendocardial ischemia of typical angina). Subepicardial ischemia is manifested by S–T-segment *eleva-*

BEFORE ANGINA   DURING ANGINA

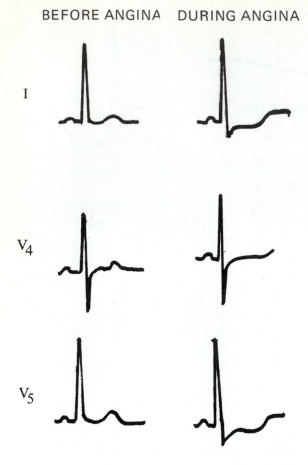

Figure 14–27. Electrocardiographic changes (diagrammatic) associated with angina pectoris. Note that the S–T segments are depressed during an episode of angina, particularly in the three leads depicted here.

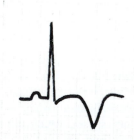

Figure 14–28. T-wave changes of myocardial ischemia. Typically, the T waves are sharply pointed, with symmetrical limbs (arrowhead shape).

tion in the leads facing the injured surface (Figure 14–29). Consequently, there is a clear electrocardiographic distinction between typical stable angina, reflected by S–T-segment depression, and variant angina, reflected by S–T-segment elevation. Moreover, instead of showing the diffuse S–T-segment depression seen with typical angina, the ECG during arterial spasm shows *localized* S–T-segment elevation in certain leads (depending on which artery is involved). This ECG pattern of localized S–T-segment elevation is very similar to the ECG pattern seen in acute transmural myocardial infarction. However, with variant angina, the S–T-segment elevation is only transient, resolving as soon as the arterial spasm abates (Figure 14–30). Indeed, S–T segments that do not return to the baseline promptly after the chest pain stops usually indicate AMI.

ELECTROCARDIOGRAPHIC CHANGES WITH EXERCISE (STRESS) TESTING

The diagnosis of angina pectoris is usually established on the basis of the patient's history alone. On some occasions, however, the history is not clear-cut, and certain diagnostic studies must be done to determine whether the chest pain is due in fact to angina pectoris. The most common test for this purpose is the exercise, or stress, test. The object of this procedure is to increase the myocardial oxygen demand through exercise. If coronary blood flow is inadequate to meet the additional demand, an ECG recorded during (and immediately after) the exercise period will usually reveal signs of myocardial ischemia, as manifested by S–T-segment depression.

After the exercise (walking on a treadmill or riding a stationary bicycle) is completed, and myocardial oxygen supply and demand are again balanced, the S–T segments return to baseline. A stress test is interpreted primarily on the basis of the behavior of the S–T segments during exercise; other criteria are of much less importance. A positive test is defined as one in which there is horizontal or downsloping S–T-segment depression of more than 1 mm in depth. A typical example of a positive exercise test is shown in Figure 14–31.

It is important to realize that exercise testing is not an entirely reliable diagnostic method. In some instances it fails to elicit S–T-segment depression despite significant coronary artery narrowing (a false-negative result). Equally disadvan-

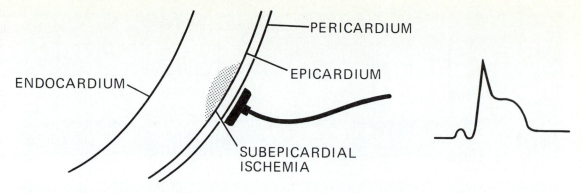

Figure 14–29. Subepicardial ischemia resulting from coronary artery spasm (variant angina). The S–T segments are elevated in leads that face the injured area.

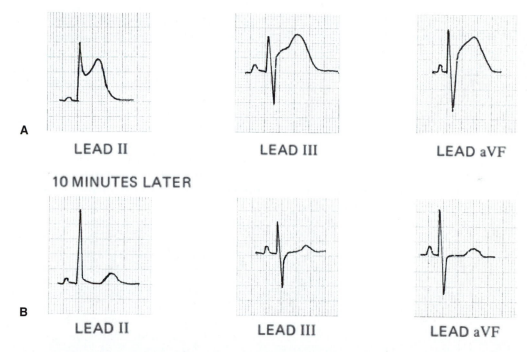

Figure 14–30. A. Transient myocardial ischemia during an episode of variant angina pectoris. Note elevated S–T segments in leads II, III, and aVF, indicating involvement of the inferior wall of the left ventricle, probably from spasm of the right coronary artery. **B.** 10 minutes later, after the pain has ended, the elevated S–T segments have returned to the baseline. Coronary artery spasm may occur with normal vessels or in conjunction with obstructive disease of the coronary arteries.

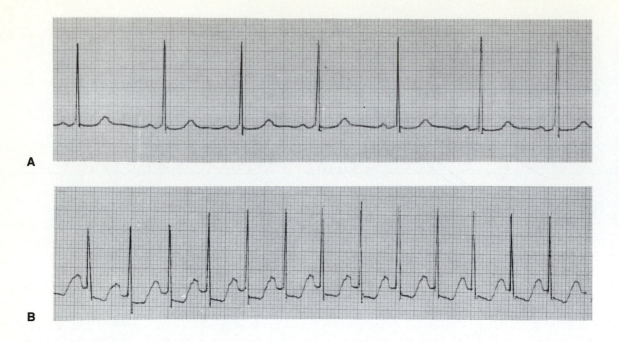

Figure 14–31. Positive exercise (stress) test. Strip **A,** which was recorded immediately before the exercise test was started, shows a heart rate of about 70/minute with normal S–T segments. After 3 minutes of exercise (strip **B**), the heart rate increased to 150/minute. Note the downsloping S–T-segment depression, 2 mm in depth, that developed at this time, defining the test as positive.

tageous is that the test sometimes appears positive despite the absence of coronary artery disease (a false-positive result). For reasons not entirely clear, women are more likely to show false-positive exercise-test results than are men. In the face of positive results, further tests are usually ordered.

Chapter 15

Cardiac Pacemakers

If the inherent electrical system of the heart does not generate impulses or fails to conduct impulses to the ventricles, it is possible to stimulate the myocardium and induce ventricular contraction by means of electrical impulses from an external source. This stimulation is achieved by using a *pacemaker,* a battery-powered device that discharges repetitive electrical impulses so that an effective heart rate can be maintained and life preserved. A pacemaker can also be used to prevent or control tachyarrhythmias. The pacemaker is set at a rate higher than the ordinary sinus rate to prevent subsequent attacks of tachycardia. In this case the pacemaker is used to suppress the ectopic focus by *overdriving* it.

Pacemakers are used in emergencies to maintain life. In such cases a noninvasive, *transcutaneous pacemaker* is usually used, since time is of the essence. If patients need temporary pacemaker support and there is sufficient time to insert a transvenous pacemaker, a temporary *transvenous pacemaker* will be used. Finally, many patients will need permanent pacing support. In such cases a *permanent pacemaker* must be inserted. Today, approximately 500,000 Americans are living with a permanent pacemaker. The following sections describe each of the three types of pacing.

TRANSCUTANEOUS PACEMAKER

The transcutaneous pacemaker (also called a noninvasive temporary pacemaker) is used in emergent situations for patients whose myocardial function is preserved but who have problems with impulse formation or conduction. It consists of two 6- to 8-inch conducting electrodes, which are applied externally to the anterior and posterior chest, and a pacemaker control box.

The impulse rate and energy output in transcutaneous pacing are regulated in the same manner as in temporary transvenous pacing (described below). If the conduction problem continues, the patient is usually prepared for the insertion of a transvenous pacemaker. The difference between the two methods is that the transcutaneous stimulus is delivered externally through the chest wall, while the transvenous stimulus is delivered directly to the endocardium by means of an electrode.

The following steps are used to apply a transcutaneous pacemaker:

1. Apply the front electrode of the pacemaker to the patient's precordium (beneath the left breast on females) and the back pacer electrode to the upper back (left of the spine).
2. Connect the pacemaker electrodes to the output cable.
3. Turn the pacemaker on and set the pacing rate to a value 10 to 20 beats/minute higher than the patient's intrinsic rate. If the patient's intrinsic rate is unknown (eg, the patient presented in asystole), set the rate at 60 beats/ minute.
4. Observe the pacing artifact on the electrocardiogram (ECG) and verify that it occurs during diastole.
5. Increase the energy output (in joules) until the stimulus is sufficient to depolarize the ventricles (ie, the pacemaker captures control of the heart).

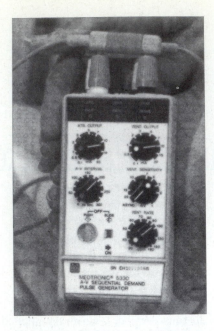

Figure 15–1. A temporary AV-sequential, battery-powered pulse generator for temporary pacing.

TEMPORARY TRANSVENOUS PACEMAKER

The impulses from a temporary transvenous pacemaker are delivered to the heart by way of one or more catheter electrodes, which are passed through the venous system into the right heart. The electrodes may be placed in the right atrium, right ventricle, or both, depending on the nature of the conduction problem and the patient's need for atrial contraction to enhance cardiac output. The electrical stimuli are furnished by a small, AV-sequential, battery-powered pulse generator. An example of the pulse generator is shown in Figure 15–1.

Indications

Temporary transvenous pacing is useful in conditions in which disturbances in the electrical conduction system are usually temporary or the patient requires support until the implantation of a permanent pacemaker. Exemplifying the former situation are conduction disturbances resulting from acute inferior myocardial infarction, which are often transient and usually disappear during the healing phase of the attack, requiring temporary cardiac pacing until this happens.

The primary purpose of transvenous pacing is to prevent primary ventricular standstill. This lethal arrhythmia seldom develops spontaneously; in most instances it is preceded by second- or third-degree heart

TABLE 15–1. INDICATIONS FOR USE OF A TEMPORARY TRANSVENOUS PACEMAKER

Symptomatic bradycardia
Asystole
Symptomatic Mobitz Type I AV block
Mobitz Type II AV block (with or without symptoms)
Irreversible complete heart block
Ventricular tachycardia unresponsive to medications

block or by bundle-branch block involving more than one fascicle of the bundle of His. Inserting a transvenous pacemaker when these advanced forms of heart block are detected can often avoid ventricular standstill.

In addition to this fundamental indication, transvenous pacing is also used in treating persistent bradyarrhythmias. It is a common practice to accelerate the heart rate deliberately by transvenous pacing when marked sinus bradycardia or a slow junctional rhythm resists customary drug therapy and compromises the cardiac output.

Temporary pacing is also used to control resistant ectopic rhythms (eg, frequent PVCs or recurrent ventricular tachycardia [VT]) that are rate-related. In such conditions, pacing the heart at a rate faster than the existing rate can often suppress premature beats. This principle of arrhythmia control is called overdriving the heart. The indications for temporary pacing are summarized in Table 15–1.

Components of Transvenous Pacing

A transvenous pacing system consists of two basic components:

1. The pulse generator (battery-operated), which serves as the source of electrical impulses. Both the rate and the intensity of these impulses can be regulated by control mechanisms.
2. An insulated wire catheter that carries the current from the pulse generator (pacemaker) to one or two small electrodes at the distal end of the catheter. The electrodes are Teflon-coated, stainless steel wires. They are placed in contact with the endocardial surface of the myocardium and permit direct stimulation of the atrium and/or the ventricle.

The Pulse Generator. There are two types of pacemakers: *set-rate* and *demand.*

The Set-rate Pulse Generator. This device, the first available for cardiac pacing, is seldom used. How-

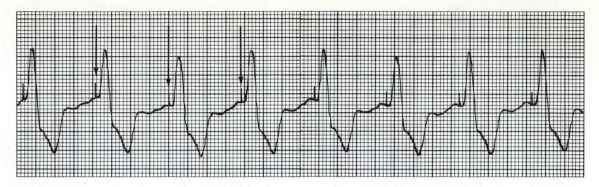

Figure 15–2. The ECG of a patient with a set-rate pacemaker. The arrows point to the pacing stimulus. The rate is set at 60 beats/minute.

ever, it is helpful to consider the design and operation of set-rate pacemakers to order to understand the advantages of the demand pacemaker. A set-rate pulse generator initiates impulses at a fixed or set rate. If, for example, the rate dial of the pacemaker is positioned at 60/minute, an impulse is fired every second. Each pacing impulse (manifested on the ECG as a "pacing spike") stimulates the myocardium to produce a QRS complex, as shown in Figure 15–2. The resulting QRS complexes are widened and have the configuration of a left bundle-branch-block pattern. (This pattern is understandable, since the electrode delivering the stimulus to the myocardium is in the right ventricle, and the impulse must be transmitted from this site to the left ventricle, creating a delay in complete ventricular activation.)

Although set-rate pacing is a dependable method for myocardial stimulation, it has one serious drawback that limits its usefulness in elective cardiac pacing: the instrument disregards the existing electrical activity of the heart and continues to discharge impulses at a fixed rate. Thus, a natural beat from the heart and an artificial pacing stimulus may occur simultaneously, as shown in Figure 15–3. This phenomenon is called *competition.*

When the natural and paced rhythms compete in this way, there is a potential threat of inducing serious ventricular arrhythmias. This is particularly true when the pacing stimulus happens to hit on the T wave of the preceding natural beat. The arrival of the pacing stimulus during the period of the T wave, the *vulnerable period,* may create repetitive firing of the heart itself in the form of VT or, worse, ventricular fibrillation (VF). In other words, set-rate pacing has the same theoretical danger of inducing VF as does a premature contraction striking a T wave. An example of VF developing as the result of a set-rate pacing stimulus striking the T wave of a preceding natural beat is depicted in Figure 15–4.

Although competition certainly does not result in ventricular arrhythmias in all or even most in-

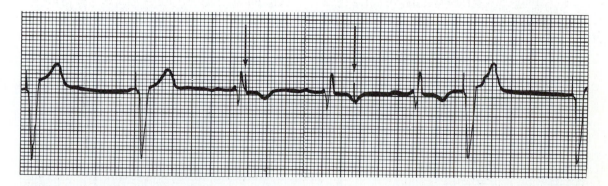

Figure 15–3. The ECG of a patient with a set-rate pacemaker. The pacemaker stimulus is competing with the patient's intrinsic cardiac impulse. Note that after two paced beats, three natural beats arise from the SA node. The pacemaker nevertheless continues to discharge impulses during this period (arrows).

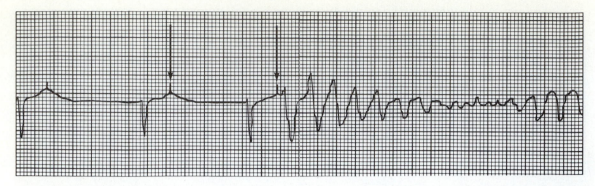

Figure 15–4. The pacing stimulus occurs during ventricular depolarization (on the T wave; arrows) and results in VF.

stances (as evident in Figure 15–5, in which the pacing stimulus hits the T wave of a PVC without provoking repetitive firing), this potential danger nevertheless exists. The risk of inducing VF is distinctly increased in the presence of myocardial ischemia, and it is for this reason that set-rate pacing is undesirable in the treatment of acute myocardial infarction (AMI).

The Demand Pulse Generator.

To avoid the potential risk of competition associated with set-rate pacing, a more sophisticated pulse generator was developed. Instead of discharging impulses at a fixed rate, irrespective of the heart's inherent electrical activity, these pacemakers are designed to be noncompetitive and to discharge only on demand.

The demand pulse generator works on the principle of demand pacemaking, which means that the pacemaker fires an impulse only if a QRS complex does *not* occur within a preset time interval. If depolarization does occur within this designated period, the pacemaker recognizes this electrical activity and deliberately withholds the pacing impulse. On this basis a pacing impulse cannot strike the T wave of a premature ventricular contraction (PVC) since the pacemaker will sense the ectopic beat (which occurs within the instrument's preset time interval) and accordingly will not discharge an impulse. On the other hand, if the pacemaker does not sense either a natural or an ectopic beat, it discharges impulses at its preset rate. An example of how a demand pacemaker functions is shown in Figure 15–6. Note that the pacemaker stops discharging impulses when a series of natural beats occur (all of which fall within the preset time interval). However, when the interval is again exceeded because a natural beat does not occur on schedule, the pacemaker again begins to discharge.

For a pacemaker to function on demand it must receive an electrocardiographic signal indicating that a natural or ectopic beat has occurred; it is this signal that inhibits the pacemaker from discharging unwanted impulses. This information is obtained by having the catheter tip of the demand pacemaker (which is in contact with the endocardial surface of the right ventricle) serve as an exploring electrode to

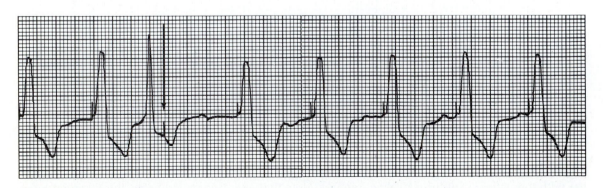

Figure 15–5. The pacing stimulus hits the T wave of a PVC (arrow) without provoking repetitive firing.

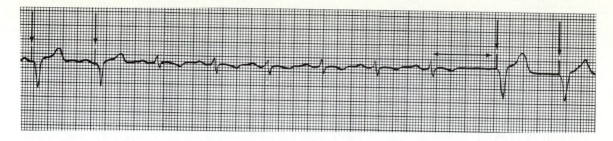

Figure 15–6. This example demonstrates how a demand pacemaker functions. The pacemaker stops discharging impulses when a series of natural beats occur (all of which fall within the preset time interval). However, when the interval is again exceeded because a natural beat did not occur on schedule (shown between the eighth and ninth complex by the horizontal arrows), the pacemaker again begins to discharge.

detect each QRS complex. The electrical activity of the heart is transmitted back through the catheter to a sensing device within the pacemaker. The pacing catheter thus serves to relay electrocardiographic signals to the pacemaker as well as to send pacing impulses from the instrument to the myocardium (Figure 15–7).

Catheter Electrodes. There are two basic types of catheter electrodes: those with a single electrode incorporated in the tip of the catheter (unipolar elec-

trode) and those with two electrodes positioned about 1 cm apart at the distal end of the catheter (bipolar electrode), as shown in Figure 15–8. As with any electrical circuit, the electrical impulse generated by a pacemaker must flow between two poles (or electrodes) in order to stimulate the heart. With a unipolar catheter only one electrode (the negative pole) is within the heart, and a second electrode (the positive pole) is required to complete the circuit. This latter electrode usually consists

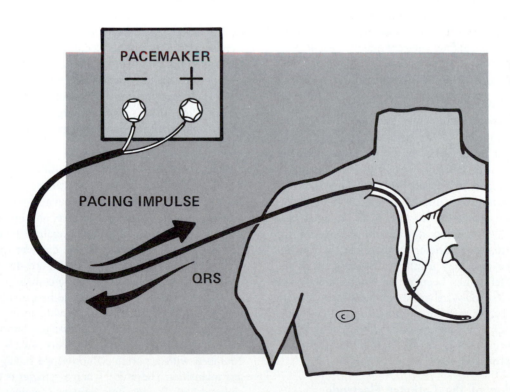

Figure 15–7. The catheter of a demand pacemaker sends pacing impulses to the myocardium as well as relaying electrocardiographic signals to the pacemaker.

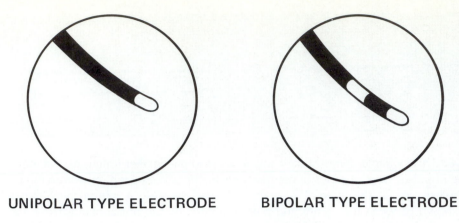

UNIPOLAR TYPE ELECTRODE   **BIPOLAR TYPE ELECTRODE**

Figure 15–8. A graphic comparison of unipolar and bipolar electrodes.

of a wire suture placed in the skin of the chest wall.

The bipolar catheter-electrode system, which is used far more commonly than the unipolar system, obviates the need for a secondary electrode, since both electrodes are incorporated into the catheter itself. Bipolar catheters are preferable to unipolar types because the presence of two adjacent electrodes within the heart enhances the likelihood of direct contact with the endocardial surface of the right ventricle, a requirement for successful pacing. With the unipolar catheter the electrode may easily become displaced from the ventricular wall and thus interrupt effective pacing.

Technique of Transvenous Pacing

Catheter Insertion. The pacing electrode of the transvenous pacemaker can be introduced into the venous system through an antecubital, femoral, jugular, or subclavian vein. Selecting the vein to be used for this purpose is essentially a matter of individual preference; there are advocates for each approach. Although an arm vein is usually the easiest to enter percutaneously, the route to the heart is long and tortuous, often making it difficult to advance the catheter into the ventricle. Furthermore, any movement of the arm may result in displacement of the catheter after it has been properly positioned. The jugular and subclavian veins, being closer to the superior vena cava, are shorter, more direct routes to the right ventricle. For this reason, and because displacement of the catheter is less likely, these latter sites are generally preferred.

Introduction of the Catheter Electrode. Once a

particular vein has been selected for insertion of the catheter electrode, the surrounding skin area must be scrupulously prepared, as for any surgical procedure. The area is draped to prevent contamination.

Several specially designed needles are available for catheter insertion. Most of these placement units consist of a large-bore needle (with a stylus) and a thin plastic sheath that fits over this cannula (Figure 15–9). After the skin is infiltrated with a local anesthetic, the catheter-placement unit is inserted into the vein; the needle (and stylus) is then removed, leaving the plastic sheath positioned in the vein.

The catheter electrode is introduced through this plastic sheath into the vein and advanced to the right ventricle. After the electrode is in proper position within the ventricle, the plastic conduit is removed so that the catheter extends directly through the skin opening. In instances in which needle penetration of the skin or vein is difficult, a small surgical "cut-down" incision can be made to facilitate entry to the vein.

Passage of the Catheter Electrode. Regardless of the site of its introduction, the catheter is advanced slowly to the superior vena cava, into the right atrium, through the tricuspid valve, and into the right ventricle, where it is positioned against the endocardial surface. The pathway of the catheter (as shown on a chest X-ray) is noted in Figure 15–10. Two methods are available to guide the catheter to its ultimate position in the ventricle. The first involves fluoroscopy, which permits direct visualization of the radiopaque catheter during its passage. Although this technique is very desirable, many CCUs are not equipped with a portable fluoroscope having an image intensifier. Therefore, when a catheter is to be positioned with fluoroscopic guidance, patients have to be moved to an X-ray department, a cardiac catheterization laboratory, or a procedure room. This separa-

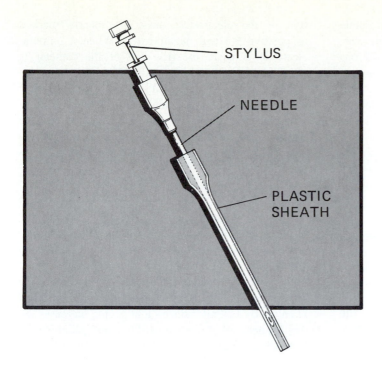

STYLUS

NEEDLE

PLASTIC
SHEATH

Figure 15–9. A placement unit for a transvenous pacemaker.

tion of the patient from the prepared setting of the CCU poses obvious risks, but is nevertheless popular because it facilitates electrode positioning.

The catheter can also be guided to the right ventricle by electrocardiographic means. This method can be used in the CCU and avoids the danger of moving the patient if portable fluoroscopy is unavailable in the unit. The principle of this "blind" technique of catheter insertion is as follows: as the electrode is being advanced to the heart, an ECG can be recorded *through* the catheter by attaching its free end to the chest-lead (V lead) terminal of the ECG machine. In other words, the catheter tip serves as an exploring electrode from within the heart. The resulting tracing is called an *intracavity* ECG. Because the ECG patterns from the vena cava, atrium, and right

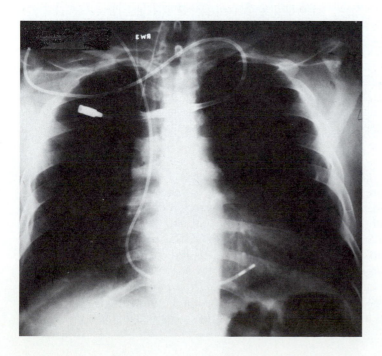

Figure 15–10. A chest X-ray demonstrating a transvenous pacing catheter in the right ventricle. Note that the catheter is bipolar.

ventricle have different configurations, it is possible to identify the position of the electrode in this way. Typical ECG patterns from these various locations are shown in Figure 15–11. Note the large, distinctive complexes recorded when the catheter enters the ventricle (Figure 15–11D). When this method of electrocardiographic guidance is used, it is necessary to connect all of the limb leads to the patient, just as if a customary ECG were to be recorded. The only difference is that the chest (V) lead, rather than being used as a skin electrode, is joined to the free end of the catheter with an alligator clamp. Temporary pacemakers are usually inserted with the guidance of fluoroscopy, but in emergency situations the changes in ECG patterns seen with electrocardiographic guidance can be used to inform the clinician about the position of the catheter tip.

Attachment of the Catheter Electrode to the Pacemaking Device.
As shown in Figure 15–1, the cardiac pacemaker has two terminals for connec-

tion of the electrodes; these are clearly marked as positive (+) and negative (−). When a unipolar electrode is used, the free end of the catheter is attached to the negative (−) terminal of the pacemaker, and the wire from the skin electrode (suture) to the positive (+) terminal. With a bipolar catheter electrode the two wires extending from the catheter can be connected to the terminals of the pacemaker without concern about positive or negative poles.

Rate of Pacing.
Several principles guide the rate at which cardiac pacing is provided. First, the number of pacing stimuli per minute must exceed the existing heart rate. In complete heart block, for example, in which the inherent cardiac rate may be 30 to 40/minute, the pacing rate would be set at 60 to 70/minute. Second, it is undesirable to pace the heart at an overly fast rate, since rapid pacing increases the oxygen demand of the myocardium, and patients with heart disease may experience angina, heart failure, or

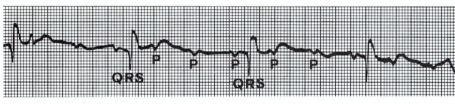

A

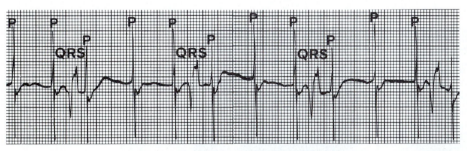

B

Figure 15–11. A. The ECG reveals complete heart block. The catheter tip is in the vena cava. The P waves are small and inverted. **B.** The catheter tip is now in the right atrium. Note the very tall, biphasic P waves recorded from this intraatrial position. **C.** As the catheter advances toward the ventricle, the P waves diminish in size while the QRS complexes become larger. **D.** The catheter tip passes from the right atrium to the right ventricle (arrow), as indicated by the sudden appearance of very large QRS complexes. **E.** The tip of the catheter is now wedged against the endocardial wall of the right ventricle. In this position the ST segment is markedly elevated. **F.** After the catheter has been properly positioned and the pacemaker turned on, a standard ECG reveals effective pacing.

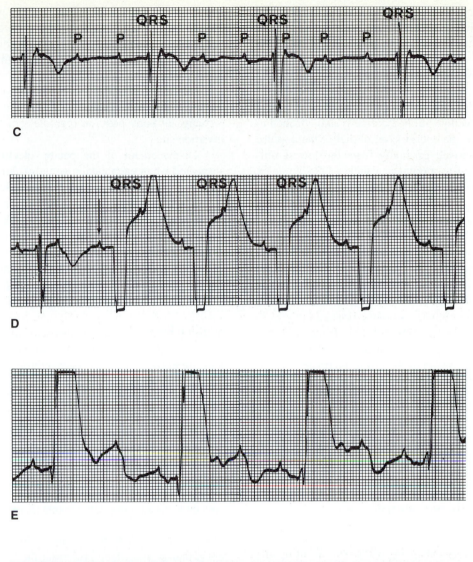

Figure 15–11 (Continued)

an extension of an acute myocardial infarction (AMI). Furthermore, when the heart is paced rapidly the time for ventricular filling is decreased and cardiac output may be adversely affected. Therefore, the pacing rate must be adjusted for each patient, so that pumping efficiency is not reduced while the underlying arrhythmia is being controlled.

Energy of Pacing. In determining the energy or intensity of the stimulus required for cardiac pacing, it is necessary to consider a fundamental characteristic of myocardial contractility: that when the heart is stimulated by an electrical impulse, it responds (contracts) either completely or not at all (the "all-or-none" law). The lowest electrical energy that will cause myocardial contraction is called the *threshold level*. If the intensity of a pacing stimulus is less than this threshold level, contraction will not occur. Conversely, a pacing stimulus exceeding the threshold level will not produce a stronger contraction, since the muscle already contracts to its fullest extent at the threshold point. In other words, there is a critical level of electrical energy below which contraction will not occur and above which it is not augmented.

Therefore, in setting the intensity of the pacing impulse, it is necessary to first determine the threshold level. This is accomplished as follows: after the catheter has been positioned correctly and attached to the pacemaker, the energy-control dial of the impulse generator is moved gradually from the lowest milliampere setting to a point at which a QRS complex is noted with each stimulus. This setting is the threshold level.

When a catheter electrode is properly positioned and its tip is in good contact with the endocardium, the threshold level of impulse energy in most patients is usually less than 2 milliamperes. If the threshold required for producing a ventricular contraction is much higher than this, such as 6 or 8 milliamperes, it is likely that the catheter is poorly situated in the ventricle and that repositioning of the tip is required. Because the threshold is not constant at all times, and varies with the contact of the electrode tip and the endocardium (as well as with other factors), it is customary to set the initial energy level for pacing at twice the threshold value in order to overcome this variation. If, for example, the threshold is found to be 1 milliampere, the final setting for the pacing stimulus should be 2 milliamperes.

Problems with Temporary Transvenous Pacing

Several difficulties may be encountered during the course of temporary pacing. The most common of these are as follows:

Displacement of the Catheter Tip. For pacing to be effective, the catheter electrode must remain proximate to the inner wall of the right ventricle. Displacement of the tip of the catheter is frequent during temporary pacing and is the most common cause of pacing failure. Displacement occurs with greater frequency when the catheter has been introduced via an arm vein (motion of the arm tends to move the entire catheter), but dislodgment of the tip may result from a change of body position regardless of the catheter-insertion site.

Displacement of the pacing electrode may be suspected when each pacing stimulus fails to produce a QRS complex. This means that the pacing impulse is ineffective and is not capturing the heartbeat. An example of loss of capture is shown in the ECG in Figure 15–12. Once displacement has occurred, the catheter usually has to be repositioned in the ventricle in order to achieve effective pacing, although changing the position of the patient in bed will occasionally restore the catheter to its proper position.

Sensing Errors. Although theoretically, competition should not develop during demand pacing, this problem can in fact occur. The competition usually results when the sensing mechanism of the pacemaker fails to recognize spontaneous heartbeats. This will happen, and will prompt the pacemaker to discharge an impulse, unless the R wave transmitted back to the sensing mechanism is of sufficient amplitude (voltage). Competition caused by improper sensing requires moving the catheter tip to a different location in the right ventricle in order to obtain a better R-wave signal for the pacemaker's sensing mechanism.

Loss of Pacing Artifact. If the pacing stimulus does not produce an artifact (spike) on the ECG, it can be presumed that one of the components of the pacing system has failed. The source of the problem is usually not difficult to identify. If the pulse indicator (on the face of the pacemaker) shows no movement, it is likely that either the batteries are exhausted or the

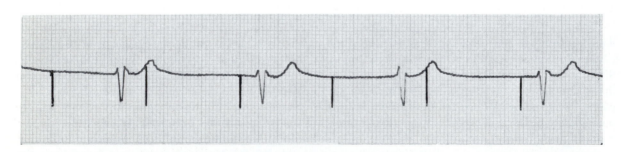

Figure 15–12. This strip demonstrates loss of capture. It is apparent that none of the pacing spikes stimulate the ventricle to produce QRS complexes.

pulse generator is broken. If, on the other hand, the pulse indicator dial shows that the pacemaker is functioning, it can be reasoned that impulses, although originating normally, are not reaching the heart. This condition may result from a broken wire within the catheter or, more simply, from disconnection of the catheter terminal from the pulse generator.

Perforation of the Ventricular Wall by the Catheter Tip.

Since the catheter electrode of the cardiac pacemaker is deliberately placed against the inner surface of the ventricular wall, it is understandable that the catheter tip may embed itself in the myocardium, particularly when the catheter remains in the heart for many days. In some patients the catheter actually burrows through the full thickness of the myocardium and finally perforates the right ventricular wall. However, this untoward event produces surprisingly few effects. Because the blood pressure within the right ventricle is normally quite low (unlike the high pressure within the left ventricle), perforation of the right ventricular chamber seldom has any hemodynamic consequences. Moreover, if there is bleeding into the pericardium, the amount of blood that enters the pericardial space is generally trivial and does not produce cardiac tamponade.

Perforation of the ventricular wall can be suspected from a sudden loss of capture after a period of successful pacing. On some occasions catheter perforation is recognized by the appearance of contractions of the diaphragm or chest wall. This muscle twitching (which is usually obvious to the patient) signifies that the catheter electrode has perforated the right ventricle and traveled to the diaphragm or intercostal muscles. The diagnosis can often be confirmed with a chest X-ray that shows the catheter tip outside the right ventricle. In the event of perforation it is necessary to withdraw the catheter gently and reposition it in the right ventricle.

Thrombophlebitis and Skin Infection.

Because pacing catheters must often remain in the venous system for prolonged periods, they create the possibility of thrombophlebitis from mechanical irritation of the vein wall. The likelihood of this inflammatory reaction is perhaps greater when smaller veins are used as insertion sites (eg, arm veins); however, other factors undoubtedly contribute to this complication. If thrombophlebitis is marked, the catheter must be removed and another one inserted in a different vein.

Because the skin puncture site for insertion of a pacemaker catheter is in effect an open wound, local infection may occur. The risk of this can be minimized (and almost excluded) by adherence to strict surgical asepsis at the time of catheter placement, and by the subsequent routine use of antibiotic (neomycin) ointment.

Nursing Responsibility in Temporary Transvenous Cardiac Pacing

Preparation of the Patient.

When a decision has been made to pace the heart temporarily, it is important to explain to the patient and family why the procedure is necessary and how it will be performed. The explanation should emphasize the preventive benefit of being able to control the heart rate as desired with pacing. The patient and family need time to ask questions or to express concerns about cardiac pacing. If the pacing is to be performed on an elective basis (eg, in a patient with second-degree heart block), the physician must obtain an informed consent signed by the patient. In emergency situations this measure can be disregarded.

A syringe containing 100 mg lidocaine should be prepared and placed at the bedside. In addition, the nurse should verify the patency of the patient's existing intravenous line. These measures are essential for combating any ventricular irritability that may develop suddenly while the catheter is being positioned within the heart. A defibrillator should be available for immediate use in the event (even though unlikely) that the catheter induces ventricular fibrillation.

Procedure.

The skin surrounding the intended site of catheter insertion is prepared with soap, alcohol, and a skin antiseptic, as with any surgical procedure. An "eye sheet" is used to drape the area, leaving only the operative site exposed. In addition, the patient's face is covered with a loose drape to prevent breath contamination of the insertion site. (Pathogens from the mouth and nose are a far greater source of wound infection than bacteria found on the skin.)

The needle placement set and appropriate catheter should be sterile and ready for use. Sterilization can be accomplished with bactericidal solutions or, preferably, a bactericidal gas technique; autoclaving should not be used because it may damage the plastic materials contained in the catheter and needle sheath. A local anesthetic (procaine or lidocaine) is used to infiltrate the skin before the large-bore needle used to introduce the catheter is inserted into the vein.

As the catheter is inserted, advanced into the heart, and positioned, the ECG must be monitored continuously and with great care to detect any premature ventricular beats occurring during these steps. This is accomplished with standard cardiac monitoring equipment (when the catheter is placed by fluoroscopy) or with an ECG machine (when placement is guided by an intracavitary electrode).

TABLE 15–2. NURSING CARE FOLLOWING INSERTION OF A TEMPORARY PACEMAKER

Check pacemaker function
  Note rate, output, and sensing
  Obtain ECG strip
  Assess patient's response to pacing
Apply occlusive dressing over catheter insertion site;
  keep dry at all times
Obtain chest X-ray to assess proper position of pacemaker
Restrict patient mobility at catheter insertion site
Administer pain medication as needed

After the physician has placed the catheter in a proper position, and effective capture of the heartbeat has been achieved, the catheter must be secured to the skin. This may be accomplished by placing a suture around the catheter and through the skin, taping the catheter to the skin with or by adhesive tape. An antibiotic ointment (neomycin or bacitracin) is then applied to the skin entry site of the catheter, and a dry dressing firmly affixed.

Nursing Care Following Pacemaker Insertion

During the course of cardiac pacing, the major responsibility of the nurse is to verify that the pacemaker system is functioning properly and effectively (Table 15–2). As noted, several problems may arise during temporary pacing, and careful observation of the patient and the monitor is essential to detect these disturbances as soon as they occur.

Loss of Capture. Should loss of capture occur, the nurse should alter the patient's position to see if this will move the electrode back into contact with the endocardium. If this simple intervention does not work, the nurse should notify the physician immediately. Depending on the underlying arrhythmia for which pacing is being used, loss of capture can have serious consequences. The failure of the pacemaker during complete heart block, for example, can result in ventricular asystole (Figure 15–13).

Absence of Pacing Artifacts. A second situation demanding emergency action is the sudden disap-

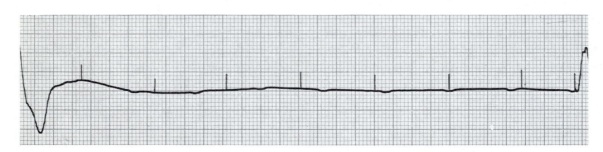

Figure 15–13. The patient had complete heart block. When the pacemaker failed to capture, ventricular asystole occurred.

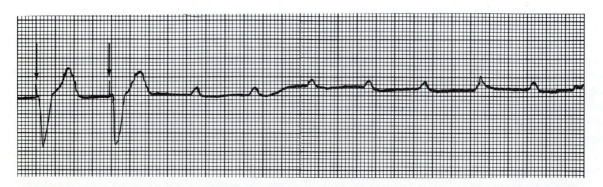

Figure 15–14. The pacing artifact (shown by arrows) suddenly disappeared when the catheter terminal became disconnected from the pulse generator.

pearance of pacing artifacts from the ECG (Figure 15–14). In many instances the nurse can promptly identify and correct the cause of this crisis. The first step in solving the problem is to make certain the catheter terminals have not become disconnected from the pacemaker device. If these connections are found to be secure, the next thing to do is to ascertain that the pacemaker battery is generating an adequate stimulus. If there is no movement of the pulse indicator, the pacemaker batteries may be exhausted and a different pacemaker should be attached. (To prevent the catastrophe of battery failure, a careful record should be kept of the number of hours each pacemaker is actually used, and batteries should be changed at the first sign of their weakening.) If pacemaker malfunction cannot be corrected instantly and the patient is in asystole, CPR should be initiated without delay.

Competition. Of less importance than loss of capture or pacemaker failure is the development of competition between the patient's paced and natural cardiac rhythms. Competition during demand pacing suggests difficulty with the sensing system of the pacemaker unit. The physician should be notified immediately of any evidence of competition.

Perforation of the Ventricle. A sudden loss of capture should lead to suspicion that the catheter tip may have perforated the right ventricle. However, this finding is not diagnostic of perforation, since loss of capture is most often the result of simple displacement of the catheter tip within the ventricular cavity. A more important indication of perforation are contractions of the diaphragm or muscles of the chest wall occurring synchronously with pacing impulses. This complication should be reported to the physician immediately and the pacemaker repositioned.

Thrombophlebitis and Skin Infection. The nurse should carefully examine the catheter-insertion site for signs of local infection. Dressings should be kept clean and dry and changed according to the protocol of the CCU. In changing the insertion-site dressing, care must be taken not to move the catheter. In addition to skin infections, signs of thrombophlebitis (redness and tenderness) should be sought, particularly when the catheter has been introduced through an arm vein or has been in place for more than three days.

PERMANENT CARDIAC PACING

The indications for permanent pacemaker implantation are summarized in Table 15–3. In some cases the indications are clear. For example, if the patient has complete heart block accompanied by symptoms and a ventricular

TABLE 15–3. INDICATIONS FOR PERMANENT PACING IN ACQUIRED ATRIOVENTRICULAR BLOCK IN ADULTS[a]

Class I: General Agreement That a Permanent Pacemaker Is Indicated.

A. Complete heart block, permanent or intermittent, with any of the following:
   1. Symptomatic bradycardia.
   2. Congestive heart failure.
   3. Ectopic rhythms and other conditions requiring drugs that suppress the automaticity of escape pacemakers and result in symptomatic bradycardia.
   4. Documented periods of asystole >3 seconds or any escape rate < 40 beats/minute in symptom-free patients.
   5. Mental confusion that clears with temporary pacing.
   6. Post-AV-junctional ablation, myotonic dystrophy.
B. Second-degree AV block, permanent or intermittent, with symptomatic bradycardia.
C. AF, atrial flutter, or supraventricular tachycardia with complete heart block or advanced AV block; bradycardia; and any of the conditions described under class I part A, above. The bradycardia must be unrelated to digitalis or drugs known to impair AV conduction.

Class II: Divergence of Opinion about the Need for a Permanent Pacemaker.

A. Asymptomatic complete heart block, permanent or intermittent, at any anatomic site, with ventricular rates >40 beats/minute.
B. Asymptomatic Mobitz Type II AV block.
C. Asymptomatic Mobitz Type I AV block at intra-His or infra-His levels.

Class III: Permanent Pacemaker Not Needed.

A. First-degree AV block.
B. Asymptomatic Type I AV block above the His-bundle (AV-node) level.

---

[a]American College of Cardiology/American Heart Association Guidelines for Implantation of Cardiac Pacemakers and Antiarrhythmia Devices
(Reprinted with permission from Dreifus LS, Fisch C, Griffin JC, et al. Special report: Guidelines for implantation of cardiac pacemakers and antiarrhythmia devices. *J Am Coll Cardiol.* 1991; 18:1–13).

rate of less than 40/minute, the patient should receive a permanent pacemaker. However, if the complete heart block is intermittent, the patient is asymptomatic, and the ventricular rate never falls below 40/minute, the indications for a pacemaker are not as convincing.

Types of Permanent Cardiac Pacemakers

The past two decades has seen an explosion of pacemaker capabilities. Initially all permanent pacemakers carried a single electrode that was placed in the

TABLE 15–4. PACEMAKER CODES

Chamber(s) Paced	Chamber(s) Sensed	Mode of Response	Programmable Functions[a]	Tachyarrhythmia Functions
A-atrium	A-atrium	I-inhibited	P-programmable	B-bursts
V-ventricle	V-ventricle	T-triggered	M-multiprogrammable	N-normal rate competition
D-dual	D-dual	D-dual[b]	C-multiprogrammable with telemetry	S-scanning
S-single chamber[c]	O-none	O-none	O-none	E-external
	S-single chamber	R-reverse		

[a]Programmable = rate and/or output.
[b]Atrially triggered, ventricularly inhibited.
[c]Single chamber = may be used for atrial or ventricular pacing.

right ventricle and provided an electrical stimulus in a fixed manner, as previously described. Over the years, pacemakers were developed to provide more physiologically appropriate support (eg, pacing of both the atrium and the ventricle in order to enhance cardiac output through a dual-chamber system) and to reduce potential complications.

When possible, the type of pacemaker chosen is one that will preserve *AV synchrony*. AV synchrony means that each ventricular contraction is preceded by an appropriately timed atrial contraction. Atrial synchrony has several advantages. First, atrial systole increases ventricular filling. This increase results in a cardiac output that is 20% to 30% greater than when atrial systole does not precede ventricular systole. Second, the atria empty more completely when they are synchronized to contract prior to ventricular contraction. This decreases atrial pressure and leads to an increased venous return to the atria.

Some pacemakers are also rate responsive. The pulse generator of these instruments is programmed to respond to changing physiologic demands (eg, as reflected by sinus rate, respiratory rate, or central venous temperature). Rate-responsive pacemakers allow for increases in heart rate during exercise and are often considered for the younger patient. A rate-modulated pulse generator with multiprogrammable capability has numerous physiologic advantages, but it is also complex and costly.

Pacemakers are usually described by three- or five-letter codes developed by the Inter-society Commission on Heart Disease. In both systems the first three letters refer to the chambers paced, the chambers sensed, and the mode of response of the pacemaker. In the five-letter-code system, the fourth and fifth letters refer to the programmable functions and special tachyarrhythmia functions of the pacemaker. The five-position pacemaker code is described in Table 15–4.

Although the various letter codes can appear confusing, they describe exactly which chamber of the heart a pacemaker is acting upon and in what manner. For example, an AAI pacemaker paces in the right atrium, senses in the right atrium, and works by inhibiting the pacing impulse if it senses an intrinsic electrical impulse occurring in the heart. This type of pacemaker is used in symptomatic SA-node dysfunction when the AV conduction system is intact. It cannot be used in patients with AV block, atrial fibrillation (AF), or atrial flutter.

In contrast, a DVI pacemaker paces both the

TABLE 15–5. CLINICAL CONDITIONS APPROPRIATE AND INAPPROPRIATE FOR VARIOUS PACEMAKER TYPES

Pacemaker Mode	Appropriate Clinical Condition	Contraindications
AAI	Symptomatic SA node dysfunction	AV block; atrial fibrillation/flutter; asystole
VVI	Symptomatic bradycardia	Heart failure; need for rate responsiveness
VDD	AV block with appropriate atrial rate and need for AV synchrony	Frequent SVT, atrial fibrillation/flutter
DVI	Symptomatic atrial bradycardia and need for AV synchrony	Frequent SVT, atrial fibrillation/flutter
DDD	Need for AV synchrony	Frequent SVT, atrial fibrillation/flutter

SVT = Supraventricular tachycardia.

atrium and the ventricle, but only senses impulses originating in the ventricle. It is inhibited by electrical impulses in the right ventricle. The DVI pacemaker is used in patients with symptomatic atrial bradycardia who need physiologic pacing (ie, atrial contraction that contributes to the cardiac output). It is inappropriate in cases of AF or atrial flutter. Examples of various clinical conditions and the type of pacemaker indicated for each are presented in Table 15–5.

Procedure of Permanent Pacemaker Implantation

Preparation. In preparing the patient and family for use of a permanent cardiac pacemaker, the nurse should carefully explain the purpose of the pacemaker, its size, and the area of the body in which it will be located. The patient and family should be told that the patient will be carefully monitored throughout the pacemaker implantation procedure. Most implants are performed without general anesthesia, but the patient is kept sedated throughout the procedure and a local anesthetic is used at the site of pacemaker implantation.

Permanent pacemakers are implanted outside the CCU in a room that provides fluoroscopy and sterile technique, since a surgical incision is required. Cardiologists often prefer the cardiac catheterization laboratory or procedure room as sites for implanting a pacemaker, while cardiac surgeons may use the operating room.

Insertion. In general, the procedure for insertion of a permanent pacemaker is similar to that for temporary transvenous pacemakers. The pacing lead is inserted through the right or left subclavian or jugular vein and positioned in the appropriate cardiac chamber. For a dual-chamber system, both leads can often be inserted in the same vein, using either the same or different puncture sites. Atrial leads are most commonly placed in the right atrial appendage or on the atrial wall. Ventricular leads are positioned in the apex of the right ventricle.

Besides preparation of the site of catheter insertion, the site of the surgical incision made for implantation of the pulse generator is also prepared. When endocardial leads are used, the pulse generator is placed in a subcutaneous pocket below the clavicle.

TABLE 15–6. TOPICS OF PATIENT AND FAMILY EDUCATION FOR PERMANENT PACEMAKER INSERTION

Purpose and function of pacemaker
Description of pacemaker
Checking for pulse rate and rhythm
Signs and symptoms of pacemaker failure (dizziness, weakness, lightheadness)
Recommended activity at home
Follow-up

In the rare case in which epicardial leads are used, the pulse generator is placed in a subcutaneous pocket of the abdominal wall. A small thoracotomy or subxiphoid incision is required for this.

The patient's oxygenation status should be monitored with a pulse oximeter throughout the procedure. Cardiac rhythm and rate, as well as blood pressure, should also be monitored. The pulse generator is programmed to the desired mode at the time of its insertion or soon thereafter.

Nursing Care Following Pacemaker Implantation

Patients are usually kept on bedrest for 24 hours after pacemaker implantation in order to prevent dislodgement of the pacemaker leads. Continuous cardiac monitoring is necessary to ensure appropriate sensing and capture. Antibiotics are usually continued for 24 hours after the procedure to prevent infection.

During this brief time in the unit, patients and their families need to be taught about the pacemaker and follow-up care (see Table 15–6). Because patients may be unable to attend to the information given them, it is critical that families be included in all education efforts, that the information be repeated, and that written materials be provided to supplement the information provided verbally. The patient and family should particularly be told about how to identify complications and what to do should symptoms develop. The patient should not be discharged from the hospital without an appointment for follow-up care.

Chapter 16

Treatment of Life-threatening Arrhythmias: Implantable Defibrillators, Radiofrequency Ablation, and Precordial Shock

Treatment of life-threatening arrhythmias has evolved over the past decade to include more than antiarrhythmic drugs and CPR. Defibrillators can be implanted inside the patient's chest to treat ventricular fibrillation (VF) as soon as it occurs, so that the patient does not have to wait for a house visit by the emergency medical service and subsequent hospitalization. Radiofrequency ablation is used to eliminate cardiac tissue responsible for abnormal myocardial conduction. In this procedure the cardiologist cauterizes abnormal areas of the myocardium that are responsible for reentrant rhythms or which serve as ectopic foci for ventricular tachycardia. The emphasis in the treatment of life-threatening arrhythmias is on their prevention, and in the unfortunate instance in which they do occur on treating them without delay.

Electrophysiologic Studies

In some cases arrhythmias cannot be identified by electrocardiography alone. Even 24-hour monitoring (Holter monitoring) or electrocardiographic monitoring during exercise (stress testing) may be insufficient to identify the nature of an arrhythmia.

An electrophysiologic study (EPS) can be performed to identify the causative electrical-conduction-system abnormality and nature of an arrhythmia. The procedure is similar to cardiac catheterization in that catheters are positioned in the right side of the heart under fluoroscopic guidance. The catheters are used to obtain intracardiac electrical recordings that provide a definitive picture of the way in which the cardiac electrical impulse is conducted in the heart. The adequacy of the sinoatrial (SA) and atrioventricular (AV) nodes, as well as the His bundle, can be evaluated and the mechanisms of supraventricular or ventricular arrhythmias can be identified.

Cardiac arrhythmias can be provoked in an electrophysiologic study. This is done by using the intracardiac catheters to deliver pacing stimuli at specific intervals in the cardiac cycle. Known as *programmed electrical stimulation,* this technique allows the electrophysiologist to identify accessory pathways and abnormal activation sequences responsible for reentrant rhythms. An arrhythmia that is induced by electrical stimulation, is sustained for more than 30 seconds, and results in altered hemodynamics, the rhythm is called an *inducible arrhythmia.* The majority of inducible arrhythmias are related to a reentry mechanism, while an arrhythmia that cannot be induced is usually related to enhanced automaticity.

Programmed electrical stimulation can be quite helpful in identifying the nature of a patient's arrhythmia and suggesting the prognosis. However, it is not infallible, and its results must be viewed in the context of the patient's clinical history and disease.

AUTOMATIC IMPLANTABLE CARDIOVERTER DEFIBRILLATORS

Automatic implantable cardioverter defibrillators (AICDs) were introduced in 1985. Their use has reduced dramatically the number of deaths caused by tachyarrhythmias. Patients with a history of cardiac arrest from ventricular tachyarrhythmias who are treated with medications have an annual mortality rate of approximately 40%; similar patients treated with an AICD have an annual mortality of less than 5%.

Patients with two types of clinical history are appropriate candidates for an AICD: (1) patients who have survived a cardiac arrest not associated with acute myocardial infarction (AMI); and (2) patients who have not experienced a cardiac arrest despite conventional drug therapy, but who have recurrent tachyarrhythmias that can be induced in the electrophysiology laboratory and which result in hypotensive ventricular tachycardia (VT) or VF.

The AICD consists of a generator implanted in a pocket in the abdominal wall that is connected to patches and sensing electrodes attached to the heart (an example is provided in Figure 16–1). The first- and second-generation implantable cardioverter defibrillators monitor cardiac activity and treat tachyarrhythmias with cardioversion or defibrillation. The shocks are delivered through electrodes implanted surgically in the endocardium or epicardium.

Most AICD units sense both the heart rate and the shape of the electrocardiographic tracing (the period during which the complex remains on the isoelectric line). This latter function is called the *probability density function* or PDF. When the electrocar-diographic complex remains off the isoelectric line for more than 50 percent of the time or the heart rate exceeds the preset rate cutoff of the device, the AICD automatically defibrillates the heart. Newer units use both criteria to identify a tachyarrhythmia. If the arrhythmia does not convert with the initial shock, four or five countershocks are delivered sequentially. An example of a sequence of four shocks given over a 2-minute period is provided in Figure 16–2.

AICD units have the ability to program in the PDF and heart-rate modes for an individual patient. Third-generation units can provide multiple or tiered regulation, including antitachycardia pacing (fast or overdrive pacing); single-chamber, ventricular demand pacing for bradycardia; and the provision of cardioversion or defibrillation shocks.

Patient preparation

Patients and their families require the same type of preparation for use of an AICD as is needed for use of a pacemaker, but also require education to prepare the patient for general surgery. Surgical placement sites for the device must be described and exercises for deep breathing and coughing reviewed. Pamphlets and booklets from the device manufacturer, as well as videotapes, can be used to facilitate learning. On the night before surgery, patients are kept off oral intake and usually receive prophylactic antibiotics. The procedure should be discussed fully with the patient, along with its risks and benefits, and an operative consent form signed.

Implantation

Implantation of an AICD can be accomplished either with a thoracotomy incision or through a transvenous technique. A median sternotomy, left lateral thoracotomy, subxiphoid, or subcostal approach may be used in a thoracotomy implantation. Historically, the lead systems of AICDs once consisted of a combination of a spring lead or epicardial patch(es) for defibrillation and two screw-in leads for sensing. Current systems use a combination of transvenous or epicardial leads for rate sensing and defibrillation. Originally, leads were placed on the heart during open-chest surgical procedures. Today, bipolar and tripolar leads or subcutaneous patches are used to achieve rate sensing, antitachycardia pacing, and defibrillation. The lead wires are connected to the generator, which is implanted in the abdominal-wall pocket (Figure 16–3).

Postoperative Care

Postoperative care of the patient who has received an AICD depends on the surgical approach used to implant the AICD. A transvenous approach results in

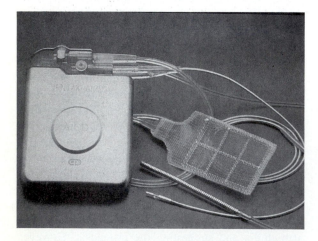

Figure 16–1. Implantable cardioverter-defibrillator with sensing electrodes and defibrillation patches.

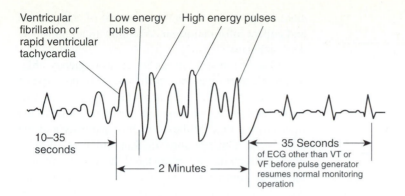

Ventricular fibrillation or rapid ventricular tachycardia

Low energy pulse

High energy pulses

10–35 seconds

35 Seconds of ECG other than VT or VF before pulse generator resumes normal monitoring operation

2 Minutes

Figure 16–2. Diagram of shock sequence in a case of VF or rapid VT. (Courtesy of Cardiac Pacemakers, Inc., St. Paul, Minn.)

minimal discomfort, while a thoracotomy or sternotomy approach requires postoperative care similar to that required with other thoracic surgical procedures. In the latter case, patients may have chest tubes for a day or two. Nursing care is focused on preventing pulmonary complications (by deep breathing and coughing, as well as the use of incentive spirometry), deconditioning (by early ambulation), and infection (by careful wound care).

Vital signs are monitored routinely. The nurse

should also be aware of the type of device implanted and the therapies required if VT or VF occur (eg, antitachycardia pacing, low- or high-energy shocks, and backup VVI pacing). The nurse should know whether the AICD has been activated postoperatively, and how to proceed if the patient receives a shock inappropriately.

Patients and family members need to be very carefully prepared for discharge. Having an implanted defibrillator can be extremely frightening for both patients and their families. Patients may become highly anxious at the thought of having another cardiac arrest or of receiving shocks from their device. Providing emotional support, correcting misinformation, and anticipating concerns and questions are all powerful interventions in this setting.

Patients who have an AICD need to carry the following information with them at all times: the model name and model number of the AICD, the telephone number of their follow-up care site, the tachycardia rate detection level of the instrument, and (in the case of AICDs with pacing capability) the pacing cutoff rate for bradycardia. Patients must also understand the potentially dangerous role of magnets in deactivating their device. Most AICD manufacturers provide a list of sources of electromagnetic interference with their devices (eg, large stereophonic speakers, wands used in playing bingo, industrial transformers, and magnetic resonance imaging machines).

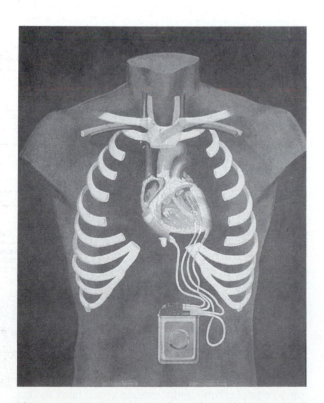

Figure 16–3. Diagram of implanted automated cardioverter-defibrillator device and lead placement. (Courtesy of Cardiac Pacemakers, Inc., St. Paul, Minn.)

RADIOFREQUENCY ABLATION

Radiofrequency ablation of ectopically conducting cardiac tissue was introduced in 1987. It is used to treat various arrhythmias and conduction problems that are unresponsive to drug therapy (Table 16–1), and is usually done in a procedure laboratory at the time of electrophysiologic study.

Radiofrequency ablation involves delivering elec-

TABLE 16–1. CLINICAL INDICATIONS FOR RADIOFREQUENCY ABLATION

Wolff-Parkinson-White syndrome
AV-nodal reentry tachycardia
Sinus node reentry tachycardia
Atrial fibrillation or flutter with a rapid ventricular response
Ectopic atrial tachycardia
Idiopathic ventricular tachycardia

trical current directly to the endocardium by way of a catheter. A low-voltage, high-frequency alternating current is sent through the catheter tip, cauterizing the abnormal conduction tissue directly beneath the tip. The patient does not feel the current because the frequencies used for ablation are so low that they do not cause muscle or nerve stimulation.

The ablation procedure usually involves the introduction of four catheters under fluoroscopic guidance. Three catheters are inserted from the femoral vein into the right atrium, His-bundle region, and right ventricle. A fourth catheter is inserted into the coronary sinus from the internal jugular or subclavian vein. If the electrophysiologist needs to place a catheter in the left side of the heart, the femoral artery is cannulated. Each ablation catheter has multiple electrodes that help identify the site of the arrhythmia.

Once the site of the arrhythmia is localized by endocardial mapping, current is sent through the ablation catheter to the causative tissue. The lesions produced by the current are small, usually only several millimeters long. The patient is observed for a short waiting period, after which the electrophysiologist once again tries to induce the patient's arrhythmia. If the offending arrhythmia occurs, more lesions are created until the arrhythmia can no longer be induced. The procedure usually lasts from 2 to 4 hours, but can last as long as 10 hours (although fluoroscopy time is kept to approximately 1 hour to prevent complications from excessive irradiation of the patient. Electrocautery of ectopically conducting endocardial tissue is highly effective in eradicating arrhythmias, with a success rate of approximately 95%.

During the ablation procedure the patient receives several medications. Anesthesia is not required, but patients are usually given a sedative to help them sleep during the procedure, since they have to lie still without moving throughout much of it. Intravenous midazolam (Versed) and meperidine can be used in combination for this purpose. Midazolam is particularly effective because of its amnesic effect. Local anesthesia is used at the site of catheterization. Heparin is given for anticoagulation. Finally, various medications (particularly isoproterenol and adeno-

sine) are given to prove the existence of arrhythmias and collect information on AV conduction and accessory pathways.

One of the indications for radiofrequency ablation is AV-nodal reentrant tachycardia. In this type of conduction disorder the patient has two pathways of conduction in the AV node and perinodal tissue of the right atrium. One of these is a fast pathway and the other slow. During sinus rhythm, impulses usually travel through the fast pathway. If, however, a premature atrial contraction finds the fast conduction pathway already depolarized, it will use the slow pathway. In the early days of radiofrequency ablation, physicians would interrupt the fast pathway, which would frequently eventuate in a complete heart block requiring a permanent pacemaker. Experience has taught that ablation of the slow pathway in cases of AV-nodal reentrant tachycardia does not create this complication.

The care of the patient following radiofrequency ablation is similar to that of the patient following coronary angiography or catheterization. Patients are immobilized, with the leg having the femoral artery access site extended. The nurse should observe the patient for bleeding from the catheter-access sites, hematoma, impaired perfusion distal to the access sites, and cardiac tamponade. Patients who have had an arterial cannulation will receive subcutaneous heparin on the evening of the day of the procedure. Patients are discharged while taking low-dose warfarin or aspirin and asked to take it for 1 month.

PRECORDIAL SHOCK

Precordial shock is used either as a lifesaving emergency method for terminating VF (defibrillation) or as an elective procedure to convert certain atrial and ventricular tachyarrhythmias to normal sinus rhythm (cardioversion). The principle of precordial shock in treating VF is straightforward: a high-voltage shock of very brief duration (only a few thousandths of a second), delivered through the chest wall, is capable of abruptly stopping the chaotic electrical activity within the heart that produced the lethal arrhythmia. Once the bizarre fibrillatory rhythm has been terminated in this way, the heart's natural pacemaker regains command and an effective beat is reestablished. This same principle is utilized in elective cardioversion, in which brief depolarization of the entire heart (at a particular time in the cardiac cycle) halts the activity of an ectopic pacemaker and allows the SA node to regain control of the heart rate.

While enormous electrical energy is required to defibrillate the heart through the chest wall, this electrical force is of such short duration that the resulting current does not injure the myocardium. The most important determinant of survival in cardiac arrest is the time that elapses between the onset of the arrhythmia and defibrillation. Therefore, time is of the essence in saving the patient's life. All efforts should be directed toward identifying the arrhythmia and, in the case of VF, giving precordial shock immediately.

Equipment for Precordial Shock

A direct-current (DC) defibrillator builds and stores thousands of volts in a capacitor within seconds, and discharges this energy on demand in less than 5 milliseconds. The stored energy is delivered to the heart through a circuit consisting of two electrodes (or paddles, as they are commonly called) which are held against the chest wall. The paddles are of large diameter (usually 3–4 inches), allowing the electrical discharge to pass through a wide area of skin and thereby preventing electrical burns. To facilitate passage of the current through the skin, a thick layer of conductive paste is applied to the skin and electrode surfaces before the energy stored in the defibrillator is discharged. The handles of the defibrillator paddles are insulated to protect the operator from leakage of current, and the operator should stand away from the bed to avoid being shocked by the electrical current delivered to the patient.

The amount of current delivered to the heart is affected by transthoracic impedance (measured in ohms, with normal impedance being 70 to 80 ohms) or resistance to current flow. The size of the electrodes, the material used to couple the electrodes to the chest wall, the distance between the electrodes and the heart (chest configuration and size), the pressure exerted on the electrodes, and the number and time interval of previous shocks all determine the degree of transthoracic impedance. If transthoracic impedance is high, a low-energy shock may fail to generate enough current to achieve defibrillation. Therefore, the nurse should always press firmly on the defibrillator paddles when delivering a precordial shock, and should use a conductive paste between the paddles and the chest wall. Saline-soaked gauze pads can also be used to ensure good conduction.

The electrical energy used for precordial shock is discharged by pressing a button switch incorporated in the handles of the defibrillator electrodes. The amount of current delivered by the defibrillator can be adjusted according to need by setting a dial on the machine. This electrical force is measured in watt-seconds (w/s) or joules (J); the scale of the force ranges from 1 to 400 J with conventional equipment.

Synchronized and Nonsynchronized Precordial Shock

When precordial shock is used electively to convert atrial and ventricular tachyarrhythmias to sinus rhythm (cardioversion), it is important that the electrical discharge be synchronized with the cardiac cycle. This is necessary because of the potential danger of inducing VF when any electrical impulse, even a premature ventricular contraction (PVC), strikes during the vulnerable period of the cardiac cycle (ie, during the time of the T wave). The same threat may exist if a precordial shock (or a pacemaker impulse) arrives during the critical interval of the vulnerable period. To avoid this hazard, precordial shock is deliberately synchronized so that the electrical force is delivered at a point during the cardiac cycle at which the heart is refractory to stimulation; this nonvulnerable (refractory) period corresponds to the time of the QRS complex.

The equipment for precordial shock is so designed that the discharge energy can be synchronized with the safe (refractory) period of the cardiac cycle. When the synchronizer switch is on and the discharge button is triggered, the instrument waits until the next R wave before delivering its energy. If on the other hand the synchronizer is off, discharge occurs the instant the machine is triggered, without reference to the cardiac cycle.

It is essential to understand clearly just when a precordial shock should or should not be synchronized with the cardiac cycle. *In terminating VF with precordial shock (defibrillation), the synchronizer switch must be in the off position.* If the synchronizer switch is on in this circumstance, the machine *will not fire,* because it waits for a QRS complex, which is nonexistent during VF. In the case of VT, synchronization may be difficult and the switch should be turned off.

Conversely, when precordial shock is employed *electively* to convert other arrhythmias (eg, atrial fibrillation [AF]), the synchronizer must be *turned on* in order to avoid the possibility of the discharge striking during the vulnerable period and inducing VF. Synchronization is recommended for supraventricular tachycardia, AF, and atrial flutter.

Asystole does not benefit from defibrillation or cardioversion. When asystole is seen, an alternate lead should be checked to make sure that the pattern is not a fine ventricular fibrillation.

Automated External Defibrillators

Automated external defibrillators have been developed in an attempt to increase the likelihood of defibrillating patients outside the hospital. Although most hospitals continue to use conventional defibrillators, automated external defibrillators will be described here, since patients with these devices may arrive at the hospital, and all Advanced Cardiac Life Support (ACLS) providers have instruction in their operation and use.

The automated external defibrillator incorporates a cardiac-rhythm-analysis system that senses and records the patient's heart rhythm. The defibrillator may be programmed to an automated or a semiautomated mode. In the automated mode the unit need only be turned on. If it senses VF it will deliver a shock through two adhesive pads applied to the patient in the same positions as the paddles used for conventional defibrillation. In the semiautomated or shock-advisory mode, the operator initiates the shock when the machine analyses the cardiac rhythm and sends a message that a shock is indicated. Most automated external defibrillators have a capacity for manual override, should it prove necessary.

Energy of Discharge

As indicated, the level of discharge energy is adjustable in all defibrillators and must be set for the particular arrhythmia being treated. The authors of the 1992 Guidelines for Cardiopulmonary Resuscitation and Emergency Cardiac Care (American Heart Association) recommend that the first defibrillation attempt be at 200 J, and that the second shock be given at an energy of 200 to 300 J. If the first two shocks fail to defibrillate, a third shock of 360 J should be delivered immediately. If defibrillation is initially successful but the patient's rhythm again degenerates into VF, shocks should be repeated at the same level that previously converted the arrhythmia. If the first three shocks fail to defibrillate the patient, CPR should be continued, epinephrine should be given in a dose of 1 mg intravenously, ventilation should be established, and the shocks should again be repeated.

Little relationship appears to exist between body size and the energy requirements for precordial shock. Consequently, larger than normal amounts of energy (ie, over 360 J) are generally not more effective in defibrillating patients with a large body mass.

In the case of elective cardioversion, the precise energy setting for defibrillation varies with the type of arrhythmia. Certain arrhythmias are more responsive to precordial shock than others, and require less energy for conversion. Atrial flutter and supraventricular tachycardia, for example, can generally be terminated with minimal electrical force (50 J), while AF is often more resistant and demands a higher energy setting (100 J). The energy required to convert VT depends on the morphologic characteristics and rate of the arrhythmia. VT that is regular in form and rate responds to cardioversion at energies beginning at 100 J. VT that is irregular in rate and rhythm responds like VF, and the initial setting should be at 200 J.

Technique of Elective Cardioversion and the Nursing Role

Preparation for Procedure

The physician must explain the procedure for elective cardioversion to the patient and family members, and obtain written informed consent for it. If the patient is taking digitalis, the dosage should be reviewed and a blood specimen drawn for assay of the serum digitalis level. Digitalis may provoke ventricular arrhythmias, although patients can be safely cardioverted with digoxin levels of 0.8 to 2.0 ng/mL. All necessary equipment and materials for cardioversion should be at the bedside: the cardioverter, syringes, antiarrhythmic drugs (including 100 mg lidocaine), anesthetic agents, and a code cart. The nurse should start an intravenous drip if one is not already running. The drip is used to administer the anesthetic agent and any antiarrhythmic drugs that may be necessary. The nurse should attach an oxygen saturation monitor (pulse oximeter) and noninvasive sphygmomanometer to the patient.

Setting the Defibrillator for Cardioversion

For elective cardioversion, the synchronizer switch of the defibrillator is turned on, so that the discharge of energy will coincide with the R wave of the cardiac cycle. Because synchronization cannot be achieved unless the patient's ventricular complexes are of sufficient amplitude to trigger the discharge, the "gain" dial may have to be adjusted to obtain R waves of adequate amplitude (as evidenced by a flashing light or other signal). If complexes of sufficient amplitude cannot be obtained by increasing the gain, a different lead must be used to obtain taller waves (eg, by changing the lead position from lead II to lead I).

For safety it is wise to verify that proper synchronization will occur when the defibrillator is discharged. This is accomplished by a test mechanism within the defibrillator that indicates where the discharge will fall in the cardiac cycle when the shock is actually delivered. The energy to be used for the cardioversion attempt is identified by the physician.

Anesthesia

Although precordial shock itself creates little pain because of the extremely short duration of the stimulus, the sensation (and the associated generalized muscle contraction) is nevertheless frightening and unpleasant for most patients. Because an analgesic effect is required for only a few seconds, very short-acting anesthetic agents are given intravenously just before the shock is delivered. Effective regimens include a sedative (eg, diazepam, midazolam, or a barbiturate) with or without an analgesic agent (fentanyl, morphine, or meperidine). In many hospitals someone from the anesthesia service is asked to attend a cardioversion.

Paddle Electrodes: Preparation and Placement

A thick layer of conducting gel is placed on the face of the defibrillator electrodes and distributed evenly.

Additional electrode paste is applied to the positions on the chest wall at which the paddles will be held.

Standard paddle placement consists of holding one paddle just to the right of the upper sternal area (below the clavicle) and the other to the left of the nipple, with the center of the electrode in the midaxillary line (Figure 16–4). An alternative position involves holding one paddle anteriorly on the left precordium and the other (a special flat paddle) under the heart posteriorly, in the right infrascapular position. The precise location of the paddles is not critical as long as the flow of current traverses the heart. The flow of current must pass directly through the heart.

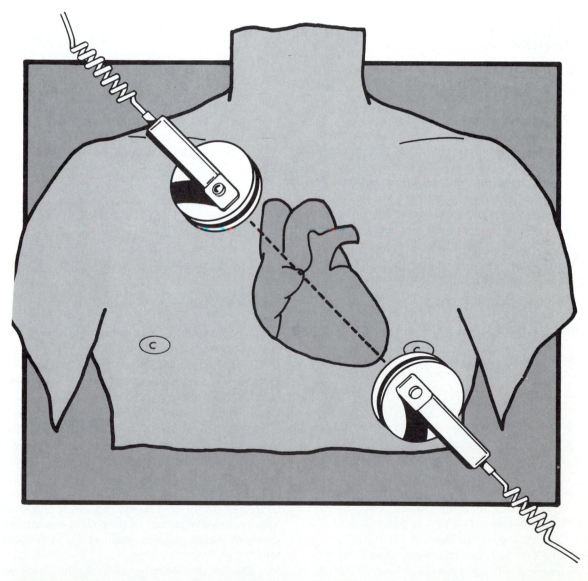

Figure 16–4. Placement of paddles for defibrillation. One paddle is in the right sternal area and the other on the left lateral chest wall.

Self-adhesive electrode pads can also be used effectively in these same locations.

Before the energy for defibrillation is discharged, it is important to ascertain that the conducting paste remains localized at the electrode sites and has not spread over the chest wall. Excess jelly should be wiped away before proceeding, or the current will flow across the skin surface (rather than through the heart).

The paddles must be pressed firmly and evenly against the chest wall; failure to preserve good contact results in dissipation of energy. Furthermore, tilting of the paddles may cause skin burns. Since there is a theoretical threat that the electrical force being delivered to the patient could pass through the bed and reach the operator or others, it is wise to have all personnel stand clear of the bed at the moment of discharge.

Cardioversion

When the discharge switch of the defibrillator is pressed, the effect is immediately evident from a sudden, generalized contraction of the patient's muscles. Observation of the cardiac monitor will confirm whether normal sinus rhythm has been restored. In some instances PVCs occur following cardioversion, and in such cases lidocaine 100 mg should be administered promptly to combat cardiac irritability. In the extremely unlikely event that the cardioversion attempt causes VF, the synchronizer switch of the defibrillator must be turned off, the energy increased to 400 J, and a second shock delivered instantly to defibrillate the patient. Remember that defibrillation cannot be accomplished if the synchronizer is turned on!

Technique of Emergency Defibrillation

Although emergency defibrillation was described in the discussion of VF (Chapter 12), it is important to review this procedure with particular emphasis on the differences between defibrillation and elective cardioversion.

1. Defibrillation is a lifesaving technique, and in order to be successful must be accomplished within a minute or so after the onset of a lethal arrythmia. This means that precordial shock must always be the *initial step* in treating such an arrhythmia (within the setting of a CCU), and that no time should be wasted with other measures, such as the administration of oxygen or closed-chest massage. The first person reaching the bedside, whether a physician or a nurse, should proceed to defibrillate the patient at once.

2. The discharge energy should be set at 200 J for the first shock.

3. It is absolutely essential that the synchronizer switch of the defibrillator be in the *off* position for defibrillation, so that the discharge will occur the instant the trigger is pressed.

4. Conductive jelly is applied to the electrode surfaces, and the paddles are held firmly against the chest wall in the same manner described for elective cardioversion.

5. If for some reason defibrillation is unsuccessful, precordial shock should be repeated immediately. Three shocks are delivered in a row, one after the other, in a stacked sequence (200 J, 200–300 J, and 360 J, respectively). No delays for delivering medications or CPR should occur between the shocks. With some defibrillation equipment it is necessary to recharge the capacitor by pressing an appropriate button before a second discharge can be delivered.

6. In both defibrillation and cardioversion *it is important that no one touch the bed, patient, or ventilatory adjuncts (eg, endotracheal tube or ventilation bags) at the time a precordial shock is delivered,* in order to avoid their receiving an electric shock.

Postresuscitation Care

The immediate goals of postresuscitative care in patients requiring defibrillation are to optimize tissue perfusion, especially to the brain, and prevent the recurrence of cardiopulmonary arrest by instituting measures to address the cause of the arrest, such as antiarrhythmic therapy. The patient requires a careful cardiovascular, pulmonary, and neurologic assessment. A urinary catheter should be inserted if the patient is comatose, and a nasogastric tube should be emplaced if bowel sounds are absent. A careful evaluation should also be done for complications of CPR, specifically rib fracture, pericardial tamponade, hemopneumothorax, and (if the patient was intubated during the arrest) misplacement of the endotracheal tube.

Emotional support is an important component of the care of patients who are alert and responsive following resuscitation from a cardiac arrest. A cardiac arrest can be extremely frightening for the patient, and many patients will recount disturbing memories surrounding it. CCU nurses and other staff members can be extremely helpful in alleviating patient's anxiety simply by listening to the patient's account of the experience and providing reassurance about the close monitoring that will be given in the CCU.

The best treatment for cardiac arrest, however, is its prevention.

References

Aberg A, Bergstrand R, Johansson S, et al. Declining trend in mortality after myocardial infarction. *British Heart Journal.* 1984;51:346–351.

Ades PA, Waldmann ML, McCann WJ, Weaver SO. Predictors of cardiac rehabilitation participation in older coronary patients. *Archives of Internal Medicine.* 1992;152:1033–1035.

Ahrens T. Changing perspectives in the assessment of oxygenation. *Critical Care Nurse.* 1993;78–83.

Akhtar M, Breithardt G, Camm AJ, Coumel P, et al. CAST and beyond: Implications of the cardiac arrhythmia suppression trial. *Circulation.* 1990;81:1123–1127.

American College of Cardiology/American Heart Association Task Force on Assessment of Diagnostic and Therapeutic Cardiovascular Procedures (Subcommittee to Assess Clinical Intracardiac Electrophysiologic Studies): Zipes DP, Akhtar M, Denes P, DeSanctis RW, et al. Heart Association Task Force Report. Guidelines for clinical intracardiac electrophysiologic studies. *Journal of the American College of Cardiology.* 1989;14:1827–1842.

American College of Cardiology/American Heart Association, Task Force on Assessment of Diagnostic and Therapeutic Cardiovascular Procedures, Subcommittee to Develop Guidelines for the Early Management of Patients with Acute Myocardial Infarction. Guidelines for the early management of patients with acute myocardial infarction. *Journal of the American College of Cardiology.* 1990;16:249–292.

Ausubel K, Furman S. The pacemaker syndrome. *Annals of Internal Medicine.* 1985;103:420–429.

Balke CW, Gold MR, Department of Medicine, Division of Cardiology, University of Maryland Hospital, Baltimore. Excitation–contraction–relaxation coupling in the normal and failing heart. *Heart Disease and Stroke.* 1993;2:150–155.

Barbiere CC, Liberatore K. Automated external defibrillators: An update of additions to the ACLS algorithms. *Critical Care Nurse.* 1992;June:17–20.

Barbiere CC, Liberatore K. From emergent transvenous pacemaker to permanent implant and follow-up. *Critical Care Nurse.* 1993;April:39–43.

Bays HE, Dujovne CA, Lansing AM. Drug treatment of dyslipidemias: Practical guidelines for the primary care physician. *Heart Disease and Stroke.* 1992;1:357–365.

Beta Blocker Heart Attack Trial. A randomized trial of propranolol in patients with acute myocardial infarction. I. Mortality results. *Journal of the American Medical Association.* 1982;147:1707–1714.

Bigger T, Multicenter Post-Infarction Research Group. The relationship among ventricular arrhythmias, left ventricular dysfunction, and mortality in the two years after myocardial infarction. *Circulation.* 1984;69:250–258.

Bigger T, Weld F, Rolinitsky M. Prevalence, characteristics and significance of ventricular tachycardia (three or more complexes) detected with ambulatory electrocardiographic recordings in the late hospital phase of acute myocardial infarction. *American Journal of Cardiology.* 1981;48:815–823.

Birman H, Haq A, Hew E, Aberman A. Continuous monitoring of mixed venous oxygen saturation in hemodynamically unstable patients. *Chest.* 1984;86:753–756.

Black L, Coombs VJ, Townsend SN. Reperfusion and reperfusion injury in acute myocardial infarction. *Heart & Lung.* 1990;19:274–285.

Blazing MA, Morris JJ, Jr. Atrial fibrillation: Conventional wisdom reappraised. *Heart Disease and Stroke.* 1992;78–84.

Blumenthal JA, Bradley W, Dimsdale JE, Kasl SV, et al. Task force III: Assessment of psychological status in patients with ischemic heart disease. *Journal of the American College of Cardiology.* 1989;14:1034–1042.

Borggrefe M, Budde T, Podezeck A, Breithardt G. High frequency alternating current ablation of an accessory pathway in humans. *Journal of the American College of Cardiology.* 1987;10:576–582.

Borriello SL, Siegel SC, Fishman RF. Directional coronary atherectomy: A new treatment for coronary artery disease. *Heart & Lung.* 1994;23:199–204.

Brannon PH, Johnson R. The internal cardioverter defibrillator: Patient–family teaching. *Focus on Critical Care.* 1992;19:41–44.

Bremner SM, McCauley KM, Axtell KA. A follow-up study of patients with implantable cardioverter defibrillators. *Journal of Cardiovascular Nursing.* 1993;7:40–51.

Bridges EJ, Woods SL. Pulmonary artery pressure measurement: State of the art. *Heart & Lung.* 1993;22:99–111.

Bubien RS, Knotts SM, McLaughlin S, George P. What you need to know about radiofrequency ablation. *American Journal of Nursing.* 1993;30–37.

Butman SM, Ewy GA, Standen JR, Kern KB, Hahn E. Bedside cardiovascular examination in patients with severe chronic heart failure: Importance of rest or inducible jugular venous distension. *Journal of the American College of Cardiology.* 1993;22:968–974.

Byra-Cook CJ, Dracup KA, Lazik AJ. Direct and indirect blood pressure readings: A correlation in critical care patients. *Nursing Research.* 1990;39:285–288.

Cannom DS, Winkle RA. Implantation of the automatic implantable cardioverter defibrillator (AICD): Practical aspects. *PACE.* 1986;9:793–809.

Cason CL, Lambert CW, Holland CL, Huntman KT. Effect of backrest elevation and position on pulmonary artery pressures. *Cardiovascular Nursing.* 1990;26:1–5.

Castelli WP, Wilson PW, Levy D, Anderson K. Cardiovascular risk factors in the elderly. *American Journal of Cardiology.* 1989;63:12H–19H.

Caunt JE. The changing role of coronary care nurses. *Intensive and Critical Care Nursing.* 1992;8:82–93.

Cavender JB, Rogers WJ, Fisher LD, et al. Effects of smoking on survival and morbidity in patients randomized to medical or surgical therapy in the Coronary Artery Surgery Study (CASS): 10-year follow-up. *Journal of the American College of Cardiology.* 1992;20:287–294.

Chen JTT. Radiographic diagnosis of heart failure. *Heart Disease and Stroke.* 1992;58–63.

Chulay M, Miller T. The effect of backrest elevation on pulmonary artery and pulmonary capillary wedge pressures in patients after cardiac surgery. *Heart & Lung.* 1984;13:138–140.

Chung EK. *Principles of Cardiac Arrhythmia.* Baltimore: Williams & Wilkins; 1983.

Cohen S, Wills TA. Stress, social support, and the buffering hypothesis. *Psychological Bulletin.* 1985;98:310–357.

Cohn JN. Future directions in vasodilator therapy for heart failure. *American Heart Journal.* 1991;121:969–974.

Cohn JN. Prevention of heart failure. *Heart Disease and Stroke.* 1994;3:5–8.

Cole PL. Thrombolytic therapy: Then and now. *Heart & Lung.* 1991;20:542–551.

Collins MA. When your patient has an implantable cardioverter defibrillator. *American Journal of Nursing.* 1994;34–38.

Connor R. Coronary artery anatomy: The electrocardiographic and clinical correlations. *Critical Care Nurse.* 1983;3:68–73.

Copeland JG, Emery RW, Levinson MM, Copeland J, et al. The role of mechanical support and transplantation in treatment of patients with end stage cardiomyopathy. *Circulation.* 1985;72:7–12.

Cragg DR, Friedman HZ, Bonema JD, et al. Outcome of patients with acute myocardial infarction who are ineligible for thrombolytic therapy. *Annals of Internal Medicine.* 1991;115:173–177.

Craney JM. Radiofrequency catheter ablation of supraventricular tachycardias: Clinical consideration and nursing care. *Journal of Cardiovascular Nursing.* 1993;7:26–39.

Cuddy TE, Pfeffer MA. Indications and value of the use of captopril after myocardial infarction. *Heart Disease and Stroke.* 1993;2:393–396.

Culpepper-Richards K, Bairnsfather L. A description of night sleep patterns in the critical care unit. *Heart & Lung.* 1988;17:35–42.

Davidson T, VanRiper S, Harper P, Wenk A. Implantable cardioverter defibrillators: A guide for clinicians. *Heart & Lung.* 1994;23:205–215.

de Vreede JJM, Gorgels APM, Verstraaten GMP, et al. Did prognosis after acute myocardial infarction change during the past 30 years? A meta-analysis. *Journal of the American College of Cardiology.* 1991;18:698–706.

Divertie MB, McMichan JC. Continuous monitoring of mixed venous oxygen saturation. *Chest.* 1984;85:423–428.

Dorian P. Electrophysiology, pacing, and arrhythmia: The implantable defibrillator and antiarrhythmic drugs—competitive and complementary treatment for severe ventricular arrhythmia. *Clinical Cardiology.* 1993;16:827–830.

Dracup K. Are critical care units hazardous to health? *Applied Nursing Research.* 1988;1:14–21.

Dreifus LS, Hessen S, Samuels F. Recognition and management of supraventricular tachycardias. *Heart Disease and Stroke.* 1993;2:223–230.

Dreifus LS, Mitamura H, Rhauda A, Vail S, et al. Effects of AV sequential versus asynchronous AV pacing on pulmonary hemodynamics. *PACE.* 1986;9:171–177.

Dreifus LS, Zinberg A, Hurzeler P, Puziak AD, et al. Transtelephonic monitoring of 25,919 implanted pacemakers. *PACE.* 1986;9:371–378.

Drew BJ. Bedside electrocardiogram monitoring. *AACN, Clinical Issues in Critical Care.* 1993;4:25–33.

Drew BJ. Continuous bedside ECG monitoring: State of the art for the 1990s. *Heart & Lung.* 1991;20:610–623.

Drew BJ, Scheinman MM. Value of electrocardiographic leads MCL_1, MCL_6 and other selected leads in the diagnosis of wide QRS complex tachycardia. *Journal of the American College of Cardiology.* 1991;1025–1033.

Dunnington CS, Johnson NJ, Finkelmeier BA, Lyons J, Kehoe RF. Patients with heart rhythm disturbances: Variables associated with increased psychological distress. *Heart & Lung.* 1988;17:381–389.

Eaker ED, Packard B, Thom TJ. Epidemiology and risk factors for coronary heart disease in women. *Cardiovascular Clinics.* 1989;19:129–145.

East TD. Computers in the ICU: Panacea or plague? *Respiratory Care.* 1992;37:170–180.

Edwards GB, Schuring LM. Sleep protocol: A research-based practice change. *Critical Care Nurse.* 1993;84–88.

Emergency Cardiac Care Committee and Subcommittees, American Heart Association. Guidelines for Cardiopulmonary Resuscitation and Emergency Cardiac Care. *The Journal of the American Medical Association.* 1992;268: 2171–2298.

Evans GT, Jr, Scheinman MM, Zipes DP, et al. The percutaneous cardiac mapping and ablation registry: Final summary of results. *PACE.* 1988;11:1621–1626.

Fabius DB. Diagnosing and treating ventricular tachycardia. *Journal of Cardiovascular Nursing.* 1993;7:8–25.

Farrar DJ, Hill JD, Gray LA, et al. Heterotopic prosthetic ventricles as a bridge to transplantation: a multicenter study in twenty-nine patients. *New England Journal of Medicine.* 1988;318:333–340.

Fisher JD, Kim SG, Mercando AD. Electrical devices for treatment of arrhythmias. *American Journal of Cardiology.* 1988;61:45A–57A.

Fishman RF, Kuntz RE, Carrozza JP, et al. Long term results of directional coronary atherectomy: Predictors of restenosis. *Journal of the American College of Cardiology.* 1992;20:1101–1110.

Francis G. Should asymptomatic ventricular arrhythmias in patients with congestive heart failure be treated with antiarrhythmic drugs? *Journal of the American College of Cardiology.* 1988;12:274–276.

Frasure-Smith N. In-hospital symptoms of psychological stress as predictors of long-term outcome after acute myocardial infarction in men. *American Journal of Cardiology.* 1991;67:121–127.

Frye RL, Collins JJ, DeSanctis RW, Dodge HT, et al. Guidelines for permanent cardiac pacemaker implantation, May 1984. *Journal of the American College of Cardiology.* 1984;4:434–442.

Fuller BF, Foster FM. The effects of family–friend visits versus staff interaction on stress/arousal of surgical intensive care patients. *Heart & Lung.* 1982;11:457–463.

Funk M. Diagnosis of right ventricular infarction with right precordial ECG leads. *Heart & Lung.* 1986;15:562–570.

Furst E, Morse W, Slye DA. Cardiovascular technology. *Journal of Cardiovascular Nursing.* 1992;6:78–83.

Gardner RM, Hollingsworth KW. Optimizing the electrocardiogram and pressure monitoring. *Critical Care Medicine.* 1986;14:651–658.

Geertsen HR, Ford M, Castle CH. The subjective aspects of coronary care. *Nursing Research.* 1976;25:211–215.

Gheorghiade M, Schultz L, Barbara T, Kao W, Goldstein S. Natural history of the first non-Q-wave myocardial infarction in the placebo arm of the Beta-Blocker Heart Attack Trial. *American Heart Journal.* 1991;122:1548–1553.

Gillum RF. Trends in acute myocardial infarction and coronary heart disease death in the United States. *Journal of the American College of Cardiology.* 1994;23:1273–1277.

GISSI. GISSI-2: A factorial randomized trial of alteplase versus streptokinase and heparin versus no heparin among 12,490 patients with acute myocardial infarction. *Lancet.* 1990;336:65–71.

GISSI. Long-term effects of intravenous thrombolysis in acute myocardial infarction: Final report of the GISSI study. *Lancet.* 1987;2:871–874.

Gist HC, Mesrobian HD, Ziskind AA. New interventional techniques for coronary revascularization. *Heart Disease and Stroke.* 1993;2:198–202.

Glantz SA, Parmley WW. Passive smoking and heart disease: Epidemiology, physiology, and biochemistry. *Circulation.* 1991;83:1–12.

Goldberg FJ, Gore JM, Alpert JS, Dalen JE. Non-Q-wave myocardial infarction: Recent changes in occurrence and prognosis—A community-wide perspective. *American Heart Journal.* 1987;113:273–279.

Goldberg R, et al. Outcome after cardiac arrest during acute myocardial infarction. *American Journal of Cardiology.* 1987;59:251–255.

Goldberg RJ, Gorak EJ, Yarzebski J, et al. A community-wide perspective of sex differences and temporal trends in the incidence and survival rates after acute myocardial infarction and out-of-hospital deaths caused by coronary heart disease. *Circulation.* 1993;87:1947–1953.

Gore JM, Sloan K. Use of continuous monitoring of mixed venous saturation in the coronary care unit. *Chest.* 1984;86:757–761.

Graham IW. Reconstructing nursing: A coronary care perspective of the primary nurse philosophy. *Intensive and Critical Care Nursing.* 1992;8:118–124.

Grines CL. Thrombolytic, antiplatelet, and antithrombotic agents. *American Journal of Cardiology.* 1992;70:181–261.

Grines CL, DeMaria AN. Optimal utilization of thrombolytic therapy for acute myocardial infarction: Concepts and controversies. *Journal of the American College of Cardiology.* 1990;16:223–231.

Groom L, Frisch SR, Elliott M. Reproducibility and accuracy of pulmonary artery pressure measurement in supine and lateral positions. *Heart & Lung.* 1990;19:147–151.

Guerci AD, Gerstenblith G, Brinker JA, et al. A randomized trial of intravenous tissue plasminogen activator for acute myocardial infarction with subsequent randomization to elective coronary angioplasty. *New England Journal of Medicine.* 1987;317:1613–1618.

Gupta K, Lichstein E, Chadda K. Heart block complications acute inferior wall infarction. *Chest.* 1976;69:599–604.

Hall WD. Treatment of systolic hypertension. *Heart Disease and Stroke.* 1992;1:271–273.

Hands M, Lloyd B, Robinson J, et al. Prognostic significance of electrocardiographic site of infarction after correction for enzymatic site of infarction. *Circulation.* 1986;73:885–891.

Hanisch PJ. Identification and treatment of acute myocardial infarction by electrocardiographic site classification. *Focus on Critical Care.* 1991;18:480–488.

Hansell HN. The behavioral effects of noise on man: The patient with intensive care unit psychosis. *Heart & Lung.* 1984;13:59–65.

Hardesty RL, Griffith BP, Trento A, Thomson ME, et al. Mortally ill patients and excellent survival following cardiac transplantation. *Annals of Thoracic Surgery.* 1986; 41:126–129.

Heater BS. Nursing responsibilities in changing visiting restrictions in the intensive care unit. *Heart & Lung.* 1985; 14:181–186.

Hebert KA, Glancy DL. Indications for Swan–Ganz catheterization. *Heart Disease and Stroke*. 1994;3:196–200.

Hill NE, Goodman JS. Importance of accurate placement of precordial leads in the 12-lead electrocardiogram. *Heart & Lung*. 1987;16:561–566.

Hillis L, Forman S, Braunwald E. Thrombolysis in myocardial infarction (TIMI) phase II co-investigators. Risk stratification before thrombolytic therapy in patients with acute myocardial infarction. *Journal of the American College of Cardiology*. 1990;16:313–315.

Hinohara T, Robertson GC, Selmon MR, Vetter JW, et al. Restenosis after directional coronary atherectomy. *Journal of the College of Cardiology*. 1992;20:623–632.

Hinohara T, Rowe MH, Robertson GC, et al. Effect of lesion characteristics on outcome of directional coronary atherectomy. *Journal of the American College of Cardiology*. 1991;17:1112–1120.

Hlatky M, Califf R, Lee K, et al. Prognostic significance of precordial ST-segment depression during inferior acute myocardial infarction. *American Journal of Cardiology*. 1985;55:325–329.

Honan MB, Harrell FE, Jr, Reimer KA, Califf RM, et al. Cardiac rupture, mortality and the timing of thrombolytic therapy: A meta-analysis. *Journal of the American College of Cardiology*. 1990;16:359–367.

Horner SM. Efficacy of intravenous magnesium in acute myocardial infarction in reducing arrhythmias and mortality: Meta-analysis of magnesium in acute myocardial infarction. *Circulation*. 1992;86:774–779.

Hudgins C, Sorenson G. Directional coronary atherectomy: A new treatment for coronary artery disease. *Critical Care Nurse*. 1994;61–66.

Humen DP, Kostuk WJ, Klein GJ. Activity-sensing, rate-responsive pacing: Improvement in myocardial performance with exercise. *PACE*. 1985;8:52–59.

Hurst JW. The renaissance of clinical electrocardiography. *Heart Disease and Stroke*. 1993;2:290–295.

ISIS-1 (First International Study of Infarct Survival) Collaborative Group. Randomized trial of intravenous atenolol among 16,027 cases of suspected acute myocardial infarction: ISIS-1. *Lancet*. 1986;2:57–66.

ISIS-2 (Second International Study of Infarct Survival) Collaborative Group. Randomized trial of intravenous streptokinase, oral aspirin, both, or neither among 17,187 cases of suspected acute myocardial infarction: ISIS-2. *Lancet*. 1988;2:349–360.

ISIS-3 (Third International Study of Infarct Survival) Collaborative Group. A Randomized comparison of steptokinase vs. tissue plasminogen activator vs. anistreplase and of aspirin plus heparin vs. aspirin alone among 41,299 cases of suspected acute myocardial infarction. *Lancet*. 1992;339:753–770.

Jain P, Vlay SC. Pharmacological management of acute myocardial infarction. *Clinical Cardiology*. 1992;15:795–803.

Kannel WB, McGee DL. Disease and cardiovascular disease: The Framingham Study. *Journal of The American Medical Association*. 1979;241:2035–2038.

Kartmann JL. Sleep and the elderly critical care patient. *Critical Care Nurse*. 1985;5:52–57.

Kaufmann MW, Pasacrtea J, Cheney R, et al. Psychosomatic aspects of myocardial infarction and implications for treatment. *International Journal of Psychiatry in Medicine*. 1986;15:371–379.

Kelly P, Cannom D, Garan H, et al. The automatic implantable cardioverter defibrillator. Efficacy, complications, and survival in patients with malignant ventricular arrhythmias. *Journal of the American College of Cardiology*. 1988;11:1278–1286.

Kennedy GT, Bryant A, Crawford MH. The effect of lateral body positioning on measurements of pulmonary artery and pulmonary artery wedge pressures. *Heart & Lung*. 1984;13:155–158.

Kessler KM, Chakko SC, Myerburg RJ. Management of premature ventricular contractions. *Heart Disease and Stroke*. 1992;1:275–280.

Kindwall KE, Brown J, Josephson ME. Electrocardiographic criteria for ventricular tachycardia in wide complex left bundle branch block morphology tachycardias. *American Journal of Cardiology*. 1988;61:1279–1283.

Kirchhoff KT, Pugh E, Calame R, Reynolds N. Nurses' beliefs and attitudes toward visiting in adult critical care settings. *American Journal of Critical Care*. 1993;2:238–245.

Kirshenbaum JM. Therapy for acute myocardial infarction: An update. *Heart Disease and Stroke*. 1992;1:211–217.

Klein LW, Helfant RH. The Q-wave and non-Q-wave myocardial infarction: Differences and similarities. *Progress on Cardiovascular Disease*. 1986;3:205–220.

Kleman M, Bickert A, Karpinski A, Wantz D, et al. Physiologic responses of coronary care patients to visiting. *Journal of Cardiovascular Nursing*. 1993;7:52–62.

Kline EM. Pharmacologic review of thrombolytic agents. *Critical Care Nursing Clinics of North America*. 1990;2:613–627.

Kolar JA, Dracup K. Psychosocial adjustment of patients with ventricular dysrhythmias. *Journal of Cardiovascular Nursing*. 1990;4:44–55.

Konstam M, Dracup K, Baker D, et al. Heart failure: Evaluation and care of patients with left-ventricular systolic dysfunction. *Clinical Guideline No. 11*. AHCPR Publication No. 94-0612. Rockville, MD: Agency for Health Care Policy and Research, Public Health Service, US Department of Health and Human Services. June 1994.

Kopecky SL, Gersh BJ, McGoon MD, Whisnant JP, et al. The natural history of lone atrial fibrillation: A population-based study over three decades. *New England Journal of Medicine*. 1987;317:669–674.

Kornfeld D. The intensive care unit in adults: Coronary care and general medical/surgical. *Advanced Psychosomatic Medicine*. 1980;10:1–29.

Krone RJ, Friedman E, Thanavaro S, Miller JP, et al. Long-term prognosis after first Q-wave (transmural) or non-Q-wave (nontransmural) myocardial infarction: Analysis of 593 patients. *American Journal of Cardiology*. 1983;52:234–239.

Kuck KH, Friday KJ, Kunze KP, Schluter M, et al. Sites of conduction block in accessory atrioventricular pathways. Basis for concealed accessory pathways. *Circulation*. 1990;82:407–417.

Kuck KH, Kunze KP, Schluter M, Geiger M, Jackman WM. Ablation of a left-sided free-wall accessory pathway by percutaneous catheter application of radiofrequency current in a patient with the Wolff–Parkinson–White syndrome. *PACE.* 1989;12:1681–1690.

Kuck KH, Kunze KP, Schluter M, Geiger M, et al. Modification of a left-sided accessory atrioventricular pathway by radiofrequency current using a bipolar epicardial endocardial electrode configuration. *European Heart Journal.* 1988;9:927–932.

Kuck KH, Schluter M, Geiger M, Siebels J, Duckeck W. Radiofrequency current catheter ablation of accessory atrioventricular pathways. *Lancet.* 1991;337:1557–1561.

Kutalek SP, Michelson EL. Cardiac pacing and antiarrhythmic devices: Newer modes of antibradyarrhythmia pacing. *Modern Concepts of Cardiovascular Disease—American Heart Association.* 1991;60:31–35.

Langberg JJ, Chin M, Schamp DJ, et al. Ablation of the atrioventricular junction with radiofrequency energy using a new electrode catheter. *American Journal of Cardiology.* 1991;67:142–147.

Lapidus L, Bengtsson C. Socioeconomic factors and physical activity in relation to cardiovascular disease and death: A 12 year follow up of participants in a population study of women in Gothenburg, Sweden. *British Heart Journal.* 1986;55:295–301.

Lasater MG. Torsade des pointes: Etiology and treatment. *Focus on Critical Care.* 1986;13:17–20.

Lavie CJ, Genton E. Hemostasis, thrombosis, and antiplatelet therapy: Implications for prevention of cardiovascular disease. *Cardiovascular Review Reports.* 1991; 12:24–47.

Lavie CJ, Milani RV, Littman AB. Benefits of cardiac rehabilitation and exercise training in secondary coronary prevention in the elderly. *Journal of the American College of Cardiology.* 1993;22:678–683.

Leon AS, Connett J, Jacobs DR, Jr. Rauramaa R. Leisure-time physical activity levels and risk of coronary heart disease and death: The Multiple Risk Factor Intervention Trial. *Journal of The American Medical Association.* 1987;258:2388–2395.

Levine PA. Physiological pacing 1988: A comparison of single- and dual-chamber pacing systems with rate adaptive single and dual-chamber pacing systems. *Journal of Electrophysiology.* 1989;3:167–222.

Lewis PS. Clinical implications of non-Q-wave (subendocardial) myocardial infarctions. *Focus on Critical Care-AACN.* 1992;19:29–33.

Lindquist RD, Jeffrey RW, Johnson A, Haus E. The stress of patient adjustment to the coronary care unit as related to perceptions of personal control and control preference. *Heart & Lung.* 1985;14:297–298.

Lipid Research Clinics Program. The Lipid Research Clinics Coronary Primary Prevention Trial results. I: Reduction in incidence of coronary heart disease. *Journal of The American Medical Association.* 1984;251:351–364.

Littrell K, Schumann LL. Promoting sleep for the patient with a myocardial infarction. *Critical Care Nurse.* 1989; 9:44–49.

Lloyd EA, Hauer RN, Zipes DP, Heger JJ, Prystowsky EN. Syncope and ventricular tachycardia in patients with ventricular preexcitation. *American Journal of Cardiology.* 1983;52:79–82.

Malan SS. Psychosocial adjustment following MI: Current views and nursing implications. *Journal of Cardiovascular Nursing.* 1992;6:57–70.

Manolis AS, Tan-DeGuzman W, Lee MA, Rastegar H, et al. Clinical experience in seventy-seven patients with the automatic implantable cardioverter defibrillator. *American Heart Journal.* 1989;118:445–450.

Marchlinski FE, Flores BT, Buxton AE, et al. The automatic implantable cardioverter defibrillator: Efficacy, complications and device failures. *Annals Internal Medicine.* 1986;104:481–488.

Markel ML, Miles WM, Zipes DP, Prystowsky EN. Parasympathetic and sympathetic alterations of Mobitz type II heart block. *Journal of the American College of Cardiology.* 1988;11:271–275.

Marriott H. *Practical Electrocardiography,* 8th ed. Baltimore: Williams & Wilkins; 1988.

Marriott HJL, Fogg E. Constant monitoring for cardiac dysrhythmias and blocks. *Modern Concepts of Cardiovascular Disease.* 1970;39:103–108.

Matrisciano L. Unstable angina: An overview. *Critical Care Nurse.* 1992;30–39.

McGovern PG, Folsom AR, Sprafka JM, et al. Trends in survival of hospitalized myocardial infarction patients between 1970 and 1985: The Minnesota Heart Survey. *Circulation.* 1992;85:172–179.

Mirowski M, Reid PR, Mower MM, Watkins L, et al. Termination of malignant ventricular arrhythmias with an implanted automatic defibrillator in human beings. *New England Journal of Medicine.* 1980;303:322–324.

Mirowski M, Reid PR, Winkle RA, Mower MM, et al. Mortality in patients with implanted automatic defibrillators. *Annals of Internal Medicine.* 1983;98:585–588.

Misinski M. Pathophysiology of acute myocardial infarction: A rationale for thrombolytic therapy. *Heart & Lung.* 1988;17:743–749.

Moise A, Theroux P, Taeymans Y, et al. Unstable angina and progression of coronary atherosclerosis. *New England Journal of Medicine.* 1983;309.

Molchany CA. Ventricular septal and free wall rupture complicating acute MI. *Journal of Cardiovascular Nursing.* 1992;6:38–45.

Morris AH, Chapman RH, Gardner RM. Frequency of wedge pressure errors in the ICU. *Critical Care Medicine.* 1985;13:705–708.

Morris DC. Early treatment of acute myocardial infarction: The myths, mystery, and magic. *Heart Disease and Stroke.* 1993;2:308–312.

Moser DK, Woo MA. Recurrent ventricular tachycardia. *Critical Care Nursing Clinics of North America,* 1994; 6:15–26.

Moser SA, Crawford D, Thomas A. Updated care guidelines for patients with automatic implantable cardioverter defibrillators. *Critical Care Nurse.* 1993;62–73.

Moss AJ, Benhorin J. Prognosis and management after a first myocardial infarction. *New England Journal of Medicine.* 1990;322:743–753.

Mower M, Nisam S. AICD indications (patient selection): Past, present and future. *PACE.* 1988;11:2064–2070.

Muller DWM, Ellis SG, Debowey DC, Topol EJ. Quantitative angiographic comparison of the immediate success of coronary angioplasty, coronary atherectomy and endoluminal stenting. *American Journal of Cardiology.* 1990;66:938–942.

National Cholesterol Education Program. Report of the National Cholesterol Education Program expert panel on detection, evaluation, and treatment of high blood cholesterol in adults. *Archives of Internal Medicine.* 1988;148:36–69.

Navas JP, Martinez-Maldonado. Pathophysiology of edema in congestive heart failure. *Heart Disease and Stroke.* 1993;2:325–329.

Naylor CD, Chen E. Population-wide mortality trends among patients hospitalized for acute myocardial infarction: The Ontario Experience, 1981 to 1991. *Journal of the American College of Cardiology.* 1994;24:1431–1438.

Nicod P, Gilpin E, Dittrich H, Polikar R, et al. Short- and long-term clinical outcome after Q-wave and non-Q-wave myocardial infarction in a large patient population. *Circulation.* 1989;79:528–536.

Nisam S, Thomas A, Mower M, Hauser R. Identifying patients for prophylactic automatic implantable cardioverter defibrillator therapy: Status of prospective studies. *American Heart Journal.* 1991;122:607–612.

O'Connor GT, Buring JE, Yusuf S, et al. An overview of randomized trials of rehabilitation with exercise after myocardial infarction. *Circulation.* 1989;80:234–244.

O'Keefe JH, Rutherford BD, McConahay DR, et al. Early and late results of coronary angioplasty without antecedent thrombolytic therapy for acute myocardial infarction. *American Journal of Cardiology.* 1989;64:1221–1230.

O'Neil WW. Mechanical rotational atherectomy. *American Journal of Cardiology.* 1992;69:12F–18F.

Ockene JK, Kuller LH, Svendsen KH, et al. The relationship of smoking cessation to coronary heart disease and lung cancer in the Multiple Risk Factor Intervention Trial (MRFIT). *American Journal of Public Health.* 1990; 80:954–958.

Orencia AJ, Hammill SC, Whisnant JP. Sinus node dysfunction and ischemic stroke. *Heart Disease and Stroke.* 1994;3:91–94.

Packer M. Sudden unexpected death in patients with congestive heart failure: A second frontier. *Circulation.* 1985;72:681–685.

Paffenbarger RS, Jr, Hyde RT, Wing AL, Hsieh CC. Physical activity, all-cause mortality, and longevity of college alumni. *New England Journal of Medicine.* 1986;314: 605–613.

Paffenbarger RS, Wing AL, Hyde RT. Physical activity as an index of heart attack risk in college alumni. *American Journal of Epidemiology.* 108;161–175.

Paolella LP, Dortman GS, Cronan JJ, Hasan RM. Topographic location of the left atrium by computed tomography: Reducing pulmonary artery catheter calibration error. *Critical Care Medicine.* 1988;16:1154–1156.

Pepine CJ, El-Tamimi H, Lambert CR. Prinzmetal's angina (variant angina). *Heart Disease and Stroke.* 1992;1:281–286.

Pfeffer MA, Braunwald E, Moy LA, Basta L, et al. On behalf of the SAVE Investigators. The effect of captopril on mortality and morbidity in patients with left ventricular dysfunction after myocardial infarction. Results of the survival and ventricular enlargement trial. *New England Journal of Medicine.* 1992;327:669–677.

Pfeffer MA, Moye LA, Braunwald E, et al. Selection bias in the use of thrombolytic therapy in acute myocardial infarction. *Journal of The American Medical Association.* 1991;266:528–532.

Phibbs B. "Transmural" versus "subendocardial" myocardial infarction: An electrocardiographic myth. *Journal of the American College of Cardiology.* 1983;1:561–564.

Pierce CD. Acute post-MI pericarditis. *Journal of Cardiovascular Nursing.* 1992;6:46–56.

Porterfield LM, Porterfield JG. Radiofrequency ablation of a left-sided free-wall accessory pathway: A case study. *Critical Care Nurse.* 1993;46–49.

Prystowsky EN. Electrophysiologic testing. In: Kelley WN, ed. *Textbook of Internal Medicine.* Philadelphia: Lippincott; 1989.

Ragland DR, Brand RJ. Type A behavior and mortality from coronary heart disease. *New England Journal of Medicine.* 1988;318:65–69.

Reddy SG, Roberts WC. Frequency of rupture of the left ventricular free wall or ventricular septum among necropsy cases of fatal acute myocardial infarction since introduction of coronary care units. *American Journal of Cardiology.* 1989;63:906–911.

Reddy JE, Ruzevich SA, Noedel NR, Vitale LJ, Merkle EJ. Nursing care of the ambulatory patient with a mechanical assist device. *The Journal of Heart Transplantation.* 1990;9:97–105.

Reinhart SI. Uncomplicated acute myocardial infarction: A critical path. *Cardiovascular Nursing.* 1995;31:1–7.

Richard C, Thuillez C, Pezzano M, Bottineau G, et al. Relationship between mixed venous oxygen saturation and cardiac index in patients with chronic congestive heart failure. *Chest.* 1989;95:1289–1294.

Roberts R. Recognition, pathogenesis, and management of non-Q-wave infarction. *Modern Concepts of Cardiovascular Disease.* 1987;56:17–21.

Rosenberg L, Kaufman DW, Helmrich SP, et al. The risk of myocardial infarction after quitting smoking in men under 55 years of age. *New England Journal of Medicine.* 1985;313:1511–1514.

Rosenberg L, Palmer JR, Shapiro S. Decline in the risk of myocardial infarction among women who stop smoking. *New England Journal of Medicine.* 1990;322:213–217.

Rosenqvist M, Brandt J, Schuller H. Long-term pacing in sinus node disease: Effects of stimulation mode on cardiovascular morbidity and mortality. *American Heart Journal.* 1988;116:16–22.

Ross R. The pathogenesis of atherosclerosis: A perspective for the 1990s. *Nature.* 1993;362:801–809.

Ruberman W, Weinblatt E, Goldberg JD, Chaudhary BS. Psychosocial influences on mortality after myocardial infarction. *New England Journal of Medicine.* 1984;311: 552–559.

Safian RD, Baim DS. New devices for coronary intervention: Intravascular stents and coronary atherectomy catheters. In: Grossman W, Baim DS, eds. *Cardiac Catheterization, Angiography and Intervention.* Philadelphia: Lea & Febiger; 1991.

Safian RD, Gelbfish JS, Erny RE, Schnitt SJ, et al. Coronary atherectomy: Clinical, angiographic and histological findings and observations regarding potential mechanisms. *Circulation.* 1990;82:69–79.

Saksena S, Parsonnet V. Implantation of a cardioverter defibrillator without thoracotomy using a triple electrode system. *Journal of the American Medical Association.* 1988;259:69–72.

Salian RD, Snyder LD, Snyder BA, et al. Usefulness of percutaneous transluminal coronary angioplasty for unstable angina pectoris after non-Q-wave acute myocardial infarction. *American Journal of Cardiology.* 1987; 59:263–266.

Sanford S. Sleep and the cardiac patient. *Cardiovascular Nursing.* 1983;19:19–24.

Saver CL. Decoding the ACLS algorithms. *American Journal of Nursing.* 1994:27–35.

Schactman M. Rhythm disturbances in patient with pulmonary disease. *Critical Care Nurse.* 1993;41–46.

Scheinman M. Catheter and surgical treatment of cardiac arrhythmias. *Journal of the American Medical Association.* 1990;263:79–82.

Scheinman MM, Morady F, Hess DS, Gonzalez R. Catheter-induced ablation of the atrioventricular junction to control refractory supraventricular arrhythmias. *Journal of the American Medical Association.* 1982;248:851–855.

Schlant RC, Forman S, Stamler J, Canner PL. The natural history of coronary heart disease: Prognostic factors after recovery from myocardial infarction in 2,789 men: The 5-year findings of the Coronary Drug Project. *Circulation.* 60;805–814.

Shapira I, Isakov A, Burke M, Almog C. Cardiac rupture in patients with acute myocardial infarction. *Chest.* 1987; 92:219–223.

Sheldon WC. Indications for Coronary Arteriography. *Heart Disease and Stroke.* 1993;2:192–197.

Sheps D. *The Management of Post Myocardial Infarction Patients.* New York: McGraw-Hill; 1987.

Sommers MS, Stevenson JS, Hamlin RL, Ivey TD, Russell AC. Mixed venous oxygen saturation and oxygen partial pressure as predictors of cardiac index after coronary artery bypass grafting. *Heart & Lung.* 1993;22:112–120.

Stamler J, Shekelle R. Dietary cholesterol and human coronary heart disease: The epidemiologic evidence. *Archives of Pathology and Laboratory Medicine.* 1988;112:1032–1040.

Stampfer MJ, Colditz GA, Willett WC, Manson JE, et al. Postmenopausal estrogen therapy and cardiovascular disease: Ten-year follow-up from the nurses' health study. *New England Journal of Medicine.* 1991;325:756–762.

Stangle K, Seitz K, Wirtzfeld A, Alt E, Blomer H. Differences between atrial single chamber pacing (AAI) and ventricular single chamber pacing (VVI) with respect to prognosis and antiarrhythmic effect in patients with sick sinus syndrome. *PACE.* 1990;13:2080–2085.

Steele JM, Ruzicki D. An evaluation of the effectiveness of cardiac teaching during hospitalization. *Heart & Lung.* 1987;16:306–317.

Stevenson L, Flower M, Schroeder J, et al. Poor survival of patients with idiopathic cardiomyopathy considered too well for transplantation. *American Journal of Medicine.* 1987;83:871–876.

Stewart RB, Bardy GH, Greene HL. Wide complex tachycardia: Misdiagnosis and outcome after emergent therapy. *Annals of Internal Medicine.* 1986;104:766–771.

Stewart S. Current theories and therapies relating to acute myocardial infarction and reperfusion injury. *Intensive and Critical Care Nursing.* 1992;8:104–112.

Stewart SL. Acute MI: A review of pathophysiology, treatment, and complications. *Journal of Cardiovascular Nursing.* 1992;6:1–25.

Surawicz B. Ventricular arrhythmias: Why is it so difficult to find a pharmacologic cure? *Journal of the American College of Cardiology.* 1989;14:1401–1416.

Sutton R, Kenny RA. The natural history of sick sinus syndrome. *PACE.* 1986;9:1110–1114.

Swan HJC, Ganz W, Forrester J, Marcus H, et al. Catheterization of the heart in man with use of a flow-directed balloon-tipped catheter. *New England Journal of Medicine.* 1970;283:447–451.

Szaflarski NL, Cohen NH. Use of pulse oximetry in critically ill adults. *Heart & Lung.* 1989;18:444–454.

Tawa CB, Raizner AE. Recognition and treatment of myocardial rupture. *Heart Disease and Stroke.* 1994;3:143–146.

The Gusto Investigators. An international randomized trial comparing four thrombolytic strategies for acute myocardial infarction. *New England Journal of Medicine.* 1993; 329:673–682.

The SOLVED Investigators. Effect of enalapril on mortality and the development of heart failure in asymptomatic patients with reduced left ventricular ejection fractions. *New England Journal of Medicine.* 1992;327:685–691.

Theroux P, Ouimet H, McCans J, et al. Aspirin, heparin, or both to treat acute unstable angina. *New England Journal of Medicine.* 1988;319:1105–1111.

Thomas AC, Moser SA, Smutka ML, Wilson PA. Implantable difibrillation: Eight years' clinical experience. *PACE.* 1988;11:2053–2058.

Tofler G, Stone P, Muller J, et al. Effect of gender and race on prognosis after myocardial infarction: Adverse prognosis for women, particularly black women. *Journal of the American College of Cardiology.* 1987;9:473–482.

Topf M, Davis JE. Critical care unit noise and rapid eye movement (REM). *Heart & Lung.* 1993;22:252–258.

Topol EJ. Rotablator to the rescue. *American Journal of Cardiology.* 1993;71:858–859.

Underhill SL, Woods SL, Froelicher ES, Halpenny CJ (eds). *Cardiovascular Medications for Cardiac Nursing.* Philadelphia: Lippincott; 1990.

Vaughn S, Puri VK. Cardiac output changes and continuous mixed venus oxygen saturation measurement in the critically ill. *Critical Care Medicine.* 1988;16:495–498.

Villanueva K. A closer look at inferior wall myocardial infarction. *Heart & Lung.* 1985;14:255–259.

Warnica JW. Pharmacologic management of acute myocardial infarction. In: Gersh BJ, Rahimotoola SH, eds. *Acute Myocardial Infarction.* New York: Elsevier; 1991.

Weilitz PB. Weaning a patient from mechanical ventilation. *Critical Care Nurse.* 1993;33–43.

Wellens HJJ. The electrocardiogram 80 years after Einthoven. *Journal of the American College of Cardiology.* 1986;7:484–491.

Winkle RA, Stinson EB, Echt DS, Mead RH, Schmidt P. Practical aspects of automatic cardioverter/defibrillator implantation. *American Heart Journal.* 1984;108:1335–1346.

Woo MA. Clinical management of the patient with an acute myocardial infarction. *Critical Care Nursing Clinics of North America.* 1992;27:189–203.

Woods SL, Grose BL, Laurent-Bopp D. Effect of backrest position on pulmonary artery pressures in critically ill patients. *Cardiovascular Nursing.* 1982;18:19–24.

Woods SL, Mansfield LW. Effect of body position upon pulmonary artery and pulmonary capillary wedge pressures in noncritically ill patients. *Heart & Lung.* 1976;5:83–90.

Yusuf S, Peto R, Lewis J, Sleight P. Beta-blockade during and after myocardial infarction: An overview of the randomized trials. *Progress in Cardiovascular Disease.* 1985;27:335–371.

Zaim B, Zaim S, Kutalek SP. Indications for use of permanent cardiac pacemakers. *Heart Disease and Stroke.* 1994;3:71–76.

Zaim S, Walter PW. Diagnosis and treatment of ventricular tachycardia. *Heart Disease and Stroke.* 1992;1:141–147.

Ziemann K, Dracup K. How well do patient–nurse contracts work in CCU? *American Journal of Nursing.* 1989;89:691–694.

Ziemann KM, Dracup K. Patient–nurse contracts in critical care: A controlled trial. *Progress in Cardiovascular Nursing.* 1990;5:98–103.

Zorb S. Care of the cardiac patient: Assessment, evaluation, and nursing implications. Part III: Fluid requirements, patient teaching, and nursing interventions. *Journal of Intravenous Nursing.* 1988;11:154–159.

Appendix **A**

Commonly Used Medications
in Intensive Coronary Care

COMMONLY USED MEDICATIONS IN INTENSIVE CORONARY CARE

Classification	Generic Drug	Common Brand Name	Usual Dose	Action
ANTIARRHYTHMIC AGENTS				
Class I				Reduce automaticity by inhibiting fast sodium channels and "stabilizing" cell membrane.
Class IA	Disopyramide	Norpace	150 mg q.i.d.[a]	Block sodium channels and delay repolarization.
	Procainamide	Pronestyl	500–1000 mg q 3–4 hr or q 6 hr sustained release capsules	Prolongs QRS, Q–T.
				Prolongs QRS, Q–T.
	Quinidine	Generic	200–600 mg q 6–8 hr	Prolongs QRS, Q–T.
Class IB				Block sodium channel and accelerate repolarization, thereby shortening action potential duration.
	Lidocaine hydrochloride	Xylocaine	50–150 mg IV bolus 1–4 mg/min IV maintenance	Shortens Q–T.
	Mexiletine	Mexitil	200–300 mg PO q 8 hr	Shortens Q–T.
	Phenytoin sodium	Dilantin	300–400 mg IV q.d.	Shortens Q–T.
			300–400 mg PO q.d. in single or divided doses	
	Tocainide hydrochloride	Tonocard	400–600 mg PO q 8 hr	Shortens Q–T.
Class IC				Block sodium channels and inhibit His–Purkinje system, thus prolonging the QRS. Little effect on repolarization.
	Encainide	Enkaid	35 mg PO t.i.d.[a]	Prolongs P–R, QRS.
	Flecainide	Tambocor	100–200 mg PO b.i.d.[a]	Prolongs P–R, QRS, and Q–T; bradycardia.
Class II **Beta-Blocking Agents)**				Decrease myocardial oxygen demand. Slow ventricular response in rapid atrial arrhythmias.
	Acebutolol	Sectral	200 mg b.i.d.	Cardioselective; prolongs P–R and shorten Q–T.
	Esmolol	Brevibloc	Loading dose 25–50 mg over 1 min Follow by infusion 2.5–5.0 mg/min up to 10–20 mg/min	Cardioselective. Slows AV conduction.
	Propranolol	Inderal	1–3 mg IV (not to exceed 1 mg/min) 10–30 mg PO 3–4 times daily[a]	Prolongs P–R. Shortens Q–T.
Class III				Prolongs action potential.
	Amiodarone	Cordarone	200–600 mg q.d.	Prolong P–R, QRS.
	Bretylium tosylate	Bretylol	5 mg/kg IV bolus for acute ventricular arrhythmias 5–10 mg/kg over 10 min q 6 hr or 1–2 mg/min IV continuous	Prolongs P–R, QRS.
Class IV **Calcium Channel Blocking Agents**				Block calcium channel entry. Prolong refractory period of AV node.
	Diltiazem	Cardizem	30–120 mg t.i.d. or q.i.d.	Prolongs P–R.
	Verapamil	Calan Isoptin	80–120 mg q 8 hr	Prolongs P–R.

ANTIHYPERTENSIVES

Adrenergic Neuronal Blocking Agents

Generic	Brand	Dosage	Action
Guanadrel sulfate	Hylorel	10–50 mg PO b.i.d.	Decreases blood pressure, heart rate, and cardiac output. Increases sodium retention.
Guanethidine sulfate	Ismelin	10–300 mg PO q.d.	Same as guanadrel sulfate but longer onset of action.
Reserpine	Serpasil Sandril	1–5 mg PO q.d.	Decreases blood pressure, heart rate, and cardiac output. Increases sodium retention.

Central-acting Adrenergic Blocking Agents

Generic	Brand	Dosage	Action
Clonidine	Catapres	0.2–0.8 mg PO q.d. in 2–3 divided doses	Directly stimulates the alpha-adrenergic receptors to inhibit sympathetic outflow. Decreases blood pressure, heart rate, and cardiac output.
Methyldopa	Aldomet	250–725 mg PO q.d. in 2–3 divided doses	Similar to clonidine.

Alpha-Adrenergic Blocking Agents

Generic	Brand	Dosage	Action
Prazosin hydrochloride	Minipres	6–15 mg PO q.d. in 2–3 divided doses	Block alpha-adrenergic receptors to decrease blood pressure. No change in heart rate or cardiac output.
Trimazosin hydrochloride	Cardovar	100–150 mg PO b.i.d.	Similar to prazosin hydrochloride.

ANTITHROMBOTIC AGENTS

Generic	Brand	Dosage	Action
Streptokinase	Kabikinase Steptase	1.5 million units IV over 60 min	Converts circulating plasminogen to plasmin.
Alteplase (rt-PA) Tissue plasminogen activator	Activase	100 mg IV over 1.5–3 hr	Clot specific—activates plasminogen.
Anistreplase (APSAC) Anisoylated plasminogen streptokinase activator complex	Eminase	30 units IV over 5 min	Clot specific—inactive until it binds with fibrin.
Urokinase	Abbokinase Breokinase Winkinase	2–3 million units over 30 min	Converts circulating plasminogen to plasmin.
Heparin sodium		800–1600 units/hr based on PTT (desired value = 1.5–2.5 times control value)	Inhibits clotting by preventing conversion of prothrombin to thrombin.

BETA-BLOCKING AGENTS

Generic	Brand	Dosage	Action
Acebutolol	Sectral	**Arrhythmias:** 200 mg PO b.i.d. **Hypertension:** 400 mg PO q.d. or 200 mg PO b.i.d.	Selectively inhibit sympathetic nervous system activity. Specific action depends on degree of cardioselectivity (beta$_1$-receptor blockade) and membrane stabilizing activity.
Atenolol	Tenormin	**Hypertension:** 5–10 mg IV bolus; 12.5–100 mg PO q.d.	Cardioselective. Prolongs P–R and shortens Q–T. Lowers blood pressure. Cardioselective. Prevents pressure response to catecholamine release, thereby lowering blood pressure.

COMMONLY USED MEDICATIONS IN INTENSIVE CORONARY CARE *(continued)*

Classification	Generic Drug	Common Brand Name	Usual Dose	Action
BETA-BLOCKING AGENTS (CONTINUED)	Esmolol	Brevibloc	**Arrhythmias (supraventricular tachycardia):** Loading dose 25–50 mg over 1 min. Follow by infusion of 2.5–5.0 mg/min up to 10–20 mg/min	Cardioselective. Slows AV conduction.
	Labetalol	Normodyne Trandate	**Hypertension:** *Severe:* 20 mg IV slowly and 2 mg/min continuous. 1.2–2.4 mg PO b.i.d. or t.i.d. *Moderate:* 200–400 mg PO b.i.d.	Lowers blood pressure but also has alpha-blocking activity.
	Metoprolol	Lopressor	**Hypertension:** 100–400 mg PO q.d. or in divided doses. **M.I. therapy:** 5 mg IV q 5 min. times 3 then 100 mg PO b.i.d. up to 3 years post M.I.	Cardioselective. Lowers blood pressure. Decreases infarct size, prevents reinfarction.
	Nadolol	Corgard	**Angina:** 40–80 mg PO q.d. up to maximum of 240 mg PO q.d. **Hypertension:** 40–80 mg PO q.d. up to maximum of 320 mg PO q.d.	Lowers blood pressure.
	Pindolol	Visken	**Hypertension and angina:** 5–30 mg PO b.i.d.	Has intrinsic sympathomimetic activity so effective in stable, exercise-induced angina.
	Propranolol	Inderal	**Angina:** 10–20 mg PO t.i.d.–q.i.d. to maximum of 320 mg PO daily	Decreases myocardial consumption by decreasing heart rate, contractility, and blood pressure. Causes coronary artery constriction so may increase coronary artery spasm. Prolongs P–R. Shortens Q–T
			Arrhythmias: 0.5 mg IV to a total of 0–1 mg/kg then 10–40 mg q 6 hr PO	.
			Hypertension: 40 mg PO b.i.d. to maximum of 640 mg PO daily	Prevents pressor response to catecholamine release with stress or exercise.
			Hypertrophic cardiomyopathy: 20–40 mg PO t.i.d.–q.i.d.	Reduces the gradient across the subaortic obstruction in hypertrophic cardiomyopathy.
			M.I. therapy: 180–240 mg PO[a]	
	Timolol	Blocadren	**Angina and hypertension:** 10–30 mg PO b.i.d. **M.I. therapy:** 10 mg PO b.i.d	Decreases myocardial consumption by decreasing heart rate, contractility and blood pressure.
CALCIUM CHANNEL BLOCKING AGENTS	Diltiazem	Cardizem	75–150 µg/kg IV; 30–120 mg PO t.i.d. or q.i.d.	Decreases myocardial contractility. Prolongs P–R.
	Nicardipine	Cardene	20–40 mg PO q 8 hr	Decreases myocardial contractility.
	Nifedipine	Adalat Procardia	3–10 µg/kg IV; 10–40 mg q 8 hr	Decreases myocardial contractility. Dilates coronary and peripheral arterioles.
	Nimodipine	Nimotop	60 mg q 4 hr	Decreases myocardial contractility.
	Verapamil	Calan Isoptin	75–150 mg/kg IV; 80–160 mg PO q 8 hr	Decreases myocardial contractility. Blocks alpha adrenergic receptors. Prolongs P–R.

Category	Drug	Brand	Dosage	Action
DIURETICS				
Thiazides and Related Agents	Chlorothiazide	Diuril	500–2,000 mg IV q.d.[a] or 125–1000 mg PO q.d.[a]	Increase the excretion of sodium, chloride, and water in the proximal portion of the distal tubule of the nephron.
	Hydrochlorthiazide	Esidrix HydroDiuril Oretic	12.5–50 mg PO q.d.	
	Indapamide	Lozol	2.5–5.0 mg PO q.d.	
	Metolazone	Zaroxolyn	2.5–10 mg PO q.d.	
	Quinethazone	Hydromox	25–100 mg PO q.d.	
Loop Diuretic Agents	Bumetanide	Bumex	0.5–1.0 mg IV repeated q 2–3 hr to maximum of 10 mg q.d.	Inhibit the absorption of sodium, chloride, and potassium in the ascending limb of the loop of Henle of the nephron.
			0.5–2.0 mg PO q.d.[a] to maximum of 10 mg	
	Furosemide	Lasix	20–40 IV over 1–2 min. Repeat in 20 mg increments every 2 hours as needed.	
			20–480 mg PO q.d.[a] to a maximum of 600 mg q.d.	
	Ethacrinic acid	Edecrin	0.5–1.0 mg/kg IV	
			25–200 mg PO q.d.	
Potassium-Sparing Diuretic Agents	Amiloride	Midamor	5–10 mg PO q.d.[a] to a maximum of 20 mg q.d.	Inhibit sodium uptake in the distal tubule and collecting ducts, causing increased excretion of sodium and water without potassium loss.
	Spironolactone	Aldactone	25–200 mg PO q.d.[a] to a maximum of 400 mg q.d.	
	Triamterene	Dyrenium	100–200 mg PO q.d. to a maximum of 300 mg q.d.	
INOTROPIC AGENTS	Amrinone	Inocor	**Initial:** 0.75 mg/kg IV bolus slowly over 2–3 min **Maintenance:** 5–10 µg/kg/min IV	Increases myocardial contractility and decreases systemic vascular resistence. Facilitates AV nodal conduction.
	Digoxin	Lanoxin	**Initial:** 0.75–1.25 mg IV divided into 3–4 doses given q 8 hr or 0.6–1.0 mg PO divided into 3–4 doses given at 4–8 hr intervals	Increases myocardial contractility. Slows sinus node firing and AV nodal conduction. Increases systemic vascular resistance.
		Lanoxicaps	**Maintenance:** 0.1–0.5 mg PO q.d. or 0.10–0.35 mg IV q.d.	
	Dobutamine	Dobutrex	2.5–10 µg/kg/min IV up to 40 µg/kg min	Increases myocardial contractility. No change or decrease in systemic vascular resistance. Enhances AV nodal conduction.
VAGOLYTIC AGENTS	Atropine sulfate		**Bradycardia:** 0.5 mg IV, may repeat once **Asystole:** 1.0 mg IV, may repeat once	Blocks the muscarinic type of acetylcholine receptors, including the parasympathetic receptors in the heart. Increases heart rate and may initiate electrical activity in asystole.

COMMONLY USED MEDICATIONS IN INTENSIVE CORONARY CARE (*continued*)

Classification	Generic Drug	Common Brand Name	Usual Dose	Action
VASOACTIVE AGENTS				
Adrenoreceptor for Agonists				Bind with adrenergic receptors to simulate the effects of sympathetic nerve stimulation.
	Dopamine hydrochloride	Intropin	1–2 µg/kg/min IV	Stimulates dopaminergic receptors in the renal and mesenteric vasculature to increase urine output.
			2–10 µg/kg/min IV	Stimulates $beta_1$-receptors to increase heart rate and myocardial contractility. Coronary artery vasodilation may occur.
			> 10 µg/kg/min IV	Stimulates alpha receptors to increase systemic vascular resistance. Effect on cardiac output is variable.
	Epinephrine hydrochloride	Adrenalin	1–4 µg/min IV infusion	**Low dose:** Excites peripheral $beta_2$-receptors in skeletal muscle and mesentary vessels to decrease blood pressure. **High dose:** Excites peripheral alpha-receptors, $beta_1$-receptors in heart, and $beta_2$-receptors in bronchioles to increase heart rate, blood pressure, and myocardial contractility and decrease bronchial smooth muscle contraction.
	Ephedrine sulfate		10–25 mg IV slowly; also available PO (15–50 mg q 3–4 hr), nasal spray, and topical cream	Stimulates the alpha- and beta-adrenergic receptors to increase heart rate, blood pressure, myocardial contractility and bronchiolar dilation.
	Phenylephrine hydrochloride	Neo-synephrine	**Paroxysmal tachycardia:** 0.5 mg IV injected rapidly **Moderate hypotension:** 0.1–0.5 mg given at 0.5 mL/min after dilution. **Severe hypotension:** 10 mg in 500 mL D_5W is infused at 100–180 drops/min	Alpha receptor stimulation leads to increased blood pressure, increased coronary perfusion, and compensatory reflex bradycardia.
Angiotensin-converting Inhibitors	Captopril	Capoten	25–100 mg PO t.i.d.	Inhibit enzyme responsible for conversion of angiotensin I to angiotensin II, reducing systemic vascular resistance. Suppress aldosterone secretion. No change in heart rate, cardiac output, or fluid volume.
	Enalapril	Vasotec	10–40 mg PO q.d.	
	Lisinopril	Zeztril Prinivil	5–40 mg PO q.d.	
	Quinapril hydrochloride	Accupril	10–20 mg PO q.d.	

Direct Vasodilators

Drug	Brand	Dose[a]	Action
Diazoxide	Hyperstat	50–150 mg IV	Relaxes arteriolar smooth muscle to decrease blood pressure in hypertensive crisis.
Ergonovine maleate	Ergotrate	50 µg IV repeated q 5 min until coronary vasospasm induced with a maximum of 400 µg	Constricts vascular smooth muscle, especially larger arteries. Administered to diagnose coronary spasm during coronary arteriography.
Hydralazine hydrochloride	Apresoline	2–20 mg IV then titrated to achieve hemodynamic goals; 10–100 mg PO q 6 hr	Relaxes both venous and arteriolar vessels, with major effect on arterioles.
Minoxidil	Loniten	10–40 mg q.d.	Relaxes arteriolar smooth muscle to decrease blood pressure.
Sodium nitroprusside	Nipride	0.5 µg/kg/min IV and titrated in increments of 1–2 µg/kg/min to obtain desired hemodynamics	Relaxes venous and arteriolar vasculature to decrease both preload (ventricular filling pressures) and afterload (systemic and pulmonary vascular resistance).

Nitrates

Drug	Brand	Dose[a]	Action
Nitroglycerin	Nitrostat, Nitrol, Nitrostat, Nitroglycerin, Nitro-Bid, Tridil	0.15–0.6 mg SL as needed	Stimulate vasodilation of veins and arteries, including collateral coronary arteries.
Parental nitroglycerin		5–200 µg/min IV infusion	Relax smooth muscle in coronary vessels narrowed by spasm or atherosclerotic lesion.
Nitroglycerin ointment 2%	Nitrol, Nitro-Bid, Nitrong	0.5–2 inches applied topically q 3–4 hr	
Transdermal nitroglycerin	Nitrodisc, Nitro-Dur, Transderm-Nitro	1 disk (2.5–15 mg q.d.) applied topically	
Erythrityl tetranitrate	Cardilate	5–10 mg SL or chewable q 3–4 hr	
Pentaerythritol tetranitrate	Peritrate	10–40 mg PO q 3–4 hr	
Isosorbide dinitrate	Isordil	2.5–10 mg SL q 2–3 hr	
	Sorbitrate	10–60 mg PO q 4–6 hr	

[a] In divided doses. PO, orally; IV, intravenously; SL, sublingually; q.d., every day; b.i.d., twice/day; q.i.d, four times/day; PTT, partial thromboplastin time; hr, hour; min, minute; M.I, myocardial infarction.

Exercises in the Interpretation of Arrhythmias

ECG 1

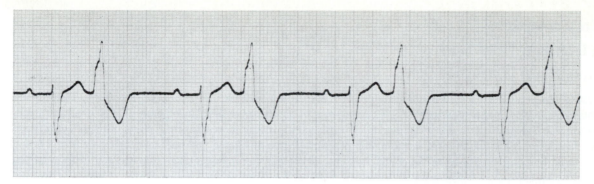

Interpretation:

_____

_____
_____
_____
_____

ECG 2

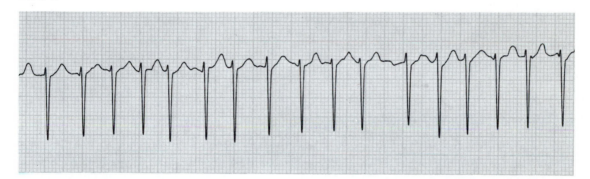

Interpretation:

_____

_____
_____
_____
_____

ECG 3

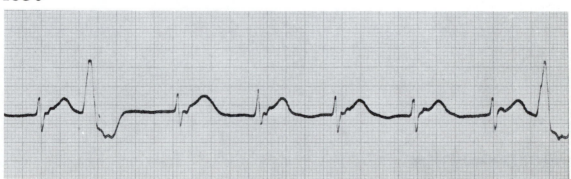

Interpretation:

_____

_____
_____
_____
_____

ECG 1

Ventricular Bigeminy
First-Degree AV Heart Block
Intraventricular Conduction Defect

This ECG shows a disorder of impulse formation in conjunction with two disorders of conduction. The impulse formation disorder is manifested by PVCs occurring every other beat (ventricular bigeminy). The conduction disorders are a first-degree AV block (P-R interval of 0.28 second) and an intraventricular conduction defect (QRS is widened to nearly 0.12 second). The combination of a first-degree block and an intraventricular conduction defect reflects widespread involvement of the conduction system—a fact that must be taken into account when selecting an antiarrhythmic drug to control the PVCs.

ECG 2

Atrial Fibrillation with a Rapid Ventricular Response

The *irregular* ventricular rhythm and the absence of P waves clearly signify atrial fibrillation (AF). The very rapid ventricular rate (180/minute) indicates that a high number of atrial impulses pass through the AV node to the ventricles. This rapid ventricular response can be slowed greatly with digitalis (or digitalis combined with verapamil), which increases the extent of AV block. AF with a fast ventricular rate is a hemodynamically inefficient rhythm and may lead to or precipitate heart failure.

ECG 3

Accelerated Junctional Rhythm
Premature Ventricular Contractions

Other than two PVCs, the remaining beats in this recording originate in the AV junction, as evidenced by P waves occurring *after* the QRS complexes. These junctional beats occur at a rate of 75/minute, which is faster than the inherent rate of an AV-junctional pacemaker (40–60/minute); consequently, the arrhythmia is designated an *accelerated junctional rhythm*.

ECG 4

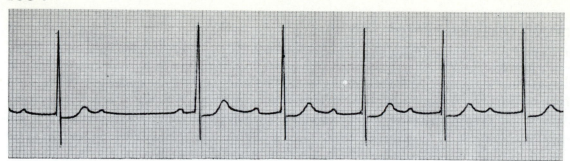

Interpretation:

_____

_____

_____

_____

ECG 5

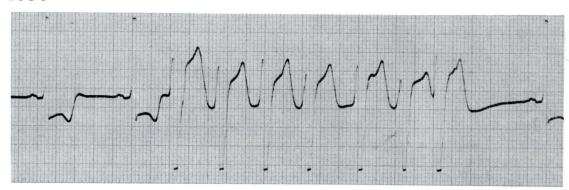

Interpretation:

_____

_____

_____

_____

ECG 6

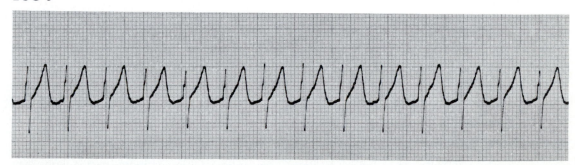

Interpretation:

_____

_____

_____

_____

ECG 4

Second-Degree Heart Block (Mobitz Type I)

The most characteristic feature of Mobitz type I second-degree AV heart block is progressive lengthening of the P-R interval until a P wave is finally blocked. This sequence is demonstrated in the accompanying ECG, which shows the end of one Wenckebach period and the beginning of another. Note that the longest P-R interval (0.40 second) occurs immediately before the blocked beat (which ends one Mobitz cycle). The shortest P-R interval (0.20 second) occurs immediately after the blocked beat, with the start of the next Mobitz cycle.

ECG 5

Ventricular Tachycardia

After two sinus beats, seven consecutive premature ventricular contractions (PVCs) occur at a rate greater than 100/minute. Any run of three or more consecutive PVCs at a fast rate represents *ventricular tachycardia (VT)*. Although the episode shown here stopped spontaneously, as is often the case with VT, lidocaine therapy was utilized subsequently to prevent further recurrences of this serious arrhythmia.

ECG 6

Supraventricular Tachycardia

From a single monitor lead recording, it is difficult to classify this arrhythmia in any more specific terms than "supraventricular tachycardia." The normal duration of the QRS complexes indicates that the tachycardia (140/minute) originated in either the atria or the junctional tissue (supraventricular) but not in the ventricles. Because of the inability to identify P waves specifically in this tracing, it cannot be determined whether the arrhythmia is paroxysmal atrial tachycardia (PAT), paroxysmal junctional tachycardia (PJT), or atrial flutter with 2:1 block. Only by using additional leads can a definite interpretation be made.

ECG 7

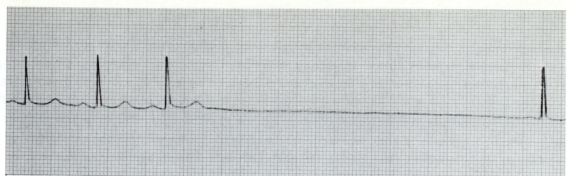

Interpretation:

_____

_____

_____

_____

ECG 8

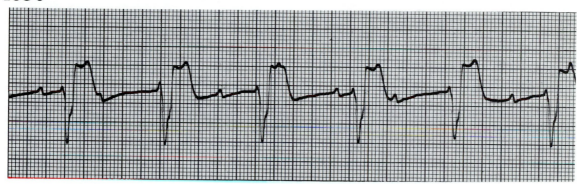

Interpretation:

_____

_____

_____

_____

ECG 9

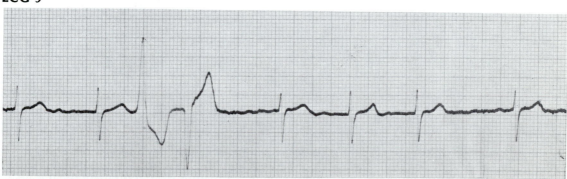

Interpretation:

_____

_____

_____

_____

ECG 7

Sinoatrial (SA) Arrest (or Block)

After two normal sinus beats, all electrical activity ceases for about 4 seconds (20 large boxes) before the next beat appears. The absence of P waves and QRS complexes during this period indicates that the SA node failed to initiate impulses (SA arrest) or that the impulses were blocked within the node (SA block). Prolonged episodes of asystole, as shown in this example, may result from ischemic injury to the SA node or from chronic disease of the SA node (sick sinus syndrome). In either case the temporary absence of a heartbeat for 4 seconds can produce syncope.

ECG 8

Complete (Third-Degree) Heart Block with Accelerated Idioventricular Rhythm

The P waves and QRS complexes bear no relationship to one another, indicating that the atria and ventricles are beating independently of each other. The atrial rate is 100/minute while the ventricular rate is 60/minute. Since none of the atrial impulses is conducted to the ventricles, the disorder can be classified as a complete (third-degree) AV heart block. That the QRS complexes are wide (more than 0.12 second) suggests that the block is below the AV-junctional area (subjunctional block) and that the ventricles are activated by a focus in the ventricles. In this circumstance the ventricular rate would be expected to be only 30 to 40/minute (the inherent rate of a ventricular pacemaker), but here the rate is 60/minute. This faster-than-anticipated ventricular rate probably reflects an accelerated idioventricular rhythm.

ECG 9

Premature Ventricular Contractions (PVCs) Occurring as a Couplet in Atrial Fibrillation

The underlying rhythm is atrial fibrillation (AF), as evidenced by the absence of P waves and an irregular ventricular response. In this setting, two PVCs occur consecutively as a couplet (or pair). Couplets are a dangerous form of ventricular ectopic activity, often warning of ventricular tachycardia (VT) or ventricular fibrillation (VF). The development of PVCs in patients with AF being treated with digitalis may be an indication of digitalis toxicity.

ECG 10

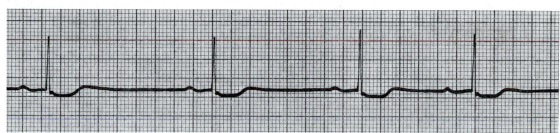

Interpretation:

_____
_____
_____
_____

ECG 11

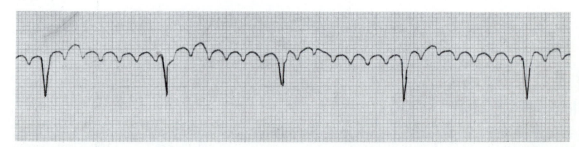

Interpretation:

_____
_____
_____
_____

ECG 12

Interpretation:

_____
_____
_____
_____

ECG 10

Premature Atrial Contractions (PACs) Occurring Consecutively as a Short Run of Atrial Tachycardia

The fourth beat in this rhythm strip occurs prematurely and is associated with an abnormally shaped P wave (partially hidden in the preceding T wave). The configuration of the QRS complex is the same as normal sinus beats. From these facts we know the beat originates in the atria and that it is a premature atrial contraction (PAC). This atrial ectopic beat triggers three consecutive PACs (a total of four PACs) at a rate of about 150/minute, after which sinus rhythm returns. This brief burst of four consecutive PACs represents a very short run of paroxysmal atrial tachycardia (PAT). Brief runs of this type are the most common form of atrial tachycardia.

ECG 11

Sinus Bradycardia
Sinus Arrhythmia
First-Degree AV Heart Block

The average heart rate is about 40/minute. Since each QRS complex is preceded by a normal P wave, this slow-rate arrhythmia is sinus bradycardia. However, the rhythm is distinctly irregular—a finding not normally anticipated with sinus bradycardia. The uneven rhythm is the result of sinus arrhythmia and is related to vagal changes during respiration. Sinus bradycardia and sinus arrhythmia often occur together because both arrhythmias are expressions of increased vagal activity. In addition, a first-degree AV block is also evident in this example (P-R interval 0.28 second). First-degree block may also be a manifestation of increased vagal tone. In other words, the combination of sinus bradycardia, sinus arrhythmia (disorders of impulse formation), and first-degree AV block (disorder of conduction) may all reflect vagal effects on the heart.

ECG 12

Atrial Flutter with Advanced AV Block

The typical sawtooth flutter waves (occurring at a rate of about 300/minute) identify this arrhythmia immediately as atrial flutter. The unusual feature of the ECG is the slow ventricular rate (about 50/minute). Most often atrial flutter is associated with a ventricular rate of 140 to 160/minute (atrial flutter with 2:1 block) or 70 to 80/minute (atrial flutter with 4:1 AV block). In this example, however, the extent of AV block is more advanced, with six flutter waves between each QRS complex (6:1 AV block). This indicates that the AV node is either injured or that the advanced block is due to drug therapy (e.g., digitalis). The administration of any drug that may increase AV block is clearly dangerous in this circumstance, and should be avoided.

ECG 13

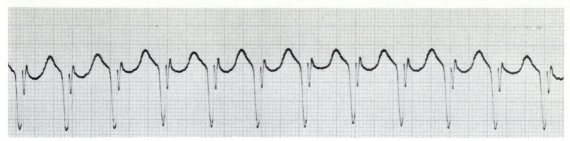

Interpretation:

_____
_____
_____
_____

ECG 14

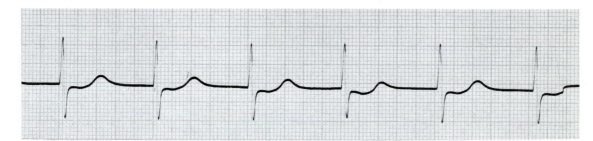

Interpretation:

_____
_____
_____
_____

ECG 15

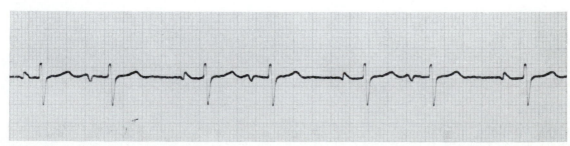

Interpretation:

_____
_____
_____
_____

ECG 13

Sinus Tachycardia
Bundle Branch Block

The lead from which this recording was made does not demonstrate definite P waves; however, it does not exclude their presence. Therefore one cannot be certain whether the arrhythmia is sinus tachycardia, an atrial or junctional rhythm, or even a ventricular tachycardia (especially in light of the wide, distorted QRS complexes). Recognizing the importance of identifying this arrhythmia precisely, the nurse changed electrode positions, after which a normal P wave became clearly visible before each QRS complex (see ECG below). On this basis, the interpretation of the arrhythmia is sinus tachycardia. In addition to this disturbance in impulse formation (sinus tachycardia), there is evidence of an unrelated disturbance of conduction. The wide, distorted QRS complexes (0.16 second in duration) reflect a bundle-branch block.

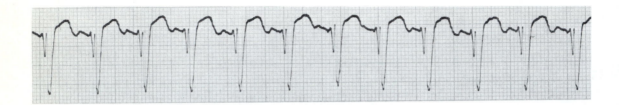

ECG 14

Junctional Rhythm

The ECG reveals a heart rate of about 60/minute, with a regular rhythm. No P waves are evident, indicating that the arrhythmia did not originate in the SA node or the atria. Since the QRS complexes are normal, it can be reasoned that impulses arise in the junctional area, and that the arrhythmia is a *junctional rhythm*. That a junctional pacemaker has assumed command means that the SA node must be discharging at a rate *slower* than the inherent rate of junctional tissue (40–60/minute). In this sense, a junctional rhythm is an escape rhythm.

ECG 15

Atrial Bigeminy
First-Degree AV Block

Every other beat is a premature atrial contraction (PAC), and this arrhythmia is therefore described as *atrial bigeminy.* Note that in this example the beats that arise in the atria are characterized by inverted P waves (in contrast to the upright P waves of the sinus beats). The P-R intervals of the sinus beats and the atrial ectopic beats are prolonged beyond 0.20 second, reflecting a delay in passage of all impulses through the AV node (first-degree AV block).

ECG 16

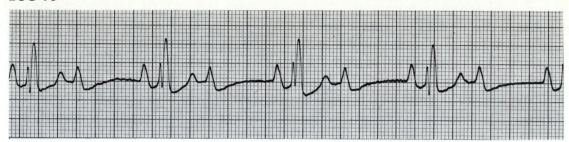

Interpretation:

_____

_____

_____

_____

ECG 17

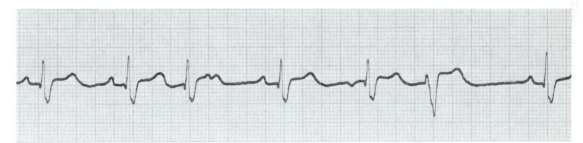

Interpretation:

_____

_____

_____

_____

ECG 18

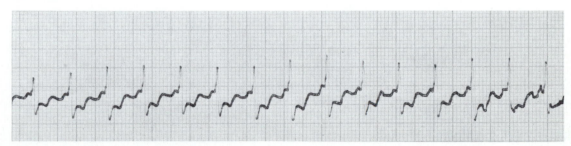

Interpretation:

_____

_____

_____

_____

ECG 16

Second-Degree AV Heart Block (Mobitz Type II)

There are two (tall) P waves between QRS complexes. Thus the atrial rate is twice the ventricular rate—a 2:1 heart block. This second-degree heart block is classified as a Mobitz Type II block because the P-R intervals are *constant* (unlike Mobitz type I second-degree AV block, in which the P-R intervals lengthen progressively before a beat is dropped). The QRS complexes are very wide because Mobitz Type II blocks occur *below* the AV node.

ECG 17

Premature Atrial Contraction (PAC)
Premature Junctional Contraction (PJC)
Premature Ventricular Contraction (PVC)
Intraventricular Conduction Disorder

This tracing demonstrates three different types of ectopic beats: atrial, junctional, and ventricular. The third beat on this strip is a PJC, with the P wave occurring after the QRS complex. The fifth beat is a PAC, as evidenced by the abnormal (inverted) P wave. The following beat (the sixth on the strip) is a PVC. In addition to these ectopic beats, the QRS complex is widened (0.12 second), reflecting an intraventricular conduction defect.

ECG 18

Atrial Flutter with 2:1 Block

As a general rule, any supraventricular arrhythmia with a regular rhythm and a heart rate between 140 and 160/minute should be regarded as atrial flutter with 2:1 block, until proven otherwise. The heart rate in this example is 150/minute, and the rhythm is regular. Two P waves (which are initially inverted) occur between QRS complexes, creating the "sawtooth" appearance that characterizes atrial flutter. The diagnosis of atrial flutter with 2:1 block can easily be missed unless its characteristic heart rate (140–160/minute) arouses suspicion of the problem.

ECG 19

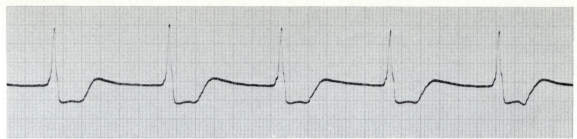

Interpretation:

_____
_____
_____
_____

ECG 20

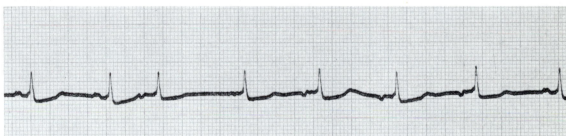

Interpretation:

_____
_____
_____
_____

ECG 21

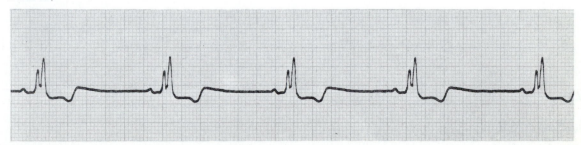

Interpretation:

_____
_____
_____
_____

ECG 19

Idioventricular Rhythm
Atrial Standstill

All of the beats in this rhythm strip originate in the ventricles, as revealed by the wide, bizarre QRS complexes and the absence of P waves before the QRS complexes. Although these ventricular ectopic beats occur consecutively, they do *not* represent ventricular tachycardia (VT), since their rate is only 50/minute. The reason that the ventricles have taken over as pacemaker is that the atria have stopped initiating impulses (atrial standstill) and the junctional tissues have not come to rescue the heartbeat. In general, the complete absence of impulses from higher centers (atria and AV-junctional area) usually indicates severe ischemia of these tissues, and is a manifestation of *downward displacement of the pacemaker (before death occurs)*.

ECG 20

Wandering Pacemaker
Premature Atrial Contraction

The main diagnostic feature of a wandering pacemaker is a changing configuration of the P waves, indicating that the pacemaker is shifting between the SA node and an adjacent site in the atria or AV-nodal area. In this particular example, the pacemaker moves temporarily from the SA node to the atria (the beats with the inverted P waves) after the occurrence of a premature atrial contraction (PAC). The last beat in the rhythm strip shows the return of a sinus pacemaker (upright P wave).

ECG 21

Bundle-Branch Block
Sinus Bradycardia

The QRS complexes are wide (more than 0.12 second) and distorted. Since each complex is preceded by a normal P wave (and constant P-R interval), we know that these beats originate in the SA node and that the abnormal ventricular complexes are due to an intraventricular conduction defect (bundle-branch block). The heart rate is only 45/minute, reflecting slow impulse formation (sinus bradycardia), which is unrelated to the bundle-branch block.

ECG 22

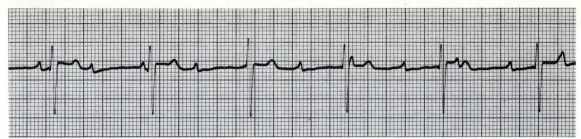

Interpretation:

ECG 23

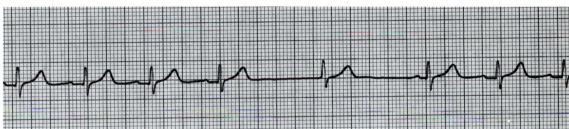

Interpretation:

ECG 24

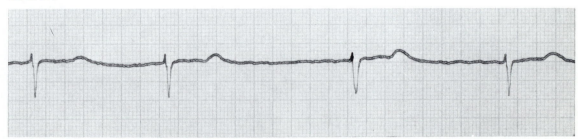

Interpretation:

ECG 22

Complete Heart Block with Narrow QRS Complexes (Junctional Pacemaker)

The diagnosis of complete heart block is based on the fact that the atria and ventricles are beating independently of each other and that no atrial impulses are conducted to the ventricles. The atria, activated by the SA node, are beating on their own at a rate of 100/minute. The ventricles are stimulated independently by a pacemaker in the AV-junctional area, as evidenced by the ventricular rate of 60/ minute along with narrow QRS complexes (with a ventricular pacemaker the anticipated heart rate would be less than 40/minute and the QRS complexes would be abnormally wide).

When the atria and ventricles beat independently, as in complete heart block, the condition is described by the broad term *atrioventricular (AV) dissociation.* However, AV dissociation is not synonymous with complete heart block, since it may also occur with several other arrhythmias.

ECG 23

Junctional Escape Beat

After four normal sinus beats, the SA node fails to discharge on schedule (probably as a result of sinus arrest or sinus arrhythmia). This causes a pause in the rhythm that finally ends when the AV junction "escapes" from SA control and produces a junctional escape beat. Unlike premature junctional contractions (PJCs) which occur before the next anticipated sinus beat, junctional escape beats occur only when sinus beats are delayed or absent. Thus, a junctional escape beat can be considered a protective mechanism to preserve the heartbeat when the SA node defaults.

ECG 24

Atrial Fibrillation with Advanced Atrioventricular (AV) Block

The rhythm is atrial fibrillation (AF), as evident from the irregular R-R intervals and the absence of P waves. The very slow ventricular response reflects advanced block in the AV node, and may be due to drugs (especially digitalis) or AV-nodal disease. In either case, AF with a ventricular rate of less than 50/minute produces serious hemodynamic consequences.

ECG 25

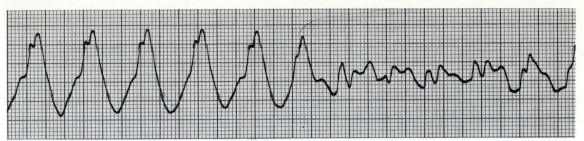

Interpretation:

_____

_____

_____

_____

ECG 26

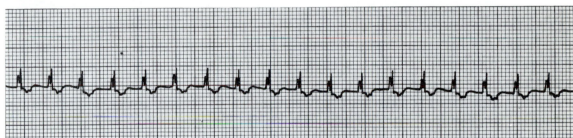

Interpretation:

_____

_____

_____

_____

ECG 27

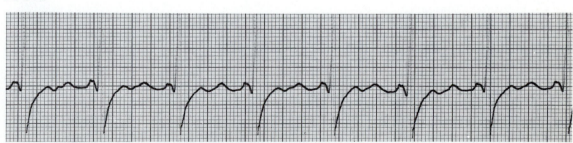

Interpretation:

_____

_____

_____

_____

ECG 25

Ventricular Tachycardia Deteriorating into Ventricular Fibrillation

The first six complexes in this strip represent a series of consecutive premature ventricular contractions (PVCs) in the form of *ventricular tachycardia (VT)*. Suddenly, the rhythm deteriorates into *ventricular fibrillation (VF)*. The onset of ventricular fibrillation after extremely widened, bizarre QRS complexes of the type demonstrated here is often seen as a terminal event in patients dying of heart failure.

ECG 26

Junctional Tachycardia

The key features of this ECG example are a very rapid ventricular rate (about 180/minute), with inverted P waves that *follow* the QRS complexes. The position of the P waves indicates that the arrhythmia originates in the AV-nodal area (rather than the atria). The low amplitude of the complexes, as recorded in this particular monitoring lead, is disadvantageous, and makes interpretation more difficult.

ECGF 27

Normal Sinus Rhythm with Prominent U Waves
Intraventricular Conduction Defect

At first glance this arrhythmia seems to resemble atrial flutter with 3:1 block. However, more careful inspection makes it evident that the three waves between each QRS complex are different in configuration and, more significantly, are not regularly spaced (as they would be with atrial flutter). The wave between the T wave and P wave is called a U wave. It is frequently associated with low serum potassium levels. Also noted in this recording is abnormal widening of the QRS complexes (greater than 0.12 second), which reflects an intraventricular conduction defect.

ECG 28

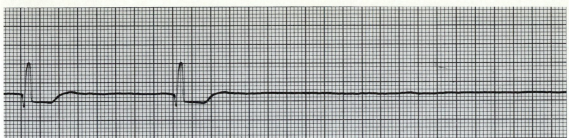

Interpretation:

_____
_____
_____
_____

ECG 29

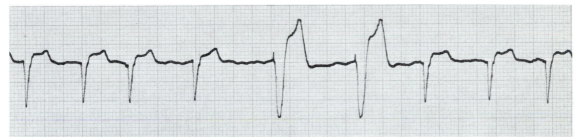

Interpretation:

_____
_____
_____
_____

ECG 30

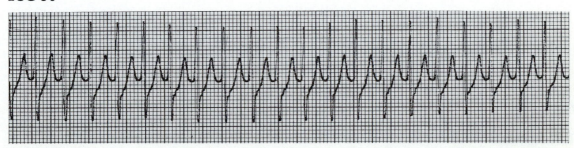

Interpretation:

_____
_____
_____
_____

ECG 28

Ventricular Standstill
Atrial Standstill

After two isolated ventricular complexes, ventricular activity stops completely (ventricular standstill or asystole). That no P waves are visible before or after the onset of ventricular standstill suggests that atrial activity has ceased (atrial standstill) even before the terminal event. The cessation of atrial activity with the subsequent development of ventricular standstill usually indicates that death is due to *downward displacement of the pacemaker.*

ECG 29

Normally Functioning Demand Pacemaker
Atrial Fibrillation

The diagnosis of atrial fibrillation (AF) is readily apparent from the grossly irregular rhythm and the absence of P waves. After four atrial beats are conducted to the ventricles, the AV node blocks the next impulses, causing the ventricular rate to fall to 68/minute (22 small boxes). The pacemaker (which had been inserted because of periods of a slow ventricular rate) correctly senses this pause and discharges an impulse to stimulate the ventricles directly. A second pacing impulse is delivered when the advanced AV block persists. AF with a faster ventricular rate then returns on its own after the two paced beats. The pacemaker functioned normally in this case: it sensed the pause created by the advanced block and discharged impulses on demand. Also, the pacing impulses produced ventricular capture.

ECG 30

Atrial Tachycardia

The heart rate is 210/minute. It is evident that this tachycardia originated *above* the ventricles (supraventricular) since the QRS complexes are normal (0.08 second). Although it is agreed that this is a supraventricular tachycardia (SVT), the arrhythmia can be recognized as atrial tachycardia (rather than junctional tachycardia or other SVT) from the unusual configuration of the T waves, which are sharp and peaked as the result of superimposed P waves.

Guidelines for Advanced Cardiac Life Support

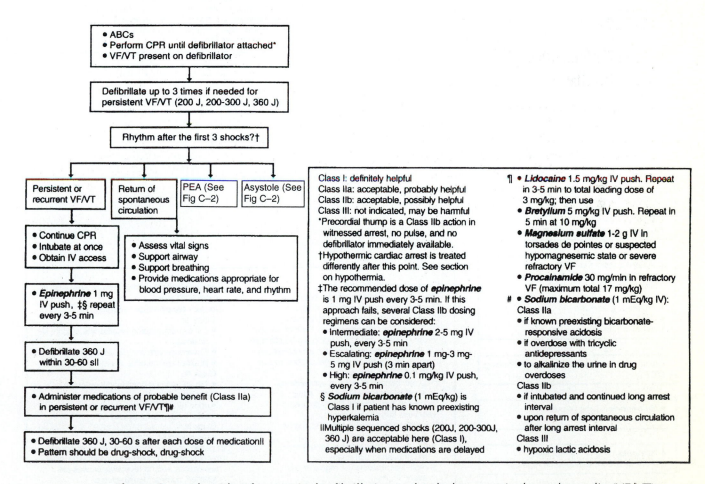

Figure C–1. Algorithm for ventricular fibrillation and pulseless ventricular tachycardia (VF/VT).

Figures in this Appendix are reproduced with permission from the American Heart Association Emergency Cardiac Care Committee's Guidelines for cardiopulmonary resuscitation and emergency cardiac care. *Journal of the American Medical Association.* 1992;268:2217–2224.

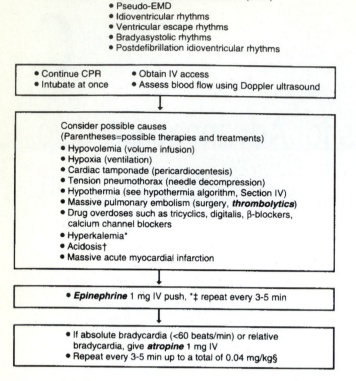

PEA includes
- Electromechanical dissociation (EMD)
- Pseudo-EMD
- Idioventricular rhythms
- Ventricular escape rhythms
- Bradyasystolic rhythms
- Postdefibrillation idioventricular rhythms

• Continue CPR   • Obtain IV access • Intubate at once   • Assess blood flow using Doppler ultrasound

Consider possible causes
(Parentheses=possible therapies and treatments)
- Hypovolemia (volume infusion)
- Hypoxia (ventilation)
- Cardiac tamponade (pericardiocentesis)
- Tension pneumothorax (needle decompression)
- Hypothermia (see hypothermia algorithm, Section IV)
- Massive pulmonary embolism (surgery, *thrombolytics*)
- Drug overdoses such as tricyclics, digitalis, β-blockers, calcium channel blockers
- Hyperkalemia*
- Acidosis†
- Massive acute myocardial infarction

- *Epinephrine* 1 mg IV push, *‡ repeat every 3-5 min

- If absolute bradycardia (<60 beats/min) or relative bradycardia, give *atropine* 1 mg IV
- Repeat every 3-5 min up to a total of 0.04 mg/kg§

Class I: definitely helpful
Class IIa: acceptable, probably helpful
Class IIb: acceptable, possibly helpful
Class III: not indicated, may be harmful
Sodium bicarbonate 1 mEq/kg is Class I if patient has known preexisting hyperkalemia.
†*Sodium bicarbonate* 1 mEq/kg:
  Class IIa
  - if known preexisting bicarbonate-responsive acidosis
  - if overdose with tricyclic antidepressants
  - to alkalinize the urine in drug overdoses
  Class IIb
  - if intubated and long arrest interval
  - upon return of spontaneous circulation after long arrest interval
  Class III
  - hypoxic lactic acidosis
‡The recommended dose of *epinephrine* is 1 mg IV push every 3-5 min. If this approach fails, several Class IIb dosing regimens can be considered.
  - Intermediate: *epinephrine* 2-5 mg IV push, every 3-5 min
  - Escalating: *epinephrine* 1 mg-3 mg-5 mg IV push (3 min apart)
  - High: *epinephrine* 0.1 mg/kg IV push, every 3-5 min
§ Shorter *atropine* dosing intervals are possibly helpful in cardiac arrest (Class IIb).

Figure C–2. Algorithm for pulseless electrical activity (PEA) (electromechanical dissociation [EMD]).

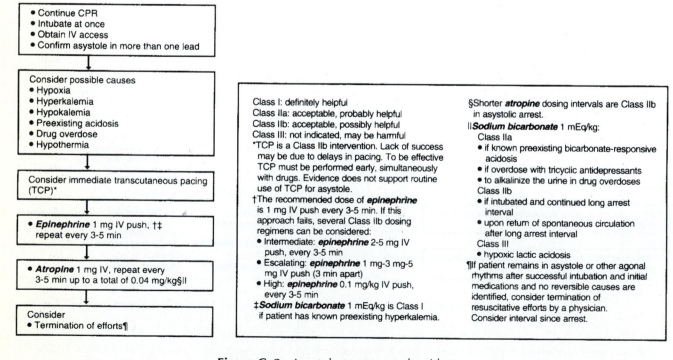

• Continue CPR • Intubate at once • Obtain IV access • Confirm asystole in more than one lead

Consider possible causes
- Hypoxia
- Hyperkalemia
- Hypokalemia
- Preexisting acidosis
- Drug overdose
- Hypothermia

Consider immediate transcutaneous pacing (TCP)*

- *Epinephrine* 1 mg IV push, †‡ repeat every 3-5 min

- *Atropine* 1 mg IV, repeat every 3-5 min up to a total of 0.04 mg/kg§||

Consider
- Termination of efforts¶

Class I: definitely helpful
Class IIa: acceptable, probably helpful
Class IIb: acceptable, possibly helpful
Class III: not indicated, may be harmful
*TCP is a Class IIb intervention. Lack of success may be due to delays in pacing. To be effective TCP must be performed early, simultaneously with drugs. Evidence does not support routine use of TCP for asystole.
†The recommended dose of *epinephrine* is 1 mg IV push every 3-5 min. If this approach fails, several Class IIb dosing regimens can be considered:
- Intermediate: *epinephrine* 2-5 mg IV push, every 3-5 min
- Escalating: *epinephrine* 1 mg-3 mg-5 mg IV push (3 min apart)
- High: *epinephrine* 0.1 mg/kg IV push, every 3-5 min
‡*Sodium bicarbonate* 1 mEq/kg is Class I if patient has known preexisting hyperkalemia.

§Shorter *atropine* dosing intervals are Class IIb in asystolic arrest.
||*Sodium bicarbonate* 1 mEq/kg:
  Class IIa
  - if known preexisting bicarbonate-responsive acidosis
  - if overdose with tricyclic antidepressants
  - to alkalinize the urine in drug overdoses
  Class IIb
  - if intubated and continued long arrest interval
  - upon return of spontaneous circulation after long arrest interval
  Class III
  - hypoxic lactic acidosis
¶If patient remains in asystole or other agonal rhythms after successful intubation and initial medications and no reversible causes are identified, consider termination of resuscitative efforts by a physician. Consider interval since arrest.

Figure C–3. Asystole treatment algorithm.

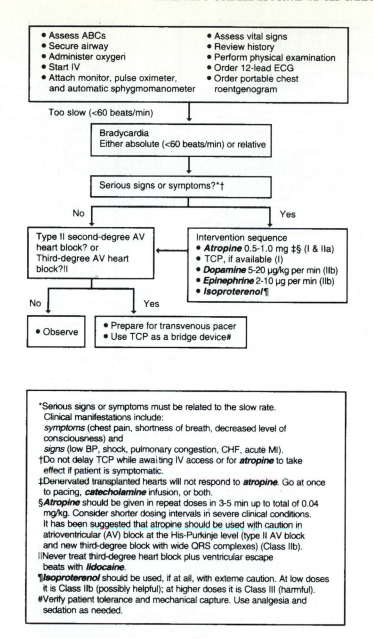

Figure C–4. Bradycardia algorithm (with the patient not in cardiac arrest).

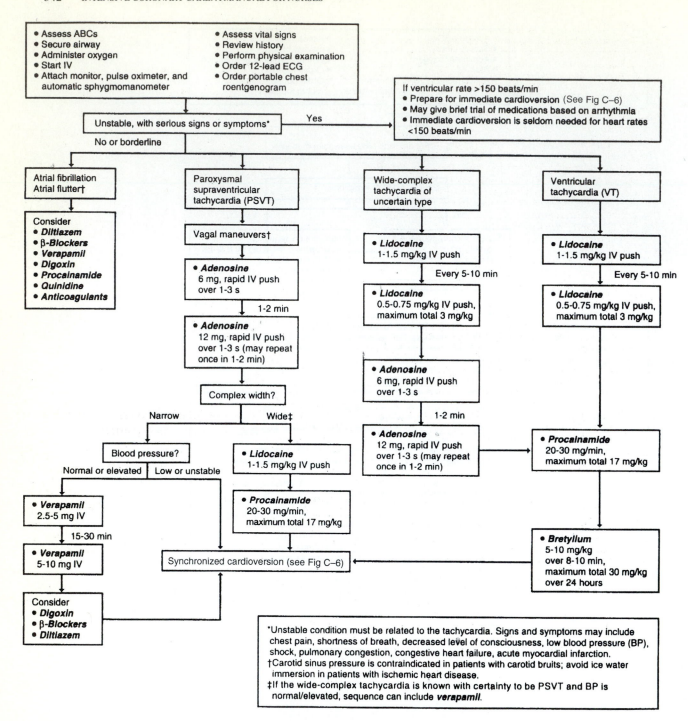

- Assess ABCs
- Secure airway
- Administer oxygen
- Start IV
- Attach monitor, pulse oximeter, and automatic sphygmomanometer

- Assess vital signs
- Review history
- Perform physical examination
- Order 12-lead ECG
- Order portable chest roentgenogram

Unstable, with serious signs or symptoms* → Yes →

If ventricular rate >150 beats/min
- Prepare for immediate cardioversion (See Fig C–6)
- May give brief trial of medications based on arrhythmia
- Immediate cardioversion is seldom needed for heart rates <150 beats/min

No or borderline

Atrial fibrillation Atrial flutter†

Consider
- *Diltiazem*
- *β-Blockers*
- *Verapamil*
- *Digoxin*
- *Procainamide*
- *Quinidine*
- *Anticoagulants*

Paroxysmal supraventricular tachycardia (PSVT)

Vagal maneuvers†

- *Adenosine*
  6 mg, rapid IV push over 1-3 s

1-2 min

- *Adenosine*
  12 mg, rapid IV push over 1-3 s (may repeat once in 1-2 min)

Complex width?

Narrow / Wide‡

Blood pressure?

Normal or elevated / Low or unstable

- *Verapamil*
  2.5-5 mg IV

15-30 min

- *Verapamil*
  5-10 mg IV

Consider
- *Digoxin*
- *β-Blockers*
- *Diltiazem*

- *Lidocaine*
  1-1.5 mg/kg IV push

- *Procainamide*
  20-30 mg/min, maximum total 17 mg/kg

Synchronized cardioversion (see Fig C–6)

Wide-complex tachycardia of uncertain type

- *Lidocaine*
  1-1.5 mg/kg IV push

Every 5-10 min

- *Lidocaine*
  0.5-0.75 mg/kg IV push, maximum total 3 mg/kg

- *Adenosine*
  6 mg, rapid IV push over 1-3 s

1-2 min

- *Adenosine*
  12 mg, rapid IV push over 1-3 s (may repeat once in 1-2 min)

Ventricular tachycardia (VT)

- *Lidocaine*
  1-1.5 mg/kg IV push

Every 5-10 min

- *Lidocaine*
  0.5-0.75 mg/kg IV push, maximum total 3 mg/kg

- *Procainamide*
  20-30 mg/min, maximum total 17 mg/kg

- *Bretylium*
  5-10 mg/kg over 8-10 min, maximum total 30 mg/kg over 24 hours

*Unstable condition must be related to the tachycardia. Signs and symptoms may include chest pain, shortness of breath, decreased level of consciousness, low blood pressure (BP), shock, pulmonary congestion, congestive heart failure, acute myocardial infarction.
†Carotid sinus pressure is contraindicated in patients with carotid bruits; avoid ice water immersion in patients with ischemic heart disease.
‡If the wide-complex tachycardia is known with certainty to be PSVT and BP is normal/elevated, sequence can include *verapamil*.

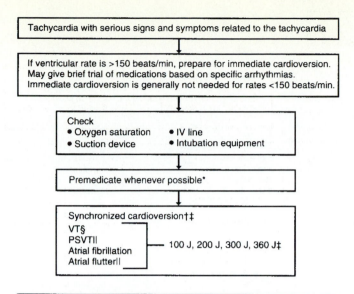

Tachycardia with serious signs and symptoms related to the tachycardia

↓

If ventricular rate is >150 beats/min, prepare for immediate cardioversion.
May give brief trial of medications based on specific arrhythmias.
Immediate cardioversion is generally not needed for rates <150 beats/min.

↓

Check
• Oxygen saturation   • IV line
• Suction device   • Intubation equipment

↓

Premedicate whenever possible*

↓

Synchronized cardioversion†‡

VT§
PSVT‖
Atrial fibrillation   —— 100 J, 200 J, 300 J, 360 J‡
Atrial flutter‖

*Effective regimens have included a sedative (eg, *diazepam,*
 midazolam, barbiturates, etomidate, ketamine, methohexital) with
 or without an analgesic agent (eg, *fentanyl, morphine, meperidine*).
 Many experts recommend anesthesia if service is readily available.
†Note possible need to resynchronize after each cardioversion.
‡If delays in synchronization occur and clinical conditions are critical,
 go to immediate unsynchronized shocks.
§Treat polymorphic VT (irregular form and rate) like VF:
 200 J, 200-300 J, 360 J.
‖PSVT and atrial flutter often respond to lower energy levels
 (start with 50 J).

Figure C–6. Electrical cardioversion algorithm
(with the patient not in cardiac arrest).

Index